Structure and Function of Domestic Animals

Structure and Function of Domestic Animals

W. Bruce Currie

Department of Animal Science
New York State College of Agriculture and Life Sciences
Cornell University

CRC Press
Boca Raton   New York   London   Tokyo

Library of Congress Cataloging-in-Publication Data

Catalog record is available from the Library of Congress.

This book contains information obtained from authentic and highly regarded sources. Reprinted material is quoted with permission, and sources are indicated. A wide variety of references are listed. Reasonable efforts have been made to publish reliable data and information, but the author and the publisher cannot assume responsibility for the validity of all materials or for the consequences of their use.

Neither this book nor any part may be reproduced or transmitted in any form or by any means, electronic or mechanical, including photocopying, microfilming, and recording, or by any information storage or retrieval system, without prior permission in writing from the publisher.

CRC Press, Inc.'s consent does not extend to copying for general distribution, for promotion, for creating new works, or for resale. Specific permission must be obtained in writing from CRC Press for such copying.

Direct all inquiries to CRC Press, Inc., 2000 Corporate Blvd., N.W., Boca Raton, Florida 33431.

© 1988 by Butterworth Publishers, a division of Reed Publishing (USA) Inc.
© 1995 by CRC Press, Inc.

No claim to original U.S. Government works
International Standard Book Number 0-8493-8766-3
Printed in the United States of America 3 4 5 6 7 8 9 10 11 12
Printed on acid-free paper

To my parents,
who never dampened curiosity despite an interminable series of:
But why?s, But how?s, and What if?s

Contents

Preface

This book is intended to provide readers of various backgrounds with a solid introduction to the structure and function of domestic animals. Emphasis is placed on function, with structure being assigned a supportive role; the latter is approached from the standpoint of what might be termed functional anatomy.

The reader who seeks a good working understanding of the biology of animals should give priority to grasping the general principles, phenomena, and mechanisms, and then support this understanding by assembling a store of factual information. Using this strategy, the reader will acquire a long-term understanding of the important issues, rather than merely remember isolated pieces of information.

The conceptual and factual components of the subject matter are not truly separable, but there is a danger that some readers may focus on the specific, detailed information at the expense of the principles; in this case, the amount of factual information may be found to be excessive.

Most students learning about animals will find the subject matter fascinating and relevant. This book will also help students of other disciplines, such as the basic sciences, because it provides real-world applications of concepts and principles learned elsewhere. I have chosen examples of an applied nature from various species. My selection was based on an expected familiarity with these animals, and the interest shown by more than a thousand animal science and pre-veterinary students over the years.

Certain of the assumptions made about the typical reader will be inappropriate for others. Some portions of the text may be overly simplistic and superficial for one reader while posing difficulty for another. I have found that the greatest variability in the science backgrounds of college students lies in the area of chemistry—especially, the fundamentals of organic chemistry. The appendices provide detail on this topic for beginning readers who do not have this preparation and for those who would benefit from a succinct review.

The technical language necessary to describe this subject occasionally causes readers some initial difficulty. Do not hesitate to make extensive use of a dictionary when reading the text. The terminology is quite precise and efforts to understand the roots of the words will be rewarded as you become comfortable with their appropriate use. Make explanatory notes on small cards coded to sections of the book or, if more convenient, in the margins.

When you have some spare moments, use them to browse ahead in the text, perhaps to examine the illustrations or to look over the main headings, and to develop a first impression about a future topic. Similarly useful would be a quick review of illustrations, legends, and your annotations or highlighted material from earlier study efforts.

Portions of the text that are beyond a core or introductory level of treatment are placed in boxes and referenced in the main text. In some cases, the boxes contain additional, detailed material that might disrupt the continuity of the main text if it were not separated from it. If the boxed material consistently causes you difficulty, skip over it and concentrate on the core text. Stronger students should include the boxed text during the second reading of a chapter. The following approach is recommended:

> When starting a new chapter, take a quick look at the headings, illustrations, and legends of the whole chapter. Spend a few minutes gauging the level of difficulty of the material.
>
> Read one or more sections. They vary in

size and complexity. Read quickly to retain the continuity. Do not labor over the difficult portions, but identify these in the margins so they can be located easily for closer examination at a later time. Examine the figures and legends in detail as they are referenced in the text. On this first pass through, skip over the boxed text.

Return to portions marked for closer study. Seek help if needed and be sure to annotate the text with explanatory notes that will be useful during any subsequent review. Examine the boxed material during this reading only if you are comfortable with the content of the core text.

Attempt the exercises provided at the end of each chapter. If you cannot easily answer the questions then you have not yet mastered the topic.

Much of the fun of studying the structure and function of domestic animals stems from the endless opportunities to apply this knowledge to the animals around you and to your own body. Most readers have some contact with animals and can experience this subject come alive by simple observation. We are reasonably normal animals ourselves and you will derive real benefit (and some amusement) from simple exercises such as counting your pulse when resting, when exercising, when excited or apprehensive, and so on. Get into the habit of thinking about this discipline at every available opportunity. Think about ways of describing some topic that has caught your interest using nontechnical language. Try out your explanation on someone who has no knowledge of our discipline. This is a legitimate approach to the subject (see Box 3–1 and Figure 9–3 for examples), and is perhaps the best test of comprehension.

Finally, this book provides merely a first exposure to a very broad subject. When you have progressed to a more advanced level, you will use specialized texts, often focused on just one of the many species or body systems described here. You will consult primary scientific literature, including scientific journal articles, specialized monographs, and conference proceedings to obtain authority for the concepts and facts that are not referenced in this book. The inclusion of references and recommended readings can be distracting and lead to unnecessary ambiguities and complexities. The omission of such references from this book is intentional; in my experience, these are not generally consulted by the beginning student who first needs an overview of the subject.

Acknowledgments

I am indebted to my teachers, colleagues, graduate assistants, and students for the part they have played in the evolution of this text. Their styles, suggestions, and criticisms have been valuable in the design and approach I have adopted, but I alone am responsible for the content, biases, and shortcomings that are inevitable in a text of this nature.

Specifically, I thank the following. Dr. George Ignotz helped by photographing much of the artwork. Dr. Murray Elliot supported me in this endeavor at all stages and minimized other burdens at work that would otherwise have posed conflicts. Professor Dr. Konrad Zerobin graciously hosted my stay in Zurich, when much of the book was written and the artwork was prepared. Finally, Jean Currie helped proofread draft versions of the book and patiently allowed disruption of all normal activities so that deadlines could almost be met.

Structure and Function of Domestic Animals

The Structural Nature of Animals

1.1 • The Form of Animals

When asked to explain the similarities and differences between pigs and horses, one would probably start by categorizing the points to be made in terms of form, structure, and function. These are the very aspects of the biology of domestic animals with which this text is concerned.

Morphology is the study of form and appearance and it is a useful place to start because structure and function underlie much of what is called form. In gross terms, an animal can be thought of as a trunk or body, to which are attached a head and neck, appendages such as legs (arms for forelimbs), and usually a tail. Further elaboration is made by distinguishing the characteristics of these parts. For example, the giraffe with its extremely long neck provides a contrast to the pig with what seems to be an almost nonexistent neck. Most breeds of sheep

have long tails, while most breeds of goat have quite short tails. Newborn animals have large heads in comparison with the rest of the body, but during growth, the trunk and the limbs are favored. Thus, the proportion of the body constituted by the head is much less in adults than in the young. Even so, newborn animals are said to be "leggy." Their limbs seem to be extraordinarily long and spindly when compared with limbs of the adult animal. This difference is much more evident in animals that are adapted for running, such as the horse and other herbivores. Such animals are called cursorial. In the wild, these species are the prey of carnivores, and there is a distinct survival advantage in the young being mobile soon after birth.

The external appearances of animals differ widely among the species and, partly because of the selection efforts of man, even within a species. The latter show up in what are called breed differences. The traditional beef breeds of cattle are quite different in overall form from the highly selected traditional dairy breeds. In sheep, there are striking differences in the appearance of the coat. During the past couple of hundred years, as distinct breeds were developed, particularly in Britain, strikingly different body shapes and wool types also emerged. Distinct shapes and degrees of wool cover are apparent in the heads of these breeds (Figure 1–1).

This adds some confusion to description because the *pelage*, or coat, of sheep is called wool and the pelage of goats is hair, yet the "wool" of some sheep breeds is quite hairlike while the "hair" of some goats has the general appearance of wool.

Some animals have horns, specialized derivatives of the skin that, like claws and hooves, are best considered to be highly modified hair structures. Horns are quite different from antlers, which are derivatives of bone.

During evolution, and to a lesser extent during breed formation when man has controlled selection, marked structural changes have accompanied speciation, and these changes show up morphologically. As quadrupeds acquired the ability to run, the distal parts of the limbs became elongated, some toes may have been lost, bones of the foot fused to increase strength, joint angles changed, and so on (Figure 1–2). In the most evolved form, cursorial animals actually stand on the equivalent of the human fingernails and toenails. At an intermediate stage of evolution the digits are used, and the least-developed cursorial animals stand on the equivalent of the palm of the hand and sole of the foot. The changes described above result in differences in stance and overall form.

As differences in structure are explored, as in the above example concerning the limb, the tools of *anatomy* are used. Anatomy, which means "to cut apart," is the study of structure of the body and the relationships between the parts making up the whole. If studied without regard for function of these parts, anatomy is truly a morbid science. Gross anatomy usually pertains

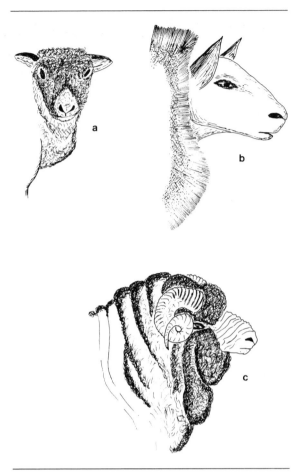

Figure 1–1. Morphologic differences between breeds. Marked differences in the shape of the head and skin folding and the extent of coat cover are obvious in the highly selected sheep breeds. *a:* Down-type breeds are compact, or blocky, and most of the head is covered with short dense wool. *b:* Cheviot-types have no wool on the head; the fleece (of 4 to 6 inches) terminates abruptly just behind the ears. *c:* Merino-type sheep have heavy neck folds and extensive skin wrinkles on the nose. The head is partly covered with dense, fine wool extending beyond the eyes.

to whole body relations and the overall nature of organ systems. At a finer level, *histology* is the study of the tissues and the cells that compose them. Finer still is *ultrastructural analysis*, a discipline that depends extensively on use of the electron microscope.

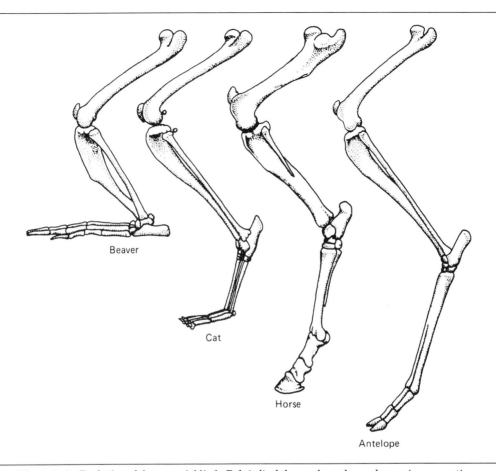

Figure 1–2. Evolution of the cursorial limb. Pelvic limb bones have been drawn in proportion using the femur as the reference length bone. (The limb bones are shown normalized to the length of the femur.) Note the marked elongation of the bones of the foot and toes and the change in the angle of the ankle. These modifications lead to altered stance and gait, along with a great increase in the length of the stride. (Reprinted by permission of the publisher. From Bone, J.F.: *Animal Anatomy and Physiology*, Reston, VA: Reston Publishing Company, 1979.)

The intimate relationship between structure and function necessitates that the two be studied in parallel. This book attempts to provide a balance between the two aspects whenever possible so the structural material may be called *functional anatomy*. At times it will seem that the treatment is unduly anatomic, with function appearing to be neglected. At other times the reverse will seem true as the emphasis falls on details of mechanism. These discrepancies are unavoidable if the material is to be grasped at anything beyond a most superficial level.

The organization of the animal body has evolved to facilitate function and regulation rather than to ease the task of the beginning student who is attempting to obtain an understanding of animals. A student interested in animal locomotion could take a very different approach to the study of anatomy than another student who plans to use the information as a foundation for meat science. The approach used here provides a basis for further study of any of the more specialized aspects of animal science.

1.2 • Cells and Tissues

Domestic animals, like all others, are made up of an amazing aggregation of simple units—the living cells. Each cell exhibits a degree of independence from all others, meaning that it is a living unit in its own right. The real beauty of function of the complex animal, however, results from the cells coexisting as a community. Individual cells support each other's needs, communicate with and protect each other. By cooperating with each other, a mixture of cells in a tissue can perform tasks that would be impossible for individual cells in isolation.

These functions of the basic units of living matter must be understood to appreciate how the whole animal functions, both in health and in disease. At this time, some descriptive information about cells is both useful and important.

At the simplest level, each cell consists of a mass of jelly-like material called *protoplasm,* which is made up of an inner *nucleus* and the surrounding *cytoplasm*. At the outer surface, the cytoplasm is contained within a cell membrane, or *plasmalemma*. There is no cell wall in animal cells. In most cells, numerous specialized structures called *organelles* can be found within the cytoplasm (Figure 1–3). In most cases the powerful resolving power of the electron microscope is needed to observe intracellular structures smaller than the nucleus. The organelles are also usually bounded by membranes, and their location within the three-dimensional space of the cell interior is determined by their attachments to a delicate intracellular latticework called the *cyto-*

skeleton. Cells are alive and dynamic but are usually killed in preparation for microscopic examination. However, it is possible to examine free-living cells and those that have been freed of their usual attachments to other cells within tissues, without killing them. Certain dyes called vital stains highlight particular features within the cell without poisoning them. Normally, the population of cells within a tissue includes young, mature, aged and deteriorating, and already dead cells. The heterogeneity of cell populations makes generalizations hazardous, but so long as it is recognized that there will always be exceptions, even if infrequent, to virtually every statement made about cells, we can begin to understand the nature of their everyday business.

One very important concept that may not be immediately apparent is the distinction between the total cellular mass of the body and the space that is made up of the regions between cells—the *intercellular, extracellular,* or *interstitial* space (these terms are used interchangeably). The extracellular space is filled with a fluid similar to blood serum, and through the extracellular space pass all materials on their way to and from the individual cells (Figure 1–4). For example, oxygen is transported from the lungs by red blood cells (or erythrocytes) to the body's cells. The oxygen passes from within the red blood cells to the blood plasma, through and between the endothelial cells that make up the walls of the capillaries, and then through the

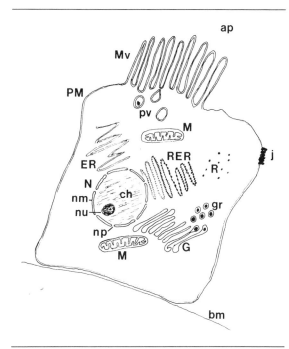

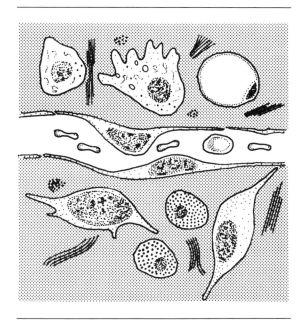

Figure 1–4. The interstitium. A relatively large proportion of solid tissue volume is extra-cellular (shaded). The lumen of the capillary (unshaded) is also an important part of the extracellular space. These spaces may be fluid or solid in nature, depending on the tissue. Inside the capillary, the space is filled with plasma; outside, the interstitium may contain collagen fibers (shown here lengthwise and in cross section).

Figure 1–3. The generalized cell. The cell is bounded by a plasma membrane (PM), which may be specialized at the apical (ap) surface and possess microvilli (Mv). At the base of the microvilli may be pinocytotic vesicles (pv). On the lateral margins, the membrane may form junctions (j) with adjacent cells. The cell may be associated at its basal surface with a basement membrane (bm), an extracellular supporting material. The nucleus (N), containing nucleolus (nu) and chromatin (ch), is bounded by a nuclear membrane (nm) with characteristic nuclear pores (np). Membranous organelles extending into the cytoplasm include smooth endoplasmic reticulum (ER) and rough endoplasmic reticulum (RER). The latter is decorated with ribosomes (R) that may also be free in the cytoplasm. The Golgi (G), a layered vesicular membrane system, forms membrane-enclosed granules (gr). These are usually secretory granules that can accumulate in the cytoplasm awaiting a secretory episode. Mitochondria (M) vary in number depending upon the metabolic activity level of the cell; they are involved in energy transformation.

Individual cells in the solid tissues of the body, which are virtually all tissues except blood and lymphlike fluids, are held together by cell-to-cell contacts or *junctions* and by structural materials, secreted by cells, that serve as a type of cell "cement" or external scaffolding.

Cells of similar characteristics, or mixtures of cells with complementary functions, are assembled as *tissues*. For example—although it is an atypical example—blood is a tissue made up of a variety of cell types that happen to be all free cells, suspended in a specialized extracellular fluid called *blood plasma*. As a more typical example, muscle is a tissue made up of arrays of muscle cells assembled in characteristic ways as bundles, which have a distinct form (Figure 1–5).

Masses of tissues, sometimes of a single type but more often a mixture, that either form dis-

extracellular fluid surrounding the cells, before it reaches its final destination. The various types of extracellular fluids will be discussed in detail later.

Figure 1–5. Tissues. Tissues are made up of a variety of cell types. These have recognizable morphologies and properties that are exposed by microscopic techniques. Three distinct types of muscle cells, or myocytes, are illustrated: skeletal, cardiac, and smooth.

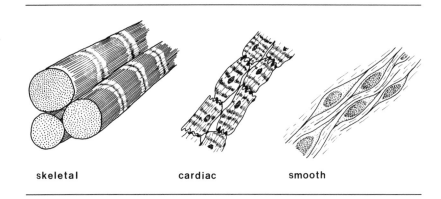

skeletal   cardiac   smooth

crete macroscopic structures or fulfill a special function in the body are called *organs*. For example, the liver is an organ of recognizable form and specialized functions. A collection of organs with complementary functions is called an *organ system*. The gut is an organ system with the obvious function of digestion and assimilation of nutrients, along with a number of other functions to be described later. The organs of reproduction constitute another organ system.

The study of large parts of the body—organ systems and organs—by observation during dissection is called anatomy. The structure and form of tissues and cells require microscopic study and fall within the discipline of histology.

This introduction will be confined to describing the five most important tissue types:

Epithelium,

Connective tissue,

Muscle,

Nervous tissue, and

Blood and lymph.

Epithelial Tissue

Epithelium characteristically covers free surfaces. In its basic form there may be a single layer of cells (simple epithelium). Alternatively, it may comprise multiple layers (stratified epithelium), as in the outer portions of the skin, or *epidermis*. Selected types of epithelia are illustrated in Figure 1–6.

Highly specialized or modified structures formed by epithelium include hair, wool, nails, claws, and horns. Many glandular structures consist largely of specialized epithelia. The form may be a series of tubules, the walls of which are epithelial, or the secretory units of the glands may be collections of flasklike structures (Figure 1–7) called *alveoli* or *acini* (*alveolus* and *acinus* are the singular forms of these words). If the glands communicate with free surfaces such as the skin, as in the case of sweat glands, or empty their contents into the lumen of the digestive tract, the glands are called *exocrine*. Others release their secretory products into the extracellular space and thence into the blood or lymph (tissue fluid); these are called *endocrine* glands. Older terminology referred to endocrine glands as glands of internal secretion, or these producing the body's hormones. The thyroid gland, which lies as two lobes on either side of the trachea or windpipe, connected by an isthmus or bridge (Figure 1–8), is an endocrine gland with important functions in the growth and development of animals. Thyroid hormones are distributed to the cells of the body by transport in the blood plasma. The biology of the thyroid and the other endocrine glands is considered in Chapter 4 of this book.

A major type of epithelium develops to line the internal or *serous* cavities, as opposed to the

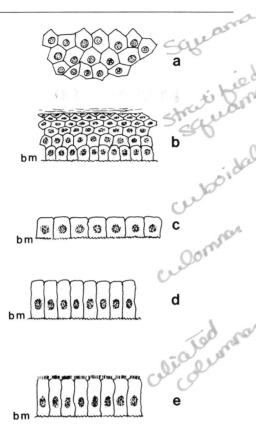

squamous
stratified squamous
cuboidal
columnar
ciliated columnar

Figure 1–6. *Epithelia.* Types of epithelia include *a:* squamous; *b:* stratified squamous; *c:* cuboidal; *d:* columnar; and *e:* ciliated columnar. Note the distinct cellular morphologies and the presence of a basement membrane (bm) in several of the types.

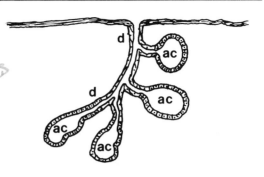

Figure 1–7. *Glandular epithelium.* This simplified gland communicates with the surface via a short duct (d). It originates in a series of acini (ac), the walls of which are made up of secretory epithelium. Glands that communicate with free surfaces are called exocrine glands.

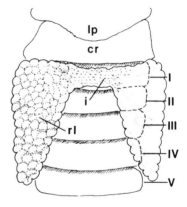

Figure 1–8. *The thyroid gland.* The thyroid is an endocrine gland, or one that internally secretes hormones. It is located ventrally and to either side of the trachea. This ventral view shows the somewhat nodular structure of the thyroid gland—detailed only for the right lobe (rl). The isthmus (i) crosses tracheal cartilaginous ring I and the two lobes lie alongside tracheal rings II to V. The ventral prominence of the larynx (lp), palpable at the throat, is shown for reference. The intervening cartilage is the cricoid (cr).

free or external surfaces. The lumen of the gut, the airways of the respiratory system, and the lumen of the genitourinary tract are external spaces, best considered as invaginations from the exterior of the developing individual. In contrast, the abdominal cavity forms from what was originally a solid mass of embryonic tissue and provides a protective environment for the abdominal viscera such as many of the organs of digestion, the organs of excretion, and the reproductive organs. All such structures are covered with a protective cellular surface of *mesothelium*. Similarly, the blood and lymphatic vessels are lined with *endothelium*. (Mesothelium

and endothelium are terms that convey information about location, *meso-* meaning intermediate and *endo-* meaning within.)

There are so many types of epithelium with such varied functions that it should be no surprise that there is also a great deal of structural variation. The cells have characteristic shapes, as illustrated in Figure 1–6. A key property of epithelial tissues relates to their serving as boundaries for free surfaces. Specialized junctions occur between adjacent cells. These connection points are hybrid structures made from portions of the plasmalemma of each of the cells in contact: their integrity is the basis for the term *epithelial barrier*.

Connective Tissues

Connective tissues function in a way that is largely implicit in the term. Two major subdivisions are the soft connective tissues and the skeletal tissues (bone and cartilage). In most cases, connective tissues have large amounts of extracellular structural material; this material in turn is a secretory product of the connective tissue cells. *Adipose*, or fat tissue, differs in having a proportionately larger intracellular volume and little extracellular structural material. This is evident in the ease with which fat depot tissues can be bluntly dissected, or torn apart. Adipose tissue is of particular interest in domestic animals because it contributes significantly to the value of meat products, both in a positive and negative sense, depending on circumstances. Fat is energetically the most costly tissue to develop when growing and finishing animals in preparation for the harvesting of meat products. Typical adipose tissue contains one or more fat droplets within the cytoplasm of the cells and serves as an important *depot*, or reserve of energy-rich molecules, of which more will be said later.

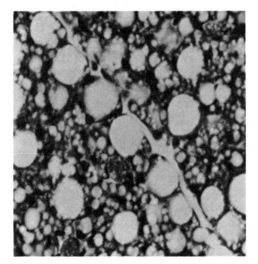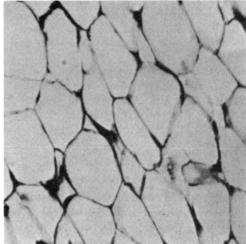

Figure 1–9. Adipose tissue in young lambs. Brown fat from the perirenal depot in a five-hour-old lamb (left) shows characteristic variation in the size of the fat droplets within a given cell. The cell boundaries are not readily discernible. The photomicrograph on the right shows white fat from the same depot tissue in a 16-day-old lamb. The brown fat has been replaced with white fat and the cells, now readily discernible, are filled with a single large fat droplet. The cytoplasm has been displaced into a thin shell near the plasma membrane. (Photomicrographs courtesy of Dr. G. Alexander, CSIRO Division of Animal Production, Prospect, NSW, Australia.)

Adipose tissue has a protective function in both a mechanical and thermoregulatory sense, but this protective function is quite secondary to the role of adipose tissue in energy metabolism. The adipocyte can undergo enormous volume expansion because of the fat droplet it contains. In its mature state, the cytoplasm is distorted into a thin shell immediately beneath the plasmalemma. Later a distinction will be made between *white adipose tissue*, which serves merely as a depot, and *brown adipose tissue*, which can oxidize fatty acids from the stored triglycerides. Because brown adipose tissue is capable of generating heat, it is called *thermogenic*, and it has important functions in meeting the needs of the newborn. The two types of fat have different forms (Figure 1–9) and quite different functions.

More usually considered to be the important connective tissues are those that secrete extracellular supportive materials. These products may be *amorphous*, or lacking obvious form, as exemplified by ground substance or intercellular matrix. Some cartilage, particularly hyaline or glassy cartilage, is of this kind, and the secreted product provides a shock-absorbing and lubricated surface to articulating bones in the mobile joints. The common soft connective tissues are spongy and flexible with numerous intertwined *fibers* lying in a fluid matrix. Great variation exists in the types and density of these extracellular fibers. The tissues lying between the skin and deeper structures have a low density of fibers and provide flexibility so the underlying tissues can move without undue tension being transferred to the relatively indistensible skin. In mature animals and obese or excessively fat younger individuals, the subcutaneous connective tissue may become dominated by enlarging adipocytes. The same spongy or areolar connective tissue makes up the *fasciae* (singular, *fascia*), or connective elements, found between muscles (Figure 1–10). Individual muscles can be bluntly separated by tearing these fasciae. As in the case of the subcutaneous tissues, the spongy fasciae within muscle masses are also sites of fat accumulation in well-nourished animals.

More structured—meaning they contain

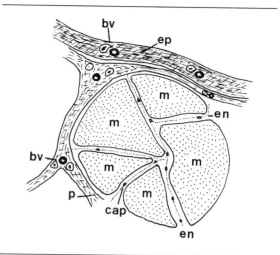

Figure 1–10. Skeletal muscle structure. In cross section, skeletal muscle cells (m), with their internal contractile filaments shown as dots, appear as bundles. They are separated by a delicate connective tissue called endomysium (en), on which are located blood capillaries (cap). The endomysium is a web-like lattice of collagen (see Figure 1–11) and elastin. The bundle of cells is enclosed by perimysium (p), a spongy connective tissue that supports larger blood vessels (bv) and may contain large numbers of adipocytes. This structural material greatly influences the texture of meat. The entire muscle is enclosed by a sheath of epimysium (ep), which becomes specialized at the ends of the muscle to form tendons.

larger numbers of extracellular fibers and are more feltlike than spongy—are the sheets of connective tissue that provide tough supporting structures such as the inner and deeper layers of the skin; the *ligaments*, which connect bones together; and the *tendons*, which attach muscles to bones. These tough tissues have mechanical functions that will be described later. Because they are tough, they adversely affect the desirability of certain cuts of meat.

The fibers that have been mentioned are specialized polymers of unusual proteins, the *collagens* and *elastin*. The polymers are of enormous size and are assembled in the fluid matrix after the component proteins have been secreted by a ubiquitous population of cells called fibrocytes. These fascinating cells are commonly viewed as primitive, yet they have the highly specialized task of manufacturing and secreting the structural framework of all soft tissues. The fibers are mixtures of different types of collagen and elastin. Collagen, after harsh processing, is encountered as gelatin, the basis of many dessert products. A fairly similar processed form has been used for centuries as glue. With some modification in processing, similar proteins in skin can be converted to leather. With skilled preparation, the connective fibers in a cut of meat can be softened and made palatable; done incorrectly, the result is a disaster and can be practically inedible. The biology of the connective tissue fibers is complex because the molecules are exceedingly large. The individual fibers are highly organized and so large they can be visualized readily with the electron microscope (Figure 1–11).

Skeletal connective tissues include cartilage and bone. The major distinction from soft connective tissue lies in the solid rather than fluid nature of the matrix. Cartilage is flexible, bone is not. Each property has a function, though it is more obvious for bone. In addition to hyaline

cartilage, some cartilage contains abundant fibers embedded in the matrix that serve to strengthen the tissue. These fibrocartilages are whitish in color and are usually associated with bony structures. For example, such cartilage is found in the pelvis, where it allows some mobility yet still provides enormous strength. Another form, having a yellowish appearance, is elastic cartilage, the flexible supporting tissue of the external ear.

The most rigid connective tissues are those making up bones. Bone is a tissue, while bones are organs. Bones may form from cartilage in many cases by a complex process of deposition of insoluble salts; calcium phosphate is the major component. The matrix is said to be ossified, but embedded within the seemingly inert tissue are dynamic living cells. The matrix itself is not stable because the salts are continuously being solubilized to enter the blood, and are being laid down in the continuing process of ossification. Cells within the bone are actively involved in both processes. Bone is best viewed as a depot tissue, similar to adipose tissue, but in this case it is an integral part of the body's mechanism

Figure 1–11. Collagen fibrils. This scanning electron micrograph of dense irregular connective tissue, as found in the dermis of skin, reveals a complex, interwoven mesh of collagen fibrils (CF). The fibrils are aggregations of enormous molecules of collagen proteins that are assembled into these structual elements after secretion from cells into the interstitium. The collagen fibrils constitute the most important structural component of most tissues. (Reproduced by permission of the publisher. From Kessel, R.G. and Kardon, R.H.: *Tissues and Organs: A Text-Atlas of Scanning Electron Microscopy,* San Francisco: W.H. Freeman and Company, 1979.)

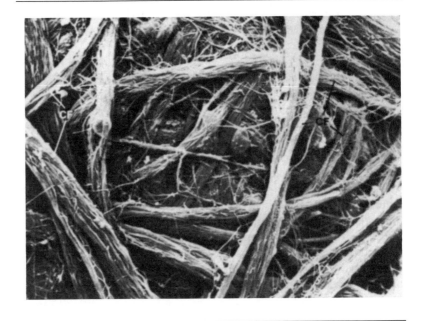

to regulate availability of the key inorganic substances, calcium and phosphate ions. This function of bone is enormously important for the productive processes of milk synthesis and egg laying. Much about the biology of bone growth and mineral metabolism will come later, in Chapters 4 and 8.

Muscle

Muscle cells are the most specialized motile cells in the body. They occur as three types: *skeletal* (or striated) muscle, *smooth* muscle, and *cardiac* muscle. Muscle cells provide the capacity for movement by shortening with great force or rapidity, or for tension development when shortening may not be apparent. Muscle cells, also called *myocytes* and, somewhat ambiguously, muscle fibers, are usually markedly elongated or spindle shaped. Skeletal muscle cells can be enormous in size, partly because during formation, many individual cells fuse together to make a compound cell called a *syncytium*. Thus nuclei and cytoplasm from an array of cells become enclosed within a single surface membrane of the "composite" cell. The prefix *sarco-* is used to indicate muscle, so the plasmalemma of muscle cells is often called the *sarcolemma*.

Skeletal Muscle

Skeletal muscle is characteristically striated or shows parallel banding at right angles to the long axis of the cell (Figure 1–12). The striations are due to the highly organized contractile elements within the cell. These elements are proteins, arranged in highly structured arrays capable of sliding upon each other to cause movement of the cell. The control of contractile events and details of the movements of these filaments are described in Chapter 3. The cells are arranged in parallel bundles held together by spongy connective tissue. The term *endomysium* denotes the connective tissue that surrounds the individual cells. The bundles of cells in turn are enclosed within tougher connective tissue, a sheathlike structure called *epimysium*. This outer structural material becomes specialized at either end of the muscle and has the appearance of cords or sheets of white fibrous connective tissue, called tendons. For most muscles, but not all, the tendons usually provide attachment to parts of the skeleton. If the muscle contracts to move a part of the skeleton relative to another part, for example, a limb moved around a joint, relative to the trunk, it is easy to consider the limb to be mobile and the trunk to be stationary. The end of the muscle attached to the mobile part is called the *insertion* and the end attached to the stationary part is the *origin* (Figure 1–13). In a formal study of anatomy, a student would be expected to learn the points of insertion and origin for all such muscles; it is not necessary at this stage in a first exposure to the biology of domestic animals. Skeletal muscles of the trunk, particularly those extending around the abdominal cavity, are of different form, being sheets or bands, and many of them terminate in flat sheets of tendons called *aponeuroses*. Muscles of the abdomen that are arranged in this fashion (Figure 1–14) serve to compress the abdominal cavity when they contract. They can be considered as supporting the visceral organs and are capable of increasing intraabdominal pressure.

Skeletal muscle is broadly and rather simplistically classified into red and white muscle. Red muscles are involved in sustained and continuous work, and the color results from high intracellular concentrations of pigmented molecules and organelles involved in energy provision. Red muscle is considered to be more resistant to fatigue. White muscle is found in areas required to perform quick but strictly intermittent movements. The requirements for energy provision and the intracellular makeup of white muscle are quite different from those of red muscle.

A typical muscle is shown dissected through the first few levels of detail in Figure 1–15. This will be taken to finer levels of dissection later. For now, note that in skeletal myocytes, the bulk

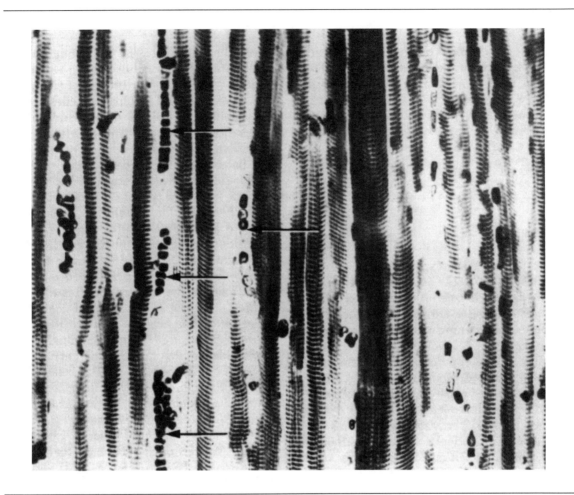

Figure 1–12. Striated muscle. This photomicrograph of a longitudinal section of striated muscle shows the characteristic banding that results from the highly organized packing of the intracellular contractile filaments, as shown in diagrammatic form in Figure 1–15. Erythrocytes (arrows) reveal the location of capillaries within the body of the muscle. (Reproduced by permission of the publisher. From Reith, E.J. and Ross, M.H.: *Atlas of Descriptive Histology*, 3rd edition, New York: Harper & Row, 1977.)

Figure 1–13. Skeleto-muscular organization. The ends of these major muscles that attach to the bones of the forearm are the insertions; the opposite ends are the origins. Complex muscles may have multiple origins or insertions. Contraction of one of these muscles will rotate the forearm around the elbow joint.

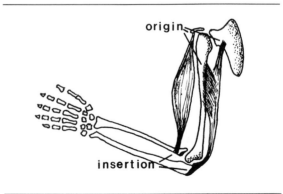

Figure 1–14. Muscle insertion into aponeuroses. A ventral, skinned dissection of the horse shows oblique muscles of the abdomen (heavy shading) terminating in broad sheets of connective tissue (light shading). These attach medially to a tough fibrous band of fused tendons called the linea alba (la).

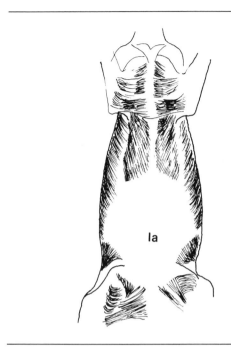

Figure 1–15. A skeletal muscle cell. This simplified diagram of skeletal muscle shows the fine internal structure of a single contractile element (myofibril) giving rise to the highly organized, banded appearance of the muscle cell or fiber. Further detail is provided in Figure 3–15. (Reproduced by permission of the publisher. From Hainsworth, F.R.: *Animal Physiology: Adaptations in Function,* Reading, MA: Addison-Wesley Publishing Company, 1981.)

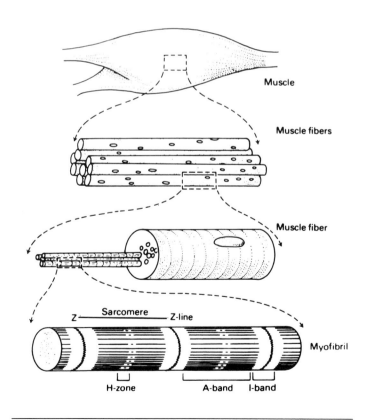

of the cell is occupied by the *myfobrils,* or the longitudinal assemblies of contractile filaments.

Cardiac Muscle

Cardiac muscle, or *myocardium,* shares some properties with skeletal muscle but has important and unique features related to its making up the circulatory pump of the body. Most of these features will be described when the physiology of the heart is considered in Chapter 5. The myofibrils of cardiac muscle are quite well organized and striations are apparent, as in skeletal muscle cells. The cells are not exclusively arranged as a mass of parallel units because that would be inappropriate for the structure of the wall of a hollow organ required to function as a pump. The cells are uninucleate and more *stellate* than spindle shaped. This means that the cells possess obliquely branching processes, which form intimate connections with similar structures on adjacent cells. The specialized contact areas are called *intercalated disks* (Figure 1–16) and they function in communication between the cells. The contractile function of myocardiocytes is highly synchronous and in large part it is achieved through the extensive intercellular contacts provided by the intercalated disks.

Cardiac cells are arranged around a matrix of connective tissue elements that fuse in selected locations as fibrous bands. There is no insertion onto any skeletal structure. Some support is obtained from the *pericardium,* a tough membrane that envelops the heart and that also provides lubrication of the surface of the myocardium. There are some more specialized subtypes of myocardiocytes to be considered. They are important for cardiac function and control of the cardiac cycle of contraction, so description of them will be deferred for now.

Smooth Muscle

Smooth muscle cells are fine, spindle-shaped units barely wider than the diameter of the single nucleus contained within. They can be very long, however, so that individual cells can be discerned by the naked eye (<0.5 mm). They

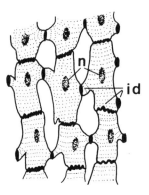

Figure 1–16. Myocardial cells. Cardiac muscle cells are uninucleate (n). They possess obliquely branching processes that abut adjacent cells in all directions. Cell–cell junctions, called intercalated disks (id), facilitate electrical communication between the cells and enable synchronous contraction to occur.

may be 50 to 100 times longer than they are wide, so shape has obvious relevance for function. For example, no part of the interior of the cell is very far from the sarcolemma.

Smooth muscle cells are suited both for tension development and for actual shortening. They may be organized into bundles of cells within a structural scaffolding of collagen and elastin fibrils, or individual cells may exist in isolation. Smooth muscle cells are found primarily in a connective tissue matrix, making up walls or parts of walls of hollow structures such as blood vessels, the gut, and the urinary duct system. In such cases, the muscle is usually organized into two distinct layers, an outer longitudinal layer and an inner circular layer, the two being separated by a thin layer of connective tissue that often provides a route of access for blood vessels and nerves to the tissue (Figure 1–17). In many cases the outer or longitudinal layer may be continuous with a ligamentous structure in which the number of smooth muscle cells is much reduced and more typical connective tissue cells such as fibrocytes predominate. Such structures often are the means by which internal organs are attached to the abdominal wall. Smooth muscles do not possess tendons

Figure 1–17. Smooth muscle organization. In this cut-away diagram, a tubular structure, such as a portion of the gut, is suspended on a ligament (lig). Blood vessels and nerves reach the gut on such structures; the ligament is continuous with the external coating, or serosal surface, of connective tissue (ect). The outer layer of smooth muscle is arranged longitudinally (lsm). At the cut surface, dots represent muscle cells cut in cross-section. Underlying the longitudinal layer is connective tissue (ct) carrying blood vessels (bv) and nerves. The circular smooth muscle (csm) lies under the connective tissue; the cut surface is a longitudinal section of this layer. The interior of the structure is made up of an epithelial lining, the mucosa (m), which encloses the lumen (lu), or space within the structure. Another connective tissue layer, the submucosa (not shown) may be located between the circular muscle and mucosa.

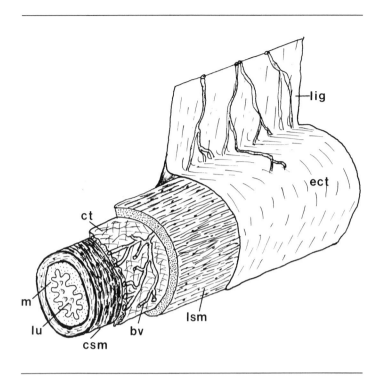

and do not have mechanical attachments to the skeleton. Microscopically, smooth muscle cells lack striations, and electron microscopy and other methods of fine analysis are needed to demonstrate the presence of myofilaments. The myofilaments are present at much reduced density than in skeletal or cardiac muscle, and they are not arranged in the strict fashion needed to appear as striations.

Nervous Tissue

Nervous tissue consists essentially of nerve cells, or *neurons*, embedded in supporting material. Each neuron typically consists of a swollen region called the *cyton*, or cell body, some short extensions or processes called *dendrites* that receive input signals, and usually one very elongated process, the *axon*, which conducts nerve impulses away from the cyton (Figure 1–18).

Neurons have structural variations and differ in size, shape, and length of the dendritic and axonal processes. In many cases the axon or nerve fiber is enclosed within a surrounding membranous sheath called *myelin*. This is a multilayered membrane that has wound itself repeatedly around the axon (Figure 1–19). It serves to insulate the axolemma, or axon membrane, from the interstitial fluid.

A peripheral nerve is composed of parallel arrays of neurons, held together with white connective tissue. There are usually no cytons except at particular locations where many occur adjacent to others to produce a swelling on the nerve called a ganglion. The gathering of cytons at particular locations is also true within the central nervous system (CNS), the brain, and the spinal cord. These masses of cytons are often called *nuclei*. They have a paucity of myelin, and such tissue is called *gray matter*. In other locations, axons and dendrites predominate over cytons and the former are associated with the whitish myelin sheath material; such tissue is called

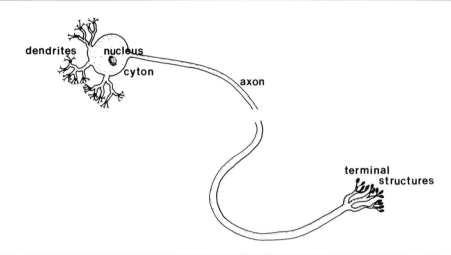

Figure 1–18. The neuron. Nerve cells typically consist of several basic structures, although the geometry varies enormously. The cyton is the cell body, and contains the nucleus. Multiple dendrites serve as inputs; a single axon, with various types of terminal structures, serves as the output arm of the cell.

Figure 1–19. The myelin sheath. The sheath is the spirally-wrapped coating of a Schwann cell, closely apposed to the axon of a neuron. In the mature form, the cytoplasm of the Schwann cell will be almost entirely excluded from the wrapping, so the sheath becomes a multilayered structure of virtually pure plasmalemma. (Reproduced by permission of the publisher. From Gordon, M.S.: *Animal Physiology: Principles and Adaptations*, 3rd edition, New York: Macmillan Publishing Co, Inc., 1977.)

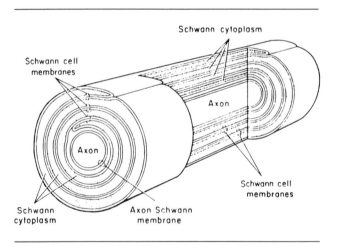

white matter. The connections between neurons, or *synapses*, will be described in detail when the function of nerve tissue is described, in Chapter 3. These communication locations are found mainly on the dendrites and near the cytons and so they occur mostly in the gray matter. The white matter is where most of the conduction of nerve impulses within the nervous system takes place. The distribution of white and gray matter in the brain and spinal cord gives these structures a characteristic appearance (Figure 1–20).

Neurons are supported by a mass of tissue of similar embryonic origin but not involved in generating, conducting, or processing information. This material is called *neuroglia* and most likely aids in a nutritive capacity. Additionally, there are minor amounts of connective tissues and, of course, blood vessels to supply the neural

Figure 1–20. *Gross structure of neural tissue.* This section of the brain has been stained to emphasize the characteristic distribution of gray matter, lying peripheral to the white matter. The white matter is extensively myelinated. In the spinal cord, white matter lies peripheral to the gray, the reverse arrangement to that of the brain. (Reprinted by permission of the publisher. From Gardner, E.: *Fundamentals of Neurology,* Philadelphia: W.B. Saunders Company, 1968.)

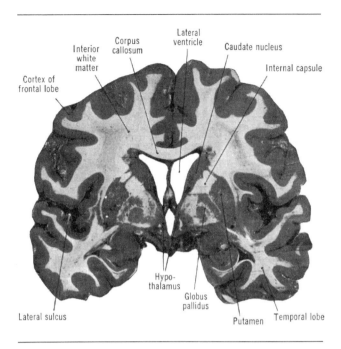

cells. Neural tissue is structurally weak because of the relative lack of connective tissue. Within the CNS, the tissues are surrounded by a series of membranes that define spaces filled with cushioning layers of fluid. The whole structure is enclosed within the protective cage of bone provided by the cranium or the spinal column (Figure 1–21).

Blood and Lymph

The last major tissue types to be considered now are unique in being fluid tissues. Blood is the liquid medium for transportation through the body of oxygen, carbon dioxide, assimilated nutrients, other products of metabolism, hormones, and so on. Like other tissues, blood consists of cells and intercellular material, but unlike

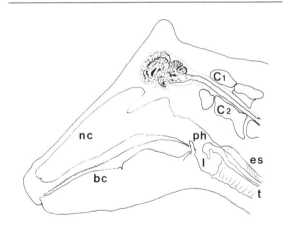

Figure 1–21. *Location of the central nervous system (CNS).* This midline section of a bovine head shows the brain and part of the spinal cord (shaded) lying within the bony neural cavity (dotted outline). Note the relatively small size of the brain. Some landmark structures include the nasal cavity (nc), buccal cavity (bc), pharynx (ph), esophagus (es), larynx (l), trachea (t), and cervical vertebrae (C1 and C2).

most tissues, blood cells are free to move about; they lack attachments to other cells. The fluid interstitial material in blood is called plasma, and the remaining components of blood are properly called the *formed elements*. These include red blood cells, or *erythrocytes*, white blood cells, or *leukocytes*, and tiny *platelets*. Erythrocytes, in mammals at least, and platelets lack nuclei so they are atypical of cells in general; they may be considered to be fragments or parts of cells. The erythrocytes are specialized for carrying oxygen because, in vertebrates, the red pigmented protein, hemoglobin, which reversibly binds oxygen, is totally confined within these cells. The cells are biconcave disks, lacking nuclei and capable of surviving in the bloodstream for only a finite period of time. Erythrocytes in birds retain their nuclei, and the cells are elliptical in shape. The erythrocytes are formed continuously throughout life by a process called erythropoiesis in tissues specialized for this function. During adult life, marrow in the cavities of bones is the site of erythropoiesis, but the liver and spleen produce the cells during fetal life.

Far less numerous than erythrocytes are the white blood cells. These are nucleated, assume various forms, and most are motile cells capable of independent movement. There are various types of leukocytes, classified according to their content of discrete granules. The major functions of these cells will be described in Chapter 9 in relation to the body's defense systems. *Granulocytes* can be stained with dyes that interact with the granules and can be distinguished from *agranulocytes*. Leukocytes are a key part of the body's defense mechanisms. Many of the cells are phagocytic, meaning that they can engulf particulate matter such as bacteria, protozoa, fragments of damaged cells, and so forth. Some of the cells have the ability to localize around sites of infection, to squeeze out of the blood vessels, and to directly attack microorganisms. They are also capable of digesting dead tissue, producing a semiliquid material known as *pus*. Many of the leukocytes participate in the immunologic defense system, either by detecting foreign materials or by actively producing antibody proteins capable of neutralizing the foreign material.

Platelets, or thrombocytes, are fragments of protoplasm a mere 2 to 4 μ in size. They are also produced in erythropoietic tissues such as marrow and in the spleen and spend just a few days in circulation. They are particularly important in hemostasis, or blood clotting, another body defense mechanism.

All tissues have interstitial fluid material; in the case of blood this is plasma. In the solid tissues, the interstitial fluid is quite similar to plasma and is formed in part by the continued leaking of a filtrate of plasma from the finest blood vessels, the capillaries. In addition, materials including water are secreted into the tissue fluid from the cell mass, and there may be formed elements such as leukocytes that have transferred out of the blood vessels and into the tissues. In Chapter 5, when the dynamics of blood circulation are considered, it will become evident that there is an enormous flux of fluid across the capillaries, largely because the blood is under hydrostatic pressure from pumping of the heart into a resistance system of fine blood vessels. The leaked fluid is also continually collected by the lymphatic system and delivered back into the blood circulation. In the process, tissue fluid becomes *lymph*. The fluid is taken up into minute blind-ended vessels like part-capillaries. These feed into progressively larger vessels called *lymphatics*, or lymph ducts, shortly before they empty into the great veins. Along their path, the lymphatics pass through lymph glands, which strain particulate matter from the lymph and add cells to the lymph. The lymph glands, or nodes, constitute part of the reticuloendothelial system.

The lymph has one special function quite distinct from those already described. Lymphatics in the wall of the intestines are the means by which fats are absorbed, and the lymph draining the gut can be very rich in fat, which confers upon it a distinctly milky appearance.

Much of the foregoing discussion will be expanded and developed in relation to the structure and function of the major body systems in subsequent chapters of this book. It is premature at this stage to probe the function of the various types of tissues and organs in great detail. Be sure to return to this introductory treatment of the basic cell and tissue types whenever starting consideration of a new major body system.

1.3 • Methods and Terminology of Anatomy

Various approaches are used in the study of anatomy, but the one that is most useful when function or physiology is studied concurrently is systematic anatomy. This is the study of the various organ groups or systems of the body. Traditionally, each organ system is studied as a unit, and then the parts are brought together for a deeper understanding of the structure and function of the whole animal. For convenience, the body is considered as consisting of 11 major systems:

Skeletal,

Muscular,

Vascular,

Digestive,

Respiratory,

Urinary,

Reproductive,

Nervous,

Endocrine,

Common integument (skin), and

Special senses.

Each of these systems is functionally related to the others, and it is artificial to select one of them for study in isolation. The nervous, endocrine, integument, and special senses systems are considered to be integrating systems, study of which gives the student opportunity to draw everything together, to appreciate the whole. Many texts depend very heavily on an anatomic approach to structure and function; in a sense they present an anatomist's views of physiology. The emphasis is placed on what is known with certainty, or the anatomic facts, and function is grafted onto this framework.

The approach taken in this book is just the reverse. Emphasis is placed on phenomena and mechanisms of function, with input from anatomy only to the extent needed to understand function. As such, factual detail is deemphasized somewhat, in favor of analysis and interpretation. Several of the *body systems* listed above will be combined in this treatment. An anatomic overview will be presented, but a detailed anatomic analysis will be avoided.

Terminology

Before we start to consider the structure of the body parts, an adequate vocabulary is needed to aid in description, location, and form. There is a voluminous terminology already in use in the discipline of anatomy. It is also complex because of frequent synonyms and the common use of the same term in two or more ways. The language of anatomy leans heavily on Greek and Latin, and those with some knowledge of classical languages will more easily grasp the meaning of seemingly complex or awkward words. When a new term is encountered, one should attempt to relate its meaning to the roots from which it is formed.

Different kinds of terms are used in anatomy. *General* terms like artery, vein, nerve, and so forth are usually qualified by an adjective or specifying term: *femoral* artery, *jugular* vein, *sciatic* nerve. *Specific* names identify given organs or parts such as *liver, spleen, forelimb, foot*. *Regional* names identify portions of the body and are used as nouns, such as *thorax* or *abdomen*, or as qualifying adjectives, such as *thoracic* or *abdominal*. *Orientation* terms are used to indicate the spatial relation of one part or organ relative to another,

or to indicate aspect. Terms of orientation are the most confusing for students of animals because of the differences between quadrupeds and bipeds such as humans.

In Figure 1–22 the quadruped is shown standing with its body straightened out in the horizontal position and the limbs also straight and vertical, although the hand and foot (or the fingers and toes) may be flat on the ground. The upper surface of the body is now *dorsal* and the lower surface is *ventral*. The sides of the body are *lateral*. The animal is facing in an *anterior* direction, and the opposite direction is *posterior*. These relational aspects do not change even if the animal changes position. For example, if the dog stands up with its forelimbs resting on a high fence, its belly surface is still ventral, and so on.

It is often convenient to substitute the terms cranial in place of anterior, and caudal in place of posterior. There is also occasional use of terms

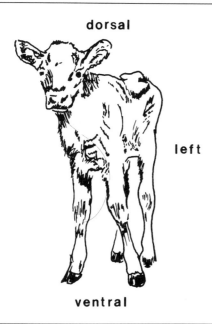

dorsal

left

ventral

Figure 1–22. Anatomical orientation. This calf is viewed from the front, its anterior end. The uppermost surface is called dorsal; the belly surface is called ventral. The lateral surface in view is the calf's left side.

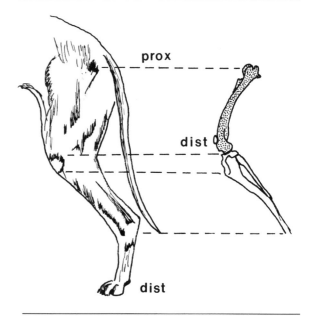

prox

dist

dist

Figure 1–23. Orientation of projecting parts. This hind limb of a greyhound illustrates the meaning of proximal (prox)—nearest the point of attachment—and distal (dist)—farthest from the point of attachment. These terms are also applied to the constituent parts, shown here for the femur, or thighbone (shaded).

adopted from human anatomy. The adjectives *ascending* and *descending* are used synonymously with *cephalad* or *caudad,* meaning directed toward the head or toward the rear, respectively. Examples of this use are: ascending aorta and descending aorta. The terms superior and inferior are additional synonyms, but these can usually be avoided.

For any projecting part, such as a limb, the attached end is described as proximal and the unattached end as distal. These adjectives are applied to parts of limbs as well (Figure 1–23). For example, the femur, a major bone of the hindlimb, has a proximal end and a distal end. The same terms are applied to parts of nerves and blood vessels. If a nerve passes from the spinal cord to a distant structure, the portion nearest the spine is called proximal and the parts farthest away are called distal. When in doubt about this, consider how the location of some structure is

described to another person. For example, we speak of the near end and the far end of a bridge with reference to where we happen to be standing. If a blood vessel is transected, we speak of the proximal cut end and the distal cut end, with reference to the major trunk vessels.

The surfaces of the projecting parts are also described using the terms applied to the trunk, although bending of the limbs often obscures the relations. For example, when the hand or its equivalent is flat on the ground, the upper surface is still dorsal while the lower surface, equivalent to the ventral surface, in this case is called *volar* or, somewhat easier to remember, *palmar.* For the foot, either volar or *plantar* is used.

This referencing can be taken further. Anatomists and morphologists describe locations on the body with reference to the long axis (Figure 1–24). The *median plane* is an imaginary plane through the center of the spinal column that

Figure 1–24. Anatomical planes. Planes are imaginary lines or cuts that section the body in various directions related to the long axis. The median plane separates the body through the length of the spinal column to give left and right halves. The transverse plane is vertically perpendicular to the median plane and serves to create cross sections. The frontal plane is perpendicular to each of the foregoing and separates the dorsal from the ventral portion.

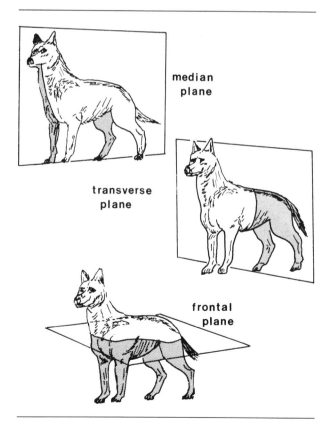

divides the body into two equal halves, the left and the right, as viewed from the animal's back. This orientation can be a little confusing during dissection, as an animal is usually placed on its back and the dissection is usually performed from the ventral surface. In this situation it is necessary to mentally transpose sides.

Imaginary planes parallel to the medial plane but dividing the body into longitudinal slices rather than halves are called *saggital planes.* *Transverse planes* are at right angles to the medial plane and transect the body into cranial and caudal portions. Transverse planes can be considered as producing cross-sections of the body. Finally, *frontal planes* are at right angles to both the medial and transverse planes and divide the body into dorsal and ventral portions.

Additionally, there is widespread use of ordinary and commonsense terms such as the opposed pairs: central and peripheral, deep and superficial, internal and external, and so forth. Finally, whenever appropriate, the foregoing terms can be combined for greater precision. For example, the area high on the flank of an animal could be described as dorsolateral.

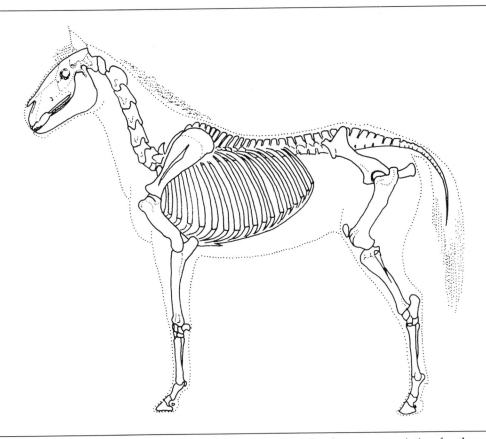

Figure 1–25. Horse skeleton. Examine this illustration to develop an appreciation for the relationships that are evident between the skull and neck, the limbs and spine, and ribs and spine. The external surface of the animal is shown in dotted outline to indicate the amount of variation in soft tissue cover of the skeleton. The portions of the skeleton which require detailed treatment are shown in subsequent figures.

1.4 • The Skeleton

The skeleton is the framework of hard structures that supports and protects the soft tissues of animals. In order of importance, skeletal structures consist of bones, cartilages, and ligaments; sometimes teeth are included in this grouping. The formal study of bones is called *osteology*, the study of cartilage is called *chondrology*, the study of joints is called *arthrology*, and the study of teeth is called *odontology*.

The skeleton (Figure 1–25) is best considered in terms of two major parts: the *axial skeleton* and the *appendicular skeleton*. In some cases a third division, the visceral skeleton, may be included.

The Axial Skeleton

The axial skeleton includes the skull, the vertebrae of the vertebral column, and the ribs and sternum (Figure 1–26). The vertebrae make up a chain, or column, of unpaired dorsomedial bones that extends from the skull to the caudal extremity of the tail. They are divided into five regions: *cervical, thoracic, lumbar, sacral,* and *coccygeal,* corresponding to the everyday terms, neck, chest, waist, rump, and tail.

The Vertebrae

The sacral vertebrae are partly fused one to another to form a rigid platelike structure that supports the pelvis. The individual bones within each region are named or numbered craniad to caudad. For example, the cervical vertebrae are labeled C-1, C-2, C-3 . . . C-7. Individual vertebrae have distinguishing features that enable a skilled anatomist to uniquely identify them. They also have some common features, and all

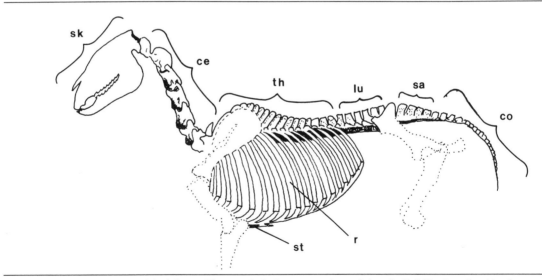

Figure 1–26. Axial skeleton. The axial skeleton consists of the skull (sk), the ribs (r), the sternum (st), and the vertebral column, divided here into cervical (ce), thoracic (th), lumbar (lu), sacral (sa), and coccygeal (co) portions. The appendicular skeletal attachments are shown in dotted outline.

can be considered to be made up of three parts (Figure 1–27): the *body*, the *arch*, and *processes*.

The body is the cylindric mass, oriented craniocaudally along its long axis, upon which all other parts are formed. The body of one vertebra is juxtaposed cranially and caudally with

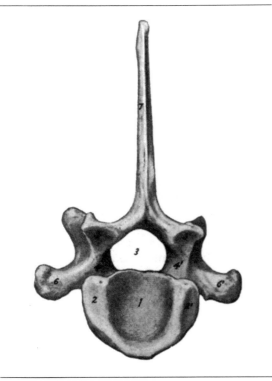

Figure 1–27. Major trunk vertebrae of cattle: C–7. The vertebra consists of a body (1) to which processes are attached. The vertebrae from different locations along the column have characteristic shapes, largely determined by the relative sizes of the processes. The last cervical vertebra (C–7) from the bovine skeleton is shown in posterior view. The arch (4) encloses the spinal canal (vertebral foramen, 3). The dorsal spinous process (7) is well developed; the transverse processes (6) are better exemplified in the lumbar vertebrae. The articular processes (5) juxtapose the first thoracic vertebra. Facets (2) provide articulating surfaces for the first ribs. (Reprinted by permission of the publisher. From Sisson, S. and Grossman, J.D.: The Anatomy of Domestic Animals, 3rd edition, Philadelphia: W.B. Saunders Company, 1938.)

bodies of adjacent vertebrae. The apposing surfaces are separated by *menisci*, or cartilaginous disks. A more detailed description is provided in Box 1–1.

Individual vertebrae within the column have distinguishing features, and there may be considerable variation between species. The least variable are the cervical vertebrae, of which there are seven in virtually all mammals. The first two are somewhat modified from the others, consistent with their special function of articulating the skull (Figure 1–28). The first (C-1), or *atlas*, articulates cranially with the *occipital condyles* of the skull (see Figure 1–30 for the location of the occipital bone) and caudally with the *axis*, or C-2. The condyles are rounded projections of bone, in this case formed as part of the occipital bone at the back of the skull. The two articulating faces of atlas are both concave in shape.

Articulation between the atlas and the skull permits dorsoventral movement of the head on the vertebral column. Articulation between atlas and axis is more pivot-like than hinge-like and so the skull and C-1 can rotate on C-2.

The vertebral column as a unit is morphologically similar across the mammalian species yet differs in function, especially in regard to flexibility. The column of herbivores such as sheep, goats, cattle, and horses is relatively rigid, at least over the thoracic, lumbar, and sacral elements. The column provides structural support for bulky and often heavy visceral contents such as the digestive tract and a heavy, pregnant uterus. The column also serves to transmit forces of the legs to the body, as required for locomotion. Carnivores, animals of prey, have very flexible spines. These animals have small, compact digestive tracts and the pregnant females exhibit strictly limited activity, using a nest or den as their base. The spinal column of carnivores, therefore, is less involved with load-bearing. Its greater flexibility is beneficial for running. Because of the flexible spinal column, the running animal adds greater distance and force to each stride; acceleration is also enhanced. These aspects of locomotion are discussed later.

Box 1–1   The Vertebrae

The orientation of the cervical, thoracic, and lumbar vertebrae can usually be deduced from the faces. With few exceptions, the cranial faces are convex and the caudal faces are concave. Coccygeal vertebrae are convex on both faces. In general, the ventral surface of the vertebra is rounded while the dorsal, or uppermost, surface of the body is flattened and forms the floor of the *foramen*, or spinal canal.

The arch has two lateral halves that extend dorsally, the two halves then fuse medially to enclose the vertebral foramen. The series of foramina, extending from C-1 to a location that varies somewhat within the sacral vertebrae, creates a longitudinal canal that encloses the spinal cord.

The processes are extensions in various directions out from the body of the vertebrae. Most obvious are the paired *transverse processes*, which project laterally or ventrolaterally; the single dorsal *spinous process*; and the paired *articular processes*, of which there are usually two anterior and two posterior, for each of the vertebrae.

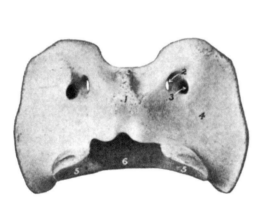 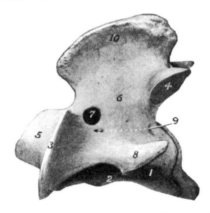

Figure 1–28. Atlas (C–1) and axis (C–2) in cattle. These specialized cervical vertebrae provide great flexibility in head movements. Atlas (C–1) is shown at left in a dorsal view. It has a slight dorsal prominence, with the tubercle (1) and large lateral wings (4). Small foramina are marked (2 and 3) but the major vertebral foramen is obscured, except for the part of the floor (6) with which the dens of axis contacts and is permitted some opportunity for rotation. The posterior articulating surfaces (5) also meet with axis. To the right, axis (C–2) is shown in left lateral view and has a quite distinct form. The body (1) is more cylindrical, and there is a more obvious ventral spine (2). The anterior articular process (3) meets with atlas; the posterior articulating facets (4) are located more dorsally. The anterior structure that fits into the vertebral foramen of atlas is the dens (5). More caudally, this merges with the arch (6), which in turn is continuous with transverse (8) and dorsal (10) processes. The minor foramina (7 and 9) are also evident in this view. (Reprinted by permission of the publisher. From Sisson, S. and Grossman, J.D.: *The Anatomy of Domestic Animals*, 3rd edition, Philadelphia: W.B. Saunders Company, 1938.)

The Ribs and Sternum

The ribs are modified long bones that articulate dorsally with the body region of two adjacent vertebrae; their ventral termini meet the *costal cartilages*. These may or may not attach directly to the *sternum*, or breastbone. Ribs are partly flattened and thinner on the cranial and caudal border, making them oval in cross-section (Figure 1–29). They have marrow cavities that function in erythropoiesis, they perform the critical function of protecting the thoracic viscera, and,

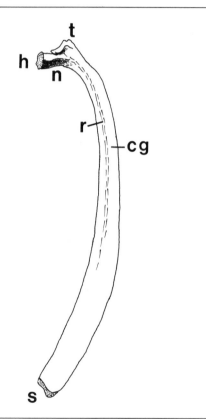

Figure 1–29. Rib. A medial view of a bovine rib is shown. The tubercle (t) articulates with a transverse process of a vertebra and is somewhat lateral to the head (h) and separated from it by the neck (n). The head articulates with parts of the bodies of two adjacent vertebrae. A ridge (r) extends down the rib and defines the costal groove (cg). The sternal end (s) is a costo-chondral junction with a costal cartilage (not shown) providing connection to the sternum.

along with their associated muscles, they are part of the respiratory mechanical apparatus. The dorsal extremity is called the *head* of the rib and is found adjacent to the intervertebral disk or meniscus. A given head articulates in part with one vertebra and in part with the next vertebra. The ventral extremity is a roughened surface, the *costochondral junction*, where bone meets cartilage. In Box 1–2 a classification of the ribs is provided for the reader seeking a more complete treatment. The spaces between the ribs are called *intercostal spaces* and are the sites of important respiratory muscles, described in Chapter 5.

The most ventral portion of the thoracic cage is the sternum, formed by fusion of unpaired bones that take various forms, depending on the species. Most caudally, the sternum terminates in a flat, triangular segment of hyaline cartilage, the *xiphoid*.

The Skull

The *skull* is the skeletal portion of the head and consists of two parts: the *cranium* and the *face*. The cranium is made up of the skull bones that immediately surround and enclose the brain, thereby forming the vault and floor of the brain cavity. Facial bones are all other bones that are not cranial (Figure 1–30).

Bones of the cranium fall into two groups: unpaired bones and paired bones. The unpaired bones can be thought of as highly specialized and modified extensions of the vertebral column. The most caudal unpaired bone is the occipital, which provides the hind wall and floor of the cranial cavity. Ventrally, a large foramen, or opening, the *foramen magnum*, provides a point of exit for the spinal cord, which then enters the spinal canal, starting at the atlas vertebra. Lateral to the foramen magnum are the processes called occipital condyles, which articulate with the face of the atlas vertebra. It is not important at this stage to have more than a general appreciation of the arrangement of the bones of the skull. A more detailed description is provided in Box 1–3.

The bones of the face similarly fall into a group of three unpaired bones and nine paired

---

Box 1–2   Classification of Ribs

Ribs can be divided into *sternal* and *asternal* groups. Sternal ribs connect via costal cartilages directly to the sternum. They are also called true ribs. The remainder are asternal, or false ribs. The most caudal ribs have free ventral ends and are known as floating ribs. In very old animals, ossification of the costal cartilages may be apparent, and there is some loss of flexibility of the thorax.

Figure 1–30. The *bovine skull*. Note the relative enormity of the mandible and the nature of the dentition. Some of the cranial bones noted in the text are obscured in this lateral view. Those shown here are occipital (a); occipital condyle (a'); frontal (b); parietal (c); temporal (d); zygomatic arch (d'); nasal (e); lacrimal (f); malar (g); maxilla (h); premaxilla (i); mandible (j); condyle of mandible (j'); coronoid process of mandible (j''); palatine (k); and paramastoid process (l).

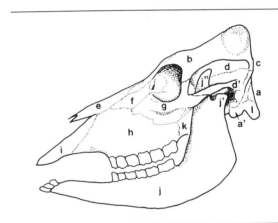

Box 1–3   The Cranial Bones

The remaining unpaired bones of the cranium, not described in the main text, are the *sphenoid* and *ethmoid*, which together make up the medial portion of the floor of the cranial cavity. All other cranial bones are paired, and individuals of pairs join medially to enclose the cranial cavity. The paired cranial bones are the *interparietal*, *parietal*, *frontal*, and *temporal* bones.

In herbivores, the bones of the cranium are difficult to depict in a lateral drawing because the massive dorsal processes of the mandible extend on either side of the temporal bones. In general terms, the parietal bones provide the dorsal shell, the frontals provide the front, the temporals the sides, the interparietals the back, and the single bones (occipital, sphenoid, and ethmoid) provide the floor, from back to front.

bones. The largest bone, the *mandible* (commonly called the jawbone), although classified as a single bone, is actually composed of two halves, fused at the forwardmost extremity. The mandible carries the lower teeth. To the rear the mandible extends into long processes that articulate around the zygomatic arches, these being lateral girdles of bone formed from the *temporal bone* and an extension of the *malar bone*. The *hyoid*, also unpaired, is a compound bone of many fused parts that supports the base of the tongue, the pharynx, and the larynx.

The many paired bones of the face form the upper jaw, supports for upper teeth, protection for the nasal cavities, sockets for the eyes, and so forth.

The Appendicular Skeleton

The appendicular skeleton attaches to the axial skeleton via the bony and ligamentous structures that make up the *pectoral girdle*, or shoulder, and the *pelvic girdle*, or hip.

The Pectoral Girdle and Limbs

In domestic herbivores, the pectoral girdle consists solely of the *scapulas*, or shoulder blades, with very pronounced suprascapular cartilages extending from the dorsal margins. There are no clavicles, or collarbones, in these animals. The forelimbs are attached to the trunk exclusively by means of fleshy and tendinous connections. In other words, there is no joint or socket between the forelimb and spine analogous to the ball-and-socket joint by which the femur articulates with the pelvis.

Using the horse as an example, the bones making up the pectoral limb, or forelimb, are shown in Figure 1–31. The bones are shown in lateral view on the left and in medial view on the right. Note the riblike tuber spinae that projects from the lateral surface of the scapula. For general equivalence, the *humerus* is the bone of

the upper arm, the *radius* and *ulna* are bones of the forearm, and the *carpus* is equivalent to the proximal part of the wrist. The *metacarpals* are equivalent to the bones of the hand.

The function of the major bones of the pectoral girdle and forelimb is described briefly below.

Scapula

The scapula transmits forces and motion of the forelimb to the body. It serves as a scaffolding to provide support and attachment for muscles and connective tissues that together support the anterior parts of the body. The flattened shape enables facile sliding without distorting the closely approximated muscles, which might otherwise impair the mechanical efficiency of the limb. The medial surface is smooth and slides back and forth against muscle and connective tissues. The lateral surface is ridged to provide attachment, at the tuber spinae, for muscles of the upper limb and shoulder and the suspending muscles and connective tissue that hold the scapula into the pectoral girdle.

Humerus

The arm bone provides connection from the scapula to the distal portions of the limb. Attachments are provided for major muscles controlling movement of the upper and lower limb. The angular articulation on the scapula, approximately 90°, has an important shock-absorbing function that cushions the body against the impact of forefeet hitting the ground.

Radius and Ulna

These two bones of the lower arm are partially or completely fused in herbivores. The fusion prevents rotation of the lower portion of the limb while allowing the back-and-forth movement required for locomotion.

Carpus

This series of bones (six to eight, varying with species) is incorrectly called the knee in animals. The bones are more equivalent to those of our

Figure 1–31. The equine pectoral limb. The major bones of the equine pectoral limb are shown from lateral (left) and medial (right) perspectives. Many of the bones have been given recognizable names. The common names for metacarpal bones are included in the figure; other more recognizable names are fetlock (j); pastern (k); navicular (l); and coffin (m). Observe the general nature of the angles at the joint areas and note that the lateral surfaces are not as smooth as the medial surfaces. The ridges and projections provide attachment sites for the muscles responsible for moving the limb.

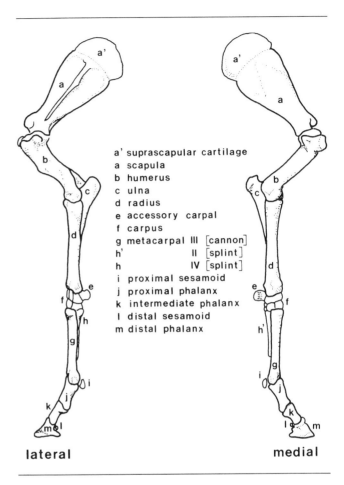

a' suprascapular cartilage
a scapula
b humerus
c ulna
d radius
e accessory carpal
f carpus
g metacarpal III [cannon]
h'   II [splint]
h   IV [splint]
i proximal sesamoid
j proximal phalanx
k intermediate phalanx
l distal sesamoid
m distal phalanx

lateral   **medial**

wrist, and use of the term ''knee'' should be restricted to the hindlimb. Equivalent to the tarsus, or hock of the hindlimb, the carpus is important in locomotion because it provides hinging and some shock absorption. Movements at this location are *flexion* in nature, which means that parts more distal to the joint can rotate toward the body. The opposite type of rotation, away from the body, is called *extension*.

It is important to distinguish between flexion and extension. Extend your arm straight out to the side and horizontal to the ground. Now bend your elbow and rotate the forearm and hand toward the front of your body. This is flexion. Now restraighten your arm. As the forearm and hand move away from your body, the distal part of the limb is undergoing extension. The terms flex and extend are often incorrectly applied to muscles. Muscles cannot flex. They can be contracted or they can relax.

The carpal bones are subject to considerable stress but are not especially resistant to compression forces. Damage to these bones is a major cause of tenderness and lameness.

Metacarpals

The number of metacarpals differs among species but corresponds to the number of visible or functional digits (Figure 1–32). In the cloven-

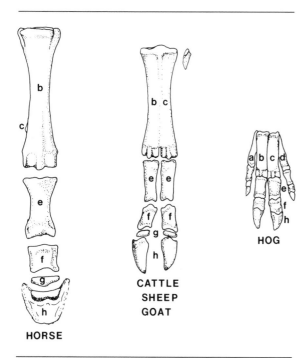

Figure 1–32. Bones of the distal limb. Front/dorsal views of comparable structures in animals with different numbers of functional digits are shown. The uppermost bones are metacarpals II to V (a–d). For the horse, metacarpal III (b) is shown; metacarpals II and IV (the splints) are partly vestigial and they lie on the posterior side. In domestic ruminants, metacarpals III and IV (b and c) are fused to form the cannon bone; metacarpal V is largely vestigial. In pigs, metacarpals II to V (a–d) are all present. Distal to the metacarpals are the phalanx bones: proximal (e), or first phalanx; intermediate (f), or second phalanx; distal (h), or third phalanx. In the exploded views, the distal sesamoids (g) are also shown. They are located on the volar side between the intermediate and distal phalanx bones.

hoofed ruminants, metacarpals III and IV are fused to form a single bone, although two separate cavities may remain. This structure is commonly called the *cannon* bone.

Digits

The digits are analogous to the fingers or toes of primates. The number of bones varies widely among species. For example, horses have a sin-

gle digit per foot, ruminants have two digits per foot, pigs have four. In addition, there may be false digits, also called *dewclaws*, but these do not articulate with a metacarpal or, in the case of the hindlimb, a metatarsal.

The Pelvic Girdle and Limb

The *pelvis* consists of a left and right innominate bone, or *os coxae*, which fuse ventrally at the *symphysis pelvis*. Each innominate bone has three major fused parts: *ilium, ischium,* and *pubis.*

Examine the illustrations in Figure 1–33 to understand the orientation of the pelvis. Note that the dorsocranial extension of the ilium, the tuber sacrale, curves upward and backward and lies medial to the tuber coxae. In the dorsal view, the broad gluteal surface faces the tail region. On the other side the pelvic surface faces forward and downward. The two pelvic faces bracket and articulate with the sacral mass of the vertebral column. The tuberacoxae (*tuber* means "swelling," *coxae* means "of the hip"), are the prominent "points" of the hip, readily discerned in the intact animal.

The pubis and ischium together form the floor of the pelvis. The anterior border of the pubis provides the lower rim of the pelvic inlet from the abdominal cavity. Laterally, the pubis, ischium, and ilium fuse at the acetabulum, a ventrolaterally facing fossa, or cavity, that encloses the articulating head of the femur. An extension of the femur, the trochanter major (see under "femur" in Box 1–4), extends dorsally beyond the lateral margin of the ischium. The floor of the pelvis includes oval-shaped openings, each of which is called an obturator foramen (plural, *foramina*).

The pelvis is superbly suited for mechanical coupling of the hindlimb and the vertebral column. This connection is made at the sacroiliac joint. The pelvis, being a massive bony girdle, efficiently transmits propulsive forces from the limb to the body.

The pelvic opening provides the rigid wall of the birth canal in the female and so is usually larger in diameter and tends to be more circular in females than in males. Knowledge of pelvic

Figure 1–33. The pelvis. This right lateral view of the bovine pelvis shows the typical angle or orientation observed in cursorial quadrupeds. The tubera coxae (d) are readily discernible as the points of the hip in most animals. The lower figure looks back through the pelvic inlet, bracketed by the shafts and wings of the ilium (a) with the sacral mass of vertebrae shown cross-hatched. Note the symphysis pelvis (i) extending caudally across the floor of the pelvis. It is the line of fusion of the pubis (nearest) and ischii which are partly obscured in this view, although the lateral processes—the tubera ischii (f)—can be seen on each side at the rear.

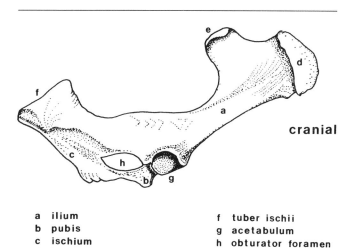

cranial

a ilium	f tuber ischii
b pubis	g acetabulum
c ischium	h obturator foramen
d tuber coxae	i symphysis pelvis
e tuber sacrale	

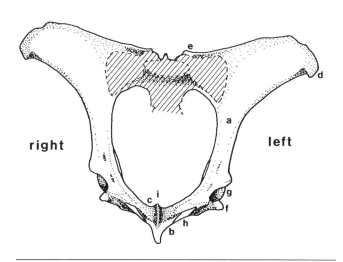

right   left

anatomy, especially of the angles and orientation of the inlet and floor, is important in obstetric management of animals.

The hindlimb bones include the *femur*, the *patella*, the *tibia* and *fibula*, the bones of the *tarsus*, the *metatarsals*, and the bones of the *digits*. The relations among these bones in cattle are shown from a lateral perspective in Figure 1–34. From this illustration it should be apparent that the angles at the major joints allow flexion rotation at all joints except the knee, that is, between the femur and the tibia-fibula. The nature of and functions of the hindlimb bones are briefly described in Box 1–4. The reader should be familiar with the names of the major bones of each limb and their relative locations.

Figure 1–34. The pelvic limb of cattle. Shown here in lateral view are the pelvic limb, the pelvis, and segments of lumbar (1), sacral (s), and first coccygeal vertebrae. Note the general similarity to the forelimb shown in Figure 1–31. You should be able to recognize the major bones or groups of bones labeled here and noted in the text. A more detailed, bone-by-bone description is provided in Box 1–4.

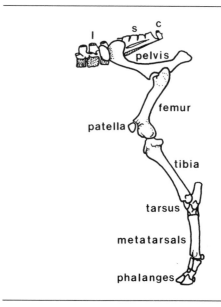

1.5 • An Introduction to Myology

Muscles are the means by which parts of the body are moved. Along with the skeleton, they provide support for the body and play a role in resisting gravity, thereby contributing to stance.

If we use the muscles supporting the neck and head as an example, there is provision for lowering and raising these structures, for moving them to the left or right, and for fixing the anterior parts in a state of rigidity. Up-and-down movement may be strictly in the medial plane, where lowering corresponds to flexing, thus bringing the head closer to the trunk; and raising is equivalent to extension, or taking the head further away from the trunk. When the neck is turned to the left or right from the medial plane, or midline, the term *abductor* is applied to the muscles responsible for this maneuver (Figure 1–35). The muscles that draw the structures back toward the midline are called *adductors*. To review an earlier definition, muscles that help straighten a limb around a joint and cause distal parts to move away from the body are extensors. Those that cause distal parts to rotate closer to the body are flexors (Figure 1–36).

Earlier, an exercise involving bending and straightening the elbow was used to illustrate flexion and extension. Now hold your right arm straight out in front and horizontal so that you are looking forward at your hand. Swing your arm so it moves 90° to the right and is now directly up

Box 1–4 The Bones of the Pelvic Limb

Femur: The massive bone of the upper leg is larger proximally than distally. The proximal articulating surface is found on the *head* of the femur; this inserts into the acetabulum of the pelvis. The distal extremity forms condyles that face ventrally and articulate with the head of the tibia. On the more ventral side, smaller bony swellings called the trochlea ("shaped like a pulley") are the points of articulation with the patella. There are considerable interspecies differences in the form and relative dimensions of the femur.

Patella: The patella, popularly called the kneecap, has no equivalent in the forelimb. It serves to increase the force and efficacy of extensor effort that can be applied to the limb distal to the knee. Hindlimb propulsion in animals is due to overall straightening of the whole leg. This is analogous to our standing from a squatting position. The patella, located somewhat dorsal to the joint and between the femur and tibia-fibula, enables more vigorous extension or kick and so adds to the velocity of movement. Note that the "kick" referred to here is different from a human kick, which involves a forward rotation that straightens the leg at the knee and rotation at the hip that allows the upper leg to flex.

Tibia: The tibia, the major bone of the lower leg, extends downward and backward from the femur to the tarsus. The bone is somewhat triangular in cross-section and proximal extremity is larger than the distal extremity.

Fibula: This small bone is considered to be becoming vestigial in the domestic mammals. It is closely apposed to and in part fused with the tibia, though considerable interspecies differences exist. Fracture of this bone, though not affecting the mechanics of hindlimb propulsion, is a common cause of lameness. The reader will most likely have encountered the fibula as a needle-sharp fine bone in a chicken's leg.

Tarsus: The tarsus does for the hindlimb much what the carpus does for the forelimb. Distal to these compound bones and joints, each limb is capable of flexing. Note, however, that rotation around the carpus is backward while flexion at the tarsus involves forward rotation (see Figures 1–31 and 1–34). These differences are quite consistent with the definition of flexion given earlier. One of the tarsal bones, the fibular tarsus, is markedly extended and serves as the insertion for the calf muscle, the gastrocnemius, by means of the Achilles tendon. The tibial tarsal, also called the trochlea, serves as the pivot for flexion and extension of the hock joint. Cattle and sheep have paired trochleae. Like the carpus, the tarsus serves in shock absorption and provides leverage to the hindfoot, thereby influencing agility and speed.

Metatarsals: These bones of the hindfoot are similar to the metacarpals but are less massive and somewhat longer. This difference is consistent with the hindlimb being mainly involved in propulsion rather than support. The reverse is true for the forelimb in cursorial animals.

Digits: The hind digits are also not remarkably different from those of the forelimb. Some animals, for example the dog and cat, usually have four digits on the hindfoot and five on the forefoot.

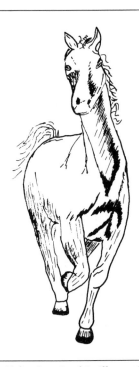

Figure 1–35. Abduction. In this illustration of an approaching horse, the head and neck are drawn to the right from the midline as the right forelimb is lifted. If only one set of the bilaterally-paired muscles (see Figure 1–38) contract, this abduction may occur to either side, depending upon whether or not the limb is supporting the animal's weight.

from your side. The muscles responsible for rotating the arm around the shoulder are abductors. Swing the arm back to where you started and you are putting the adductors to work. If you have the flexibility, reach back with your left hand onto your right shoulder blade and attempt to palpate the abductor while repeating the exercise. The adductor can be palpated on the front of the shoulder.

Quadrupeds have less ability for such extreme limb rotation as was just described for the human forelimb. Even so, our pelvic limb is much less mobile than the arm and shoulder in terms of adduction and abduction. In animals that splay

their forelimbs to bring the shoulders closer to the ground to aid in drinking (Figure 1–37), a similar abduction is used. In addition, the legs are usually extended forward and outward rather than simply splayed, to increase the efficiency of this maneuver.

Another general principle to grasp with regard to the distribution of muscles is the grouping of the more massive muscles close to the trunk, or their location on the proximal portions of the limbs. The more distal limb joints such as those of the carpus and those between the metacarpals and digits are, by and large, rotated by long tendinous extensions of muscles located much more proximally than the joint. This is well illustrated by our forelimb.

Sit with your arm bent at the elbow so your forearm and the palmar surface of the right hand are flat on a table surface in front of you. Carefully examine the dorsal surface of your hand and the lateral surface of your forearm (this should presently be uppermost). Now elevate each of your fingers an inch or so off the table (an extensor exercise) and note the extensor tendons becoming rigid, just beneath the skin. You will be able to palpate some of these tendons crossing the carpus, or wrist, and you should be able to discern the general location of the tendons or the corresponding extensor muscles through the length of the forearm, right up as far as the elbow. Now roll over your arm, wrist, and hand so that the hand rests on its dorsal surface. It is difficult to completely turn the wrist and forearm in this sitting position but, as described earlier, it is quite impossible for an animal with its ulna fused to the radius.

Now flex your fingers, drawing the fingertips towards the wrist. Do this for each finger in turn while palpating the palmar surface. Again, tendinous extensions of the flexor muscles will be felt lying over the metacarpals. They will probably be more difficult to discern at the wrist and the flexor muscles themselves

Figure 1–36. *Flexion and extension.* This leaping horse illustrates simultaneous flexion of the forelimb—bringing the distal extremity closer to the body—and extension of the hindlimb—providing thrust to the trunk. Note that these terms are descriptive of the limbs, not the muscles.

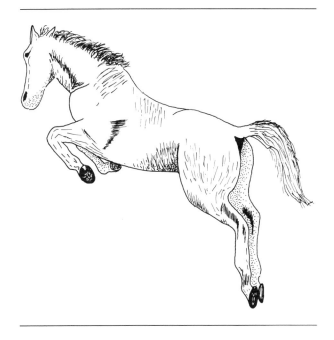

Figure 1–37. *Abduction and extension.* A newborn animal (such as the foal shown here) uses abduction and extension of all four limbs to help stabilize itself upon standing for the first time. Later, abduction and extension of the fore-limbs enable animals to lower their shoulders and may be used to aid drinking when the source of water is at a level lower than the feet.

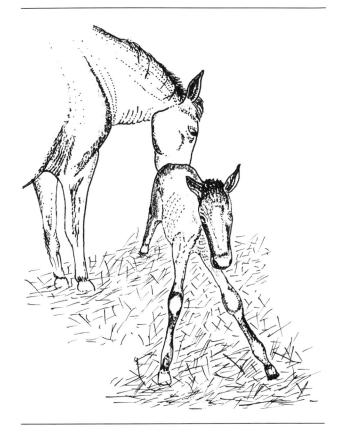

can be located only approximately in the forearm.

The same principle of the massive muscles being located proximally applies to the muscles controlling rotation of the upper limbs at the pectoral and pelvic girdles. Look for this general principle in the two diagrams in Figures 1–38 and 1–39 which show some of the muscles of the horse. In addition, examine the distribution of the more massive muscles in any animal.

Selected views of the location of certain major muscles are presented in the accompanying diagrams. Some names are provided but no attempt is made to deal with nomenclature in any comprehensive fashion. It is not intended that the reader acquire a detailed understanding of the formal names and the classification of the muscles. There are in excess of 400 muscles, and it is unrealistic to expect students to learn about them without the benefit of detailed dissection. In the figures, legends are provided giving some of the names, and an abbreviated treatment of the major functions of certain of the muscles follows. The reader should attempt to learn the major muscles responsible for movement of the foreparts of the body. Some of these are superficial muscles that are readily palpable through the skin. When handling animals in laboratories and demonstrations, one should take the opportunity to try and locate at least some of the major muscles.

Superficial Muscles

The superficial muscles of the neck and shoulder region illustrate yet another principle. When

Figure 1–38. Muscles of the neck and shoulder. This sketch shows most superficial muscles of the ventral surface of the neck and the front of the shoulders. Many of these can be discerned in a live animal. Compare this figure with the lateral view shown in Figure 1–39.

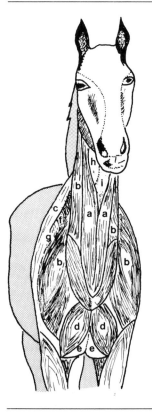

a **sternocephalicus**

b **brachiocephalicus**

c **trapezius**

d **ant. superficial pectoral**

e **post. superficial pectoral**

f **ant. deep pectoral**

g **supraspinatus**

h **omohyoideus**

i **sternothyrohyoideus**

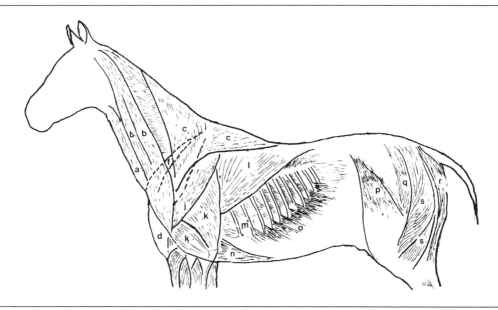

Figure 1–39. *Superficial muscles.* The major superficial muscles are illustrated in this lateral view of the horse. Note the general arrangement by comparing this figure to Figure 1–38. The muscles shown are sternocephalicus (a); brachiocephalicus (b); trapezius (c); anterior superficial pectoral (d); anterior deep pectoral (f); deltoid (j); triceps (k); latissimus dorsi (l); serratus thoracicus (m); posterior deep pectoral (n); oblique external abdominal (o); tensor fascia lata (p); superficial gluteus (q); semitendinosus (r); biceps femoris (s).

muscles occur as pairs, and most do with a member of the pair on each side of the median plane, the result of contraction varies depending on whether one or both contract. The muscles controlling the position of the head and neck illustrate this principle well.

The elongated *sternocephalic* muscle runs along the near ventral midline of the lower neck on either side and inserts on the posterior border of the mandible. If both muscles contract, the head is drawn back and the neck flexes.

Just slightly more lateral to these muscles, the *brachiocephalic* muscle has its origins at the rear of the cranium and on the processes of the first few cervical vertebrae; it inserts at the crest of the humerus. If the muscles on both sides contract when the forelimbs are supporting the animal's weight, the head and neck are extended. For both the sternocephalic and the brachiocephalic muscles, when contraction occurs only on one side, the head and neck are moved

to one side. If the forelimb is not carrying the animal's weight, contraction of the brachiocephalic muscle draws the limb forward.

The broad *trapezius* muscle fans out to have origins over the neck and the thorax and comes together at the insertion on the lateral spine of the scapula. The two portions, originating over the neck and over the thorax, are shown in Figure 1–39. The trapezius muscle elevates the shoulder. The cervical portion draws the scapula up and forward, while the thoracic portion draws the scapula up and back.

The *anterior superficial pectoral* and the *posterior superficial pectoral* muscles, short, thick, prominent muscles in the front of the thorax, are forelimb adductors. They insert onto the crest of the humerus, close to the insertion of the brachiocephalic muscle, and also serve to advance the limb. The anterior deep pectoral and the posterior deep pectoral muscles share some actions with the superficial pair but differ in other respects. These deeper muscles are also adductors (see Figure 1–40), but they draw the limb back rather than forward. If the limb is fixed and carrying the weight of the animal, these muscles serve to pull the body forward over the limb.

The *deltoid* muscle contracts to flex the shoulder and abduct the limb. It is located much more laterally than the pectorals, passing over the shoulders, and so is ideally suited for the task of moving the limb out from the medial plane.

The *triceps* muscle, another fan-shaped muscle wrapping round the shoulder, flexes the shoulder joint and extends the elbow joint. It is particularly important in conferring rigidity to the limb, as in load-bearing, by opposing the action of the flexors of the elbow.

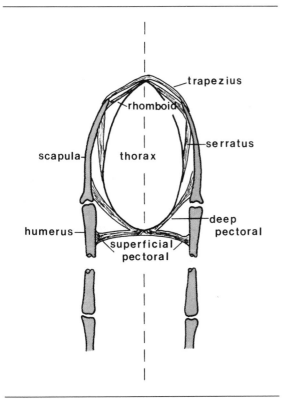

Figure 1–40. *Adductor muscles of the forelimb.* The pectoral muscles (adductors) are ideally located to aid in drawing the limb in towards the midline. In contrast, the trapezius muscle is located superficially; it serves to lift the limb and contributes to abduction (see description in the text).

Tense your arm with the elbow locked, then use your other hand to palpate the muscles of the upper arm on both the ventral and dorsal aspects. The biceps is ventral and the triceps is dorsal. Both will be firm if the elbow is locked really tightly.

The description of these muscles is by no means a formal comprehensive treatment, but it should give an indication of the important principles. A complete description would include, for each muscle of the body: name, general description of morphology, point or points of origin, point or points of insertion, action or actions, structure (including tendons and details of the nature of connections to ligaments or bones), relation to other structures around it, blood supply, and innervation. This degree of detail is inappropriate for the present overview. Readers with a specific, deeper interest in the muscles should consult any of a number of major anatomy texts for a comprehensive treatment. There are texts on general veterinary anatomy, human anatomy, and more specific books dealing with individual species.

Summary of Muscle Action

- The reader should understand abduction, adduction, flexion, and extension.

- The more massive muscles are located proximally, even though their important actions may be quite distal and brought about via long tendons.

- Action varies depending on which part of the body is fixed or immobilized.

- A joint can be "fixed" or "locked" by simultaneous contraction of the appropriate flexor and extensor.

- Bilaterally paired muscles provide for movement in one direction or another, or confer rigidity.

1.6 • The Visceral Organs

The visceral organs are described briefly here to indicate regional organization. More information will be provided in later chapters, when structure and function are discussed in greater detail.

It is convenient to consider these internal organs as making up two groups (Figure 1–41): the *thoracic viscera* and the *abdominal viscera*. For the present purposes, it will suffice to describe the viscera from a ventral approach, but to aid in orientation, some diagrams are provided that show lateral constructs and, on occasion, transverse sections of the body. The descriptions used here apply to mature ruminant animals.

The ventral surface of the body wall, immediately beneath the skin and any subcutaneous adipose tissue, consists of the ventral face of the sternum extending caudad to the *xiphoid* cartilage. Continuing back, a tough ligamentous band, the *linea alba*, provides the ventral fusion, or aponeurosis, of the abdominal wall (shown for the horse earlier in Figure 1–14). This extends caudad to the pelvic region. For this introduction

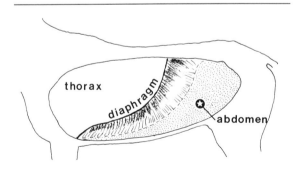

Figure 1–41. The thoracic and abdominal cavities. Note the relative location and dimensions of the visceral compartments. The diaphragm is shown with its cranial limit (solid line) fanning out to its peripheral limit (dotted line). The abdominal cavity extends farther forward medially and ventrally while the thoracic cavity extends back laterally and dorsally.

the pelvic viscera such as the bladder, uterus, and cervix in females will be included in the abdominal group.

Thoracic Viscera

If the sternum is split lengthwise and the ribs are retracted laterally to expose the *thoracic cavity*, the latter appears to be roughly triangular with a caudal base formed by the *diaphragm*. The cavity is shallower anteriorly and deeper posteriorly. The diaphragm is the caudal limit to the thoracic cavity. It is a broad, flat or cranially domed muscle that is part of the respiratory apparatus in mammals. It attaches laterally to the rear of the rib cage and lies obliquely backward to the dorsum, at the junction of the thoracic and lumbar vertebral regions.

The bulk of the thoracic cavity is occupied by the right and left *lungs*, the *major airways*, the *heart* with the *major blood vessels*, and the *esophagus* in transit from the neck to the abdominal cavity. The lungs are *lobular* and each lobe communicates with others on the same side by *bronchi*, which come together and join with those from the other lung to form the common *trachea*. The trachea then passes cranially, exits the thorax, and passes up the midventral line of the neck. The lungs collapse immediately when the thorax is opened, as will be discussed later under respiratory mechanisms.

In the absence of pneumothorax, or air in the thorax, the lungs expand to occupy most of the thoracic space. A membrane, the *pleura*, provides a continuous cover over the surface of the lung (the *visceral pleura*) and extends to provide a lining for the internal surface of the thoracic wall (the *parietal pleura*). Between these portions of the membrane is the pleural cavity. It is an example of a serous cavity, or one formed from what was originally a solid mass of embryonic tissue. The pleura is an example of a mesothelium.

The heart is located centrally, or slightly to the left side, and toward the apex of the thoracic cavity lying between the lungs. In a living animal, the heart changes its orientation to the rest of the body within each cycle of beating. The mass of the heart, the myocardium, is suspended within a tough membrane called the pericardium that provides attachment to the dorsal wall and apex of the thorax. The major blood vessels enter or exit the *base* of the heart at a craniodorsal location. The pulmonary vessels pass bilaterally to and from the lungs. The major trunk vessels pass more dorsally, forward and back, along the dorsal wall of the thorax. The esophagus, the thoracic part of the digestive tract, lies just ventral to these vessels. A cross-section at midthorax (Figure 1–42) should aid in placing these structures relative to each other.

Abdominal Viscera

The overwhelming impression obtained when the linea alba of a ruminant animal is opened is that the cavity is filled with stomach and little else (Figure 1–43). In late pregnancy, the *uterus* expands to displace much of this compound

Figure 1–42. Transverse section of the ovine thorax. This cross section, looking forward, shows the location of the thoracic viscera and the structures of the body wall on the right side. Many of the muscles are shown in lateral view in Figure 1–39. Bones are heavily shaded. The rib is sectioned obliquely and portions of two thoracic vertebrae are included in this section.

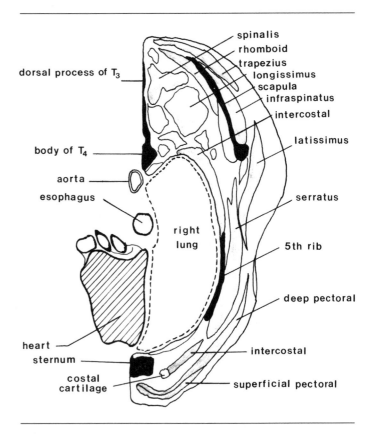

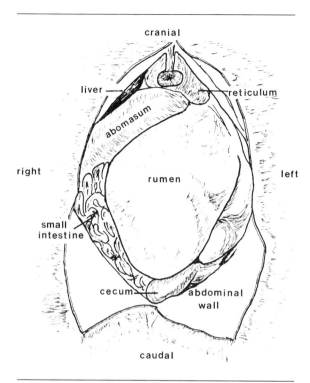

cranial

liver

reticulum

abomasum

right

rumen

left

small
intestine

cecum

abdominal
wall

caudal

Figure 1–43. Abdominal viscera. A ventral dissection from the xiphoid to the pelvis of a sheep shows the relative positions of the abdominal viscera. Note that in a ventral view, left and right are transposed. Compare this drawing with the lateral views of the viscera of cattle shown in Figure 1–44.

stomach. Later in the text, in the discussion of digestion, some comparative information will be provided that will confirm the relative enormity of the ruminant's stomach system. In very crude terms, the *liver* lies closest to the diaphragm with its curved parietal surface closely approximating the curvature of the muscle. The liver is most obvious on the right side and is lobular in many species. The *gallbladder* (Figure 1–44) lies within the fissures separating the lobes. Not all species have gallbladders. In a similar plane to that of the liver, but more evident on the left side, the *spleen* lies between the stomach and the diaphragm.

Caudally, the next structure is the *stomach*.

In ruminants, the compound stomach is made up of four portions, *reticulum, rumen, omasum,* and *abomasum,* and occupies a major portion of the volume of the abdominal cavity. The lateral views provided in Figure 1–44 show the most voluminous portion, the rumen, lying displaced somewhat to the left side. The reticulum is also more evident on this side. The omasum and abomasum are seen from the right side, lying ventral to the liver. More detail will be provided in Chapter 6.

In ruminants, the *small intestine* and *large intestine* are displaced to the right. The first portion of the small intestine, the *duodenum,* loops back from the abomasum dorsally within the abdominal cavity. The *pancreas,* a gland with both exocrine and endocrine functions, is located in the first loop of the duodenum, just behind the liver. Immediately dorsally, the right *kidney* lies close to the major blood vessels and the left kidney slightly to the rear. *Adrenal glands* are just cranial to each kidney, in close proximity to the major blood vessels passing along the dorsal wall of the abdominal cavity. Most of the remaining small intestines are ventral. The large intestine and *cecum* are coiled midway on the right side and the *rectum* is most dorsal. Note the location of the *bladder,* just anterior to the abdominal inlet to the pelvic cavity.

In females, the nonpregnant uterus lies just cranial and dorsal to the bladder. Ovaries are just dorsolateral to the uterus. In both sexes, the rectum and portions of both the reproductive and excretory systems pass through the pelvic opening.

In nonruminant herbivores, a ventral dissection would reveal a relatively small stomach and a mass of intestines occupying the abdominal space. Instead of the rumen being the most obvious organ, the enlarged cecum is the most prominent structure in these animals when viewed from a ventral dissection.

This description will be enlarged in Chapter 6, "Digestive Mechanisms," when emphasis will be placed on the structure and function of the digestive tract. The nongut viscera are described in a number of chapters.

Figure 1–44. *Thoracic and abdominal viscera in cattle.* These cutaway views of a mature cow are from the right *(a)* and left *(b)*. Recall that the domed shape of the diaphragm (Figure 1–41) means that abdominal viscera press forward in the midline, well within the thoracic cage. For a more detailed description of the individual viscera, see the text.

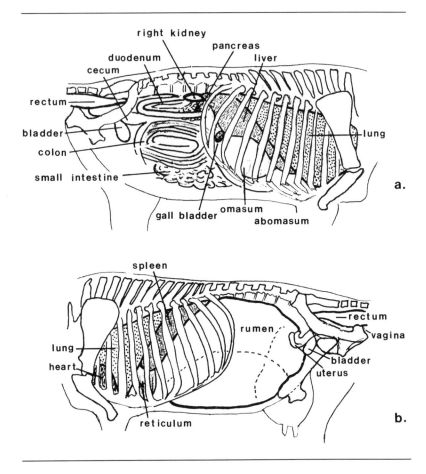

1.7 • Anatomy and Morphology of the Chicken

Some features of the domestic chicken (*Gallus domesticus*) will be noted to highlight the similarities and, more importantly, the differences between this avian species and the mammals with which most of this book is concerned. There is considerable anatomic variation among the domesticated birds, including chickens, turkeys, ducks, and geese, but the domestic chicken is by far the most important agricultural species and hence is chosen as the type species for this brief treatment of comparative anatomy.

External Anatomy and Morphology

The external form of the mature chicken (fowl) is very obviously different from that of the mammals that have been described. Disregarding for the moment those features that differ between sexes *(sexual dimorphisms)* the major regions and appendages of the chicken (Figure 1–45) include the head, neck, crop, breast, wing (forelimb), back, abdomen, uropygium, and leg. Because the leg (hindlimb) is relatively massive it is further classified into thigh, leg, hock, shank, and foot with the spur and claws. The body's additional appendages include combs, wattles, and ear lobes, which are highly vascularized, thick folds of skin; and the beak, spurs, claws, and plates on the shank, which are horny derivatives of the skin.

Most striking in contrast to mammals is the complete absence of hair and its replacement over much of the body with feathers. Feathers take several distinct forms with differences in structure related to their function, and they are found in quite distinct tracts on the body. The skin lying between feather tracts is naked. The quill is the main supporting structure of the feather and is intimately associated with dermal specializations within a follicle along with associated muscles, somewhat similar to, but more highly developed than the erector pilus muscles associated with hair follicles in mammals. The quill has a pulp cavity and is vascularized from the follicle via an opening in its proximal ex-

Figure 1–45. Morphology and external anatomy of the chicken. The external surface of the chicken is covered with an elaborate feather pattern that obscures the relationship between portions of the body, such as the neck, thorax, and abdomen. Note the accessory structures—comb, wattle, and spur—and the feather-free surface of the lower leg.

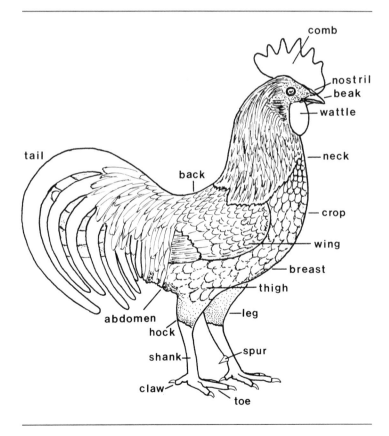

tremity. Distally, the quill merges into the shaft from which the vanes arise, one on each of opposite sides of the shaft. Vanes are compound structures made from barbs, barbules, and hooklets. The structure traps air thus aiding the insulative properties of the plumage. In addition, by providing resistance to air flow, certain feathers contribute to the aerodynamic properties of the wings thereby enabling flight.

The skin of the chicken is essentially devoid of glands, the exception being the oil gland in the pygostyle. Sudoriferous (sweat) glands are absent and there are no mammary glands.

The Skeleton

The skeleton of the chicken is markedly different from that of the quadruped mammals described in Section 1.4. A number of the bones are structurally specialized by their medullary cavities being occupied by air spaces rather than solely by marrow. Such bones are *pneumatic* and in chickens the posterior cervical and most of the thoracic vertebrae, pelvis, humerus, coracoid, and sternum (Figure 1–46) take this form. The air spaces function as part of the external respiratory apparatus (described in Chapter 5) and they aid in reducing density of the skeleton of large flying birds. Many of the bones have soft medullary bone in place of marrow in the cavities and this material may serve as a labile depot for calcium, especially in laying birds.

The skeleton is classified into axial, appendicular, and visceral portions. The axial skeleton consists of the skull, the vertebral column, the ribs, and sternum, as in mammals. The appendicular skeleton includes the pectoral and pelvic limbs, but, in contrast to the quadrupeds, a pectoral girdle is included and a portion of the pelvis is fused into a compound structure involving lumbar and sacral vertebrae and the ilium. The visceral skeleton consists solely of a bony ring in the eye.

Axial Skeleton

A vertebral formula C-14, T-7, LS-14, Cy-6 applies to the chicken. Major differences from mammals are the much greater number of cervical vertebrae, the partially fused thoracic vertebrae (the *notarium*), and the complex, fused mass of lumbar and sacral elements along with the ilium of the pelvis (the *synsacrum*). These fused vertebral structures provide rigidity and presumably aid in transmitting forces from the wings and legs to the vertebral column. The cervical vertebrae collectively form an S-shape (Figure 1–46), which, if straightened forcibly, severs the spinal cord and causes death.

Bones of the skull are classified as cranial and facial, as in mammals. The occurrence and form of the bones differ from those of mammals, but need not be considered in detail. For example, anterior bones of the face come together to form part of the beak, the maxilla is poorly developed, there are no teeth, there is a single occipital condyle, a single bone substitutes for the triad found in the middle ear of mammals, and there is no hard palate.

Chickens have two pairs of floating or asternal ribs anteriorly then five pairs connected to the sternum. The ribcage is inflexible and strong in order to support a massive sternum, the largest bone in the body. Portions of the marrow cavities of the ribs, sternum, and the thoracic vertebrae serve in an erythropoietic capacity. The ventral margin of the sternum (the keel) is originally a strictly cartilaginous structure that tends to ossify in older individuals.

Appendicular Skeleton

The pectoral girdle, consisting of the scapulae, the coracoids, and a pair of clavicles that fuse ventrally to form the "wishbone," provides a bony connection between the pectoral limb and the vertebral column. This contrasts with the fleshy connection described earlier for quadrupeds. As shown in Figure 1–46, the pectoral limb consists of the humerus, radius and ulna, and partially fused distal bones with rudimentary phalanges. The carpals and metacarpals are

Figure 1–46. Skeleton of the chicken. In this skeleton, the right leg is in mid-stride and the wing is elevated from its resting position. Selected structures include the premaxilla (a); nasal (b); mandible (c); orbit (d); frontal (e); parietal (f); tympanic cavity (g); atlas (h); axis (i); cervical vertebrae (j); coracoid (k); clavicle (l); scapula (m); humerus (n); ulna (o); radius (p); carpometacarpal (q); phalanges (r); synsacrum (s); pygostyle (t); ilium (u); ischium (u'); pubis (u"); ribs (v); femur (w); tibia (x); fibula (y); tarsometatarsals (z); oblique process (1); xiphoid process (2); sternum (3); keel (4); and first, second, third, and fourth toes (I, II, III, IV).

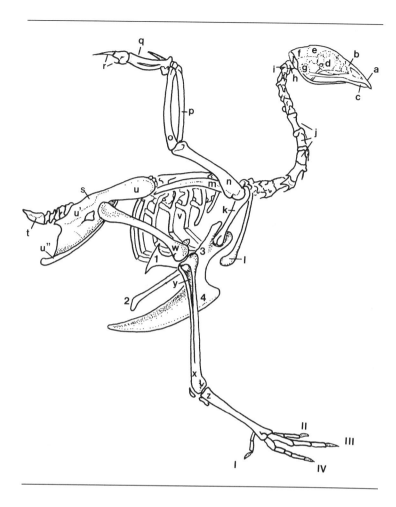

largely fused into a single mass (the *carpometacarpal* bone).

The pelvic limb, like the mammalian hindlimb, has a femur, tibia and fibula (the needle-like bone noted in Box 1–4), and patella. Distally, the tarsals and metatarsals are fused into the *tarsometatarsus*, comparable to the analogous structure in the pectoral limb. There are four digits, one of which is oriented posteriorly, and each consists of three to five phalanges (I and II have three phalanges; III has four; and IV, the most lateral, has five). In contrast to the usual mammalian form, the tibia rather than the femur is the larger bone. The pelvis is also different than that of mammals. As noted, the ilium is fused into the synsacrum. The two ischia form

a broad plate-like structure with the pubis located on the ventral margin on each side. There is no ventral fusion of the pelvis, equivalent to the symphysis pelvis in mammals, and hence there is no pelvic opening. Two obturator foramina (openings) are present as in mammals and are located toward the medial margin of the ischia.

Myology

Muscles exist as striated, cardiac, and smooth types as in mammals and, with a few specific muscles that are unique to birds (such as those of the pectoral girdle related to flying), they are generally analogous to those already described. Muscles in the chicken are structurally simpler because the amount of connective tissue between the bundles is reduced. Some of the long tendons may be ossified. The diaphragm is incomplete, even rudimentary, so the thoracic and abdominal cavities are not separated and there is no device for selectively reducing thoracic pressure for inspiratory activity. As in mammals, muscle masses of the limb are found proximally and the limb lacks any muscle covering distal to the joint between the tibia and the tarsometatarsus. Locomotor activity of the chicken's leg is fairly simple and essentially involves forward movement below the knee as the femur is rotated forward and upward and the reverse during the propulsion phase when the femur is rotated backward and downward. The dominant gait is walking or strutting and is exaggerated by involvement of the digits.

The muscles of the chicken vary in color depending on the intracellular composition and degree of vascularization.

Viscera

The internal organs concerned with digestion, circulation, respiration, excretion, and reproduction in the chicken are markedly different from those of mammals. The structural specializations will be described along with function in the chapters that focus on these body systems.

1.8 • Exercises

1. Rank the three following statements in terms of their accuracy and information content:

_____ Cells, with their interstitial fluid, make up organs if they are enclosed in epithelium.

_____ Tissues comprise populations of cells with complementary functions. Each cell contains, or has previously contained, one or more nuclei.

_____ Cells are nucleated units of protoplasm having organelles, suspended in the cytoplasm, and bounded by a sarcolemma.

2. Provide the antonym (word with opposite meaning) for the following terms:

Extensor	_____
Superficial	_____
Caudal	_____
Adductor	_____
Distal	_____
Cellular	_____

3. Name three types of muscle and note one distinguishing feature of each.

_____

_____

_____

4. Identify the bone that is misplaced in the following set:

pubis   ilium   femur   patella
tibia   fibula   humerus   ischium

5. True or false:

The diaphragm separates the abdomen and the thorax.

In mature ruminants, the rumen occupies most of the left side of the abdominal cavity.

The first cervical vertebra, the axis, articulates with the occipital condyles.

The esophagus is to the stomach as the bronchi are to the lungs.

Saggital sections are cut perpendicular to the median plane.

The tuber spinae articulate with fused vertebrae, forming the pectoral girdle.

The pericardium is not an example of mesothelium because it is on the outside, not the inside, of the heart.

The old term *suprarenal glands* is informative about the location of the adrenals.

The cytoskeleton is a framework of collagen fibrils upon which cells are held together in the form of tissues.

Morphologic changes accompany aging.

6. Sketch a rear-end view of a quadruped lying on its back with legs extended and the head and neck abducted to the animal's right.

The Basis of Animal Function

2

2.1 • Body Composition

About 70% of the adult human weight is water. Of this, 45% is intracellular, 17% is interstitial, and some 6% is in the circulatory system. Water has superb solvent properties, it is an ionizing medium, it is a good conductor, and it has a high specific heat and a high latent heat of vaporization. Water exchanges readily between body compartments, mainly by a process called diffusion, but filtration, which is pressure-driven exchange, contributes as well. Water flux rates are very high: 100 times the volume of a cell may be moving in transit through that cell every second. A complete section of this chapter will be devoted to the properties of water that are of physiologic consequence.

Chemical Composition

A great deal of information is available about the chemical composition of the bodies of animals and humans. The following data, provided for illustrative purposes, apply to a healthy, 70-kg adult man.

In addition to these macroelements, depicted in Figure 2–1, there are trace quantities of magnesium, iron, manganese, iodine, zinc, cobalt, copper, selenium, molybdenum, fluorine, and many others.

It is important to appreciate that muscle is

Elemental Composition

Oxygen	46 kg
Carbon	12 kg
Hydrogen	8 kg
Nitrogen	2 kg
Calcium	0.9 kg
Phosphorus	0.5 kg
Potassium	0.2 kg
Sulfur	0.2 kg
Sodium	0.1 kg
Chloride	0.1 kg

Organ and Tissue Masses

Muscle	29 kg
Adipose	13 kg
Skeleton	11 kg
Blood	5 kg
Skin	5 kg
CNS	1.7 kg
Liver	1.6 kg
GI tract	1.3 kg
Lungs	1.0 kg
Heart	0.3 kg
Kidneys	0.3 kg
Spleen	0.1 kg
CSF	0.1 kg
Pancreas	0.1 kg
Other	0.5 kg

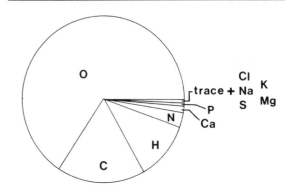

Figure 2–1. *Elemental composition.* Oxygen is by far the most abundant element in the body. Oxygen, carbon, hydrogen, and nitrogen make up about 97% of the body. The remaining macroelements, a host of microelements, and those present only in trace quantities are, however, qualitatively very important.

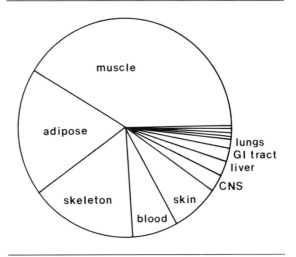

Figure 2–2. *The organ masses.* In adults, muscle is usually the major organ system; adipose tissue and the skeleton ranked second and third. In animals selected for growth rate and large mature size, adipose tissue can become dominant over muscle. Note that the carcass—comprised of muscle, adipose, and parts of the skeleton—accounts for somewhat less than the 75% shown here.

the largest organ mass and that muscle, along with the skeleton and adipose tissue, make up about 75% of body weight (Figure 2–2). It is not always recognized that skin and blood contribute as much as they do, or that the brain and spinal cord are larger than any of the visceral organs.

The dry weight of lipids in the body represents about 10% of body weight, or 7 kg of a 70-kg adult man. This leaves 63 kg as *lean,* or non-fat, body weight. The term *fat-free body* is frequently used and it is of particular importance in considerations of growth and the efficiency of growth. The nature and patterns of growth are described in Chapter 8. Of special importance now is that the water content of the lean body is remarkably constant, approximately 73% by weight. This property means that the fat-free body, and the amount of fat, can be estimated fairly readily, even in the intact living animal. The methods are outlined below.

Comparative data on body composition are available for virtually all species of agricultural importance and at various stages of maturity. Direct comparison of mature animals with the human is not of much value because, in animal science, interest is focused on animals at less mature stages. For example, Table 2–1 indicates the range of gross compositions exhibited by pigs during growth. Data of this kind will be interpreted in detail in Chapter 8 when patterns of growth are considered. For now, examine Figure 2–3 to see just how striking are the changes in relative proportions of these major body components during growth. The most dramatic changes occur in fat, from virtually none at birth to its being the dominant component in the mature animal.

The foregoing comments apply to chemically, or anatomically, well-defined body components. Because much of the physiologic support of these components is common for all types of tissues, other methods of grossly compartmentalizing the body are of value. The term *compartment* is more correct physiologically than it is anatomically, and it will be used quite frequently in the remainder of this text. For example, the introductory description of tissues described the extracellular space as an integral part of a tissue. It is now appropriate to distinguish between the fluid volume inside cells, the intracellular space, and the total volume that is extracellular (see Figure 1–4).

Analysis of Body Compartments

The volumes of several of the compartments already mentioned can be measured or estimated in vivo, meaning in the living animal. For example, total body water, extracellular water, plasma volume, and body fat can all be measured fairly easily. The methodology involves dilution of appropriate *marker* compounds, the distribution of which is confined to the compartment or compartments of interest. The principle is simple and will be described for the measurement of total body water (TBW). This parameter is particularly valuable in estimating body composition.

Total Body Water

The indicator compound antipyrine, a mild analgesic and antipyretic drug with actions similar to those of aspirin, is freely diffusible and attempts to mix uniformly through all exchangeable body water pools.

A known quantity, say I gm, of antipyrine is injected into the blood and allowed to come to equilibrium in the various water compartments in the body. At periodic intervals samples

Table 2–1. Gross Body Compositional Changes in Growing Pigs

Live Wt. (kg)	Muscle (%)	Fat (%)	Bone (%)	Skin (%)
1.0	48.6	0	31.8	19.3
9.0	57.1	11.6	19.8	11.2
44.6	57.9	15.5	16.3	9.4
62.5	51.3	27.4	14.0	7.3
89.3	46.9	35.2	11.5	6.7
134.0	42.3	41.7	10.0	5.9

Figure 2–3. Compositional changes with growth. These four diagrams depict changes in the relative amounts of the major organ masses as a pig grows. The data, from the tabulation in the text, applies to a very young piglet at 1 kg *(a)*, an animal at about 9 kg *(b)*, at 62.5 kg *(c)*, and at 134 kg *(d)*. The increase in fat leads to a reduction in the proportion of the whole made up from skin and bone, before finally affecting the proportion of muscle in the body. Of course, the actual weight of these components does not decrease; in most instances each component continues to increase in mass but at a much slower rate than fat tissue.

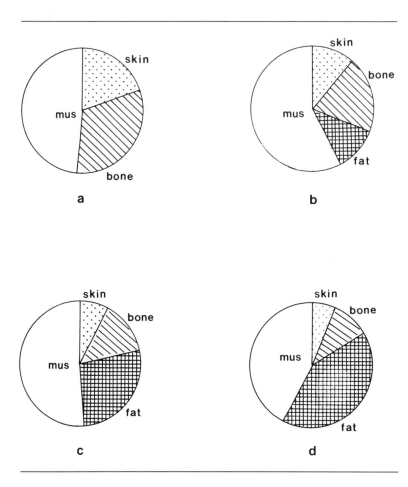

of blood are drawn and the concentration of antipyrine is determined. When the concentration stabilizes, it can be assumed that equilibrium has been reached and no further mixing time is needed. The distribution of the injected dose of *I* gm throughout the exchangeable pools of water results in an equilibrium concentration of, say, *C* gm/L in the samples that were collected and analyzed. If really uniform mixing indeed has occurred, then the concentration in blood, or blood plasma, will be typical of all water pools. When the mass of the injected dose *I* is divided by the resultant concentration (mass/volume), which is determined to be *C*, the result is an estimate of the total volume of distribution of the marker compound in liters.

Many assumptions about the marker are made, or can be corrected for, when this approach is used:

1. It mixes evenly throughout the pool.

2. It mixes rapidly, relative to removal.

3. It should not be metabolized.

4. It should be nontoxic.

5. It should be easily measured.

In reality, some water pools are not freely exchangeable in the duration of such a test. For example, much of the water of hydration of some structural proteins (described below) is so intimately associated with the protein that it is essentially "bound" and unable to be freely exchanged during brief periods of time.

Other indicator compounds suitable for measuring the total body water pool are deuterated or tritiated water; both are isotopic forms of water. Tritiated water is particularly easy to measure, although it is subject to radioisotope use restrictions. Deuterated water has two non-radioactive isotopic forms, DHO and D_2O, and these isotopes can be measured accurately, though requiring more elaborate equipment than in the case of tritiated water. These isotopes of water are not handled in the body in exactly the same way as H_2O because of their slightly heavier mass (molecular weight = 19 or 20 daltons, compared with 18). This problem is greater with tritiated water (molecular weight = 20 or 22 daltons), but measurement convenience outweighs the error factor.

Extracellular Water

The extracellular water (ECW) volume can be estimated by the same dilution principle and using any compound or ion that is restricted to pools outside of cells. Nearly a dozen markers exhibiting this property are used. They have various advantages and disadvantages. For example, inulin, a starchlike polymer from dahlias, cannot penetrate cells but it diffuses relatively slowly. This gives rise to prolonged mixing times, a problem because inulin is subjected to rapid filtration by the kidneys. Sucrose, sulfate, thiosulfate, and thiocyanate are a few of the other substances used. Exactly the same principle as that described for antipyrine and TBW is used to estimate ECW volume.

Plasma Volume

The most frequently used marker for the estimation of plasma volume (PV) is a dye known as T-1824, or Evan's blue, which rapidly binds to serum proteins on injection and so can diffuse only extremely slowly out of the vascular system and into the interstitial space. Equilibration and mixing in the plasma is rapid and the dilution can be estimated before effusion out of the circulation proceeds significantly. This is due to the movement of plasma proteins, now coupled to the dye, across capillary walls. In animals, the progress of this loss to the interstitial fluid can be assessed by the animal taking on a faint blue appearance. The dye is eliminated from the animal within a couple of days.

Serum albumin, labeled with any of several radioisotopes, can also be used, but radioisotope use considerations have largely eliminated it from the toolbox of animal scientists.

Red Blood Cell Volume

Washed erythrocytes, obtained from an animal, can be readily "tagged" or labeled with CrO_4^{2-}, injected and allowed to mix, then used to estimate dilution by the total circulating red blood cell (RBC) mass. For most purposes, knowledge of blood or plasma volume and the proportion of blood made up by the RBCs is quite adequate. In Chapter 5 it will be noted that substantial numbers of RBCs, or erythrocytes, are stored outside the general circulation, so none of the dilution-type approaches to quantifying RBC volume is entirely satisfactory.

Fat-Free Body Mass (Lean Body Mass)

Because the content of water in the lean body mass is nearly constant at 73%, as noted above, an estimate of TBW allows calculation of lean body mass:

LBM (kg) = [**TBW** (liters) × 100] / 73

By definition,

%Fat = 100 − **%LBM**

This approach has been used extensively in the past to assess body fat changes in growing animals by repeated TBW measurements using tritiated water. Radioisotope disposal problems currently limit the use of this method to just a few research laboratories.

The Body Fluid Compartments

The fluid compartments, which include intracellular fluid and a variety of extracellular components, have characteristic dimensions. These are typically expressed as percentages of body weight, and it is acceptable to equate weight in kilograms with volume in liters. Such conversions are less simple in nonmetric measurement systems. Some values are provided for the relative volumes of the major fluid compartments in Table 2–2 and Figure 2–4. The data are important for developing an understanding of the distribution of various solutes in the compartments of the body.

The solutes are distributed nonuniformly throughout these compartments. In part the differences in distribution of various solutes are due to the nature of the capillary wall separating blood from the interstitial fluid. In addition, selective permeability and other transport phenomena evident at the level of the cell membrane regulate the distribution of substances within and without the cell. The most striking differences between the compositions of these compartments (Table 2–3) are the following:

- Sodium ions are mostly extracellular.

- Chloride ions are mostly extracellular.

- Potassium ions are mostly intracellular.

- Protein is present in high concentrations in intracellular fluid, in intermediate concentrations in the blood plasma, and in relatively low concentrations in the interstitial fluid.

The major cations are sodium (Na^+) and potassium (K^+), though the quantitatively minor cations such as calcium (Ca^{2+}) and magnesium (Mg^{2+}) are of great importance. Chloride is obviously the major extracellular anion, while protein serves as the most important intracellular anion. At typical physiologic pH, there is a net negative charge on most proteins, so they can reasonably be considered to be anions.

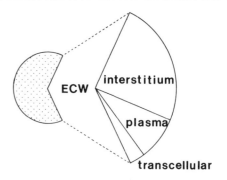

Figure 2–4. Body fluid distribution. About 65% of total body water is found inside cells, in the intracellular compartment. Of the remainder,—the extracellular water (ECW)—most is found in the interstitium, the fluid bathing the cells. Less than 10% is present in the blood plasma, although this seems to be the most obvious fluid compartment in the body. Transcellular fluid includes the secretions present at any time in the ducts of glandular systems and in fluids such as urine.

Table 2–2. The Body Fluid Compartments

Body Fluid	% of Body Wt.	
Intracellular	45	
Extracellular	25	
Interstitial fluid		17
Blood plasma		6
Transcellular fluid		2
Total water content	70	

Table 2–3. Comparison of Intracellular and Extracellular Concentrations of Key Charge Carriers in Mammalian Skeletal Muscle

Carrier	Intracellular (mEq/L)	Extracellular (mEq/L)
K^+	150	5
Na^+	12	145
Cl^-	4	125
HCO_3^-	8	28
Protein$^-$	150	0.5

The distribution of cations across the membranes of certain types of cells will be shown in Chapter 3 to be the basis for generation of action potentials. These are the electrochemical impulses that carry information in the nervous system and trigger contractile events in muscle cells.

It is important to become familiar with the magnitude of the differences in concentrations of these charged species across membranes. Both Table 2–3 and Figure 2–5 show these differences, expressed in charge quantities rather than mass quantities. If the reader is unsure why this choice was made, he or she should consult Appendix A for an explanation of why ionizable substances are often described in terms of the charges they contribute. In physiology, the commonly used unit for this purpose is milliequivalents per liter (mEq/L) or per kilogram (mEq/kg). A shorthand way of distinguishing between intracellular and extracellular concentrations is by use of the subscripts i, for inside, and o, for outside. For the sodium ion, Na_o^+ at about 145 mEq/L is about 12-fold higher than Na_i^+, at about 12 mEq/L. For potassium ions, the gradient is reversed, with K_o^+ at 5 mEq/L being about 30-fold less than K_i^+, at about 150 mEq/L. This considerably greater gradient for K^+ results in some passive loss of K^+ from inside cells and a relative negativity within cells, when compared to the

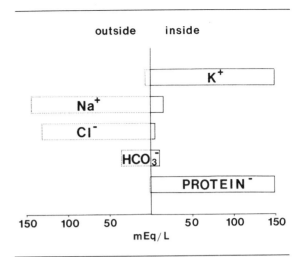

Figure 2–5. *Distribution of the major charge carriers between intracellular and extracellular compartments.* This diagram shows the relative distribution of charged species across the membrane of mammalian skeletal muscle cells. The solid bars to the right represent the intracellular concentrations and the dotted bars to the left, the extracellular concentrations for the same ions or protein anions. As in the text, these quantities are expressed in mEq/L.

outside of cells. This subject will be discussed in detail in the next chapter.

2.2 • Properties of Water of Importance in Physiology

Approximately 70% of the mass of higher animals is water. About two thirds of this water content is intracellular, and the remainder includes the solvent of interstitial fluids (17% of body weight), plasma (6% of body weight), and secretions in the ducts of the exocrine glandular system (approximately 2% of total). Water is so important to the function of cells and the body in general that a brief review of the physical chemistry of this molecule is in order. A reader lacking background in chemistry will benefit from reading Appendix A, or by consulting a high school or introductory college chemistry text for a description of the nature of atoms, ions, electron shells, and molecules.

Water molecules exhibit a high degree of charge dipole because the oxygen atom is more electronegative than are the hydrogens. Both hydrogen atoms exhibit weak positive charges, making them mutually repulsive around the oxygen, as represented in Figure 2–6. The charge asymmetry is referred to as *dipole*, and the charge distribution leads to the bonding between each hydrogen atom with the oxygen atom in water being about 60% covalent and 40% ionic. Because of this, the residual positivity on the hydrogen atom leads to its being attracted to the surplus negativity on the oxygen of an adjacent water molecule. This attractive force, which is termed *hydrogen bonding*, may be so great that the hydrogen covalently binds to the second oxygen atom. As illustrated in Figure 2–7, this colligative phenomenon results in formation of the hydronium (H_3O^+) ion and hydroxyl (OH^-) ion. The dissociation of multiple molecules of water

to hydronium and hydroxyl ions occurs reversibly with great lability. However, at a given time, water is predominantly in the associated form (H_2O).

Pure water at 25 C contains a mere 10^{-7} moles each of H_3O^+ and OH^- per kilogram (55.5 moles). Thus the ratio of dissociated to associated water is 0.0000000018 to 1; water therefore does not readily dissociate. The degree of dissociation, or content of H_3O^+, is conveniently expressed as pH, the negative $\log_{10}$ of $[H_3O^+]$, the concentration of hydronium ions. In shorthand notation, concentration is indicated by use of square brackets [ ]. In pure water pH = 7, and a pH change of 1 unit represents a tenfold increase or decrease in $[H_3O^+]$.

Like all other liquids with distinct charge dipoles, water exhibits a high *dielectric constant*. Because of the dipole, water molecules are highly organized and readily separate other charged species within a solution. This property is called the dielectric effect. The high degree of water-water organization is best exhibited in ice, with its formal crystalline structure, but there is good reason to believe that icelike aggregates of water are continually forming and breaking down, even in water in the liquid state. These water "clusters" are labile aggregates of hydrogen-bonded water molecules.

The ability to decrease the attractive forces between charged species is the basis for water serving as a powerful ionizing medium. The extensive ionization then dispersion of ions by water results in formation of solutions (Figure 2–8). Thus, for ionizable molecules, water possesses powerful solvent power. The solute ions exist in a state in which they are surrounded by a shell of oriented water molecules. This complex is referred to as a *hydrated ion* and has a characteristic size. Ions formed from the alkali metals (Li^+, Na^+, K^+, in order of increasing atomic weight) are particularly important as carriers of current across biologic membranes. This will be developed in relation to the generation of potentials across membranes in Chapter 3. Whereas the ionic radii (nonhydrated) calculated from crystallography follow this same rank order, the reverse is true of the hydrated ions. This

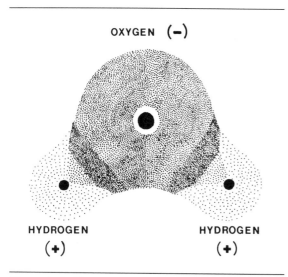

OXYGEN (–)

HYDROGEN
(+)

HYDROGEN
(+)

Figure 2–6. The water dipole. Shading has been used to give a general impression of electron density around the three atomic nuclei. The figure shows the hydrogens to be relatively electron deficient because of the electrophilic behavior of the oxygen. This asymmetry of charge is the basis for using the term dipole.

Figure 2–7. Hydrogen bonding in water. Water dipoles associate with one another through hydrogen bonding. The negativity of the oxygen atom attracts a hydrogen atom, with its relative positivity, from other water molecules. If the attracted hydrogen leaves its parent molecule to form a hydronium ion (H_3O^+), the remainder becomes a hydroxyl ion (OH^-).

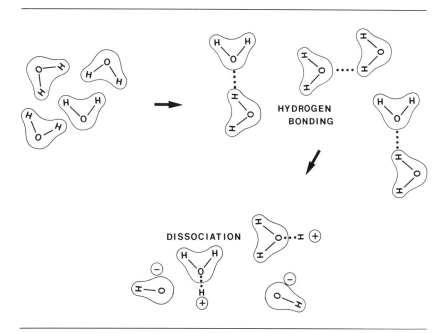

Figure 2–8. Ionization and solution. The upper diagram depicts a crystalline structure of sodium chloride, an ionizable salt. In the lower figure, the ions have dispersed and have been separated by water, a dielectric solvent. The dissociation of such a solute is complete; no sodium chloride molecules remain associated.

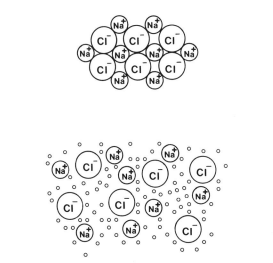

behavior results from less shielding of the nuclear positivity by a smaller shell of electrons surrounding the nucleus of smaller mass. Therefore, a larger number of water dipoles are attracted and remain associated with the ion. The relative sizes of the three hydrated and non-hydrated ions (Li^+, Na^+, K^+) are reversed in order.

Somewhat similar to the foregoing is the interaction of charged water molecules (dipoles if associated, H_3O^+ and OH^- ions if dissociated) with charged macromolecules such as proteins. If the reader has no knowledge of the chemical nature of proteins, a very brief introduction can be found toward the end of Appendix B. Dissociable functional groups on proteins result in highly charged regions (Figure 2–9) that are responsible for many protein-protein interactions, including those providing conformational stability. These are the complex higher order structures needed for the normal function of macromolecules.

Water forms highly oriented layers or shells

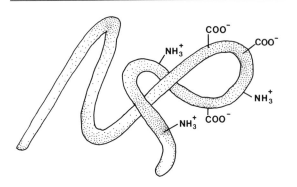

Figure 2–9. Major dissociable groups on proteins. The most important charged groups on proteins are the $-NH_3^+$ groups of basic amino acids, and the $-COO^-$ groups of the acidic amino acids. Any concentration of such charged groups within the three-dimensional structure of the molecule is called a polar domain.

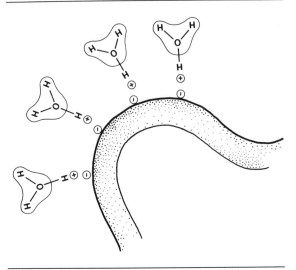

Figure 2–10. Water clusters near charged residues. The negatively charged domain on this highly stylized protein attracts positively charged hydronium ions. The water in the hydronium ion forms a hydration shell over this portion of the macromolecule. The shell reduces the degree of protein–protein associations that could occur if oppositely charged regions of the proteins were allowed to interact extensively.

around the charged areas of macromolecules (Figure 2–10) which shield the coulombic forces of the protein charges. Protein-protein and protein-ion interactions alter as a result of this shielding, and protein solubility may result. The highly charged surface regions, also called domains, on proteins are termed *hydrophilic*, or water attracting, while the noncharged domains are termed *hydrophobic*, or water repelling; the latter regions do not attract charged water molecules. If the shielding of protein charges by water is abolished, as for example when the dielectric strength of the solvent is markedly reduced, protein-protein interactions are enhanced and precipitation will result. This phenomenon is commonly exploited in preparative biochemistry when water-miscible organic solvents of lower dielectric constant are used to remove proteins from extracts of tissues. This precipitation is often performed with ethanol or acetone and can provide considerable selectivity during isolation and purification of macromolecules.

These general properties of water as a solvent are of critical importance for the behavior of ions in physiologic situations, particularly in determining their interactions with other solutes and with macromolecules in the particulate bio-

phases such as the membranes of cells and organelles.

Other characteristics of water will be elaborated upon throughout the remainder of this text. Of particular interest are specific heat, latent heat of vaporization, thermal conduction, and surface properties.

Specific Heat

Water absorbs a substantial load of thermal energy, or heat, without drastic change in temperature. The converse is also true: substantial amounts of heat can be given up without a major fall in temperature. Many physiologic processes, discussed later in detail, are exquisitely temperature sensitive, and water serves in several ways to buffer potentially devastating thermal fluctuations. In addition, because the water content of living tissue is high, the total storage of heat energy is also high.

Latent Heat of Vaporization

The amount of energy required to vaporize water is substantial. Depending on the circumstances, this can be either advantageous or potentially costly to animals. Relief of excessive thermal loads can be achieved by the thermoregulatory processes of sweating and panting, in which energy is expended to vaporize water. This topic is developed in Chapter 9 in the analysis of interactions between animals and their environment. Often overlooked is the corollary that heat is continually expended in maintaining mucosal surfaces in the moist state. Every incoming breath of air is warmed to body temperature and humidified to saturation in the upper respiratory tract to protect the alveolar exchange membrane of the lungs (see Chapter 5).

Water as a Thermal Conductor

In addition to the specific heat of water and the consideration that some 6.5% of total body water at any moment is rapidly circulating in the cardiovascular system, water in the form of interstitial fluid also bathes all cells and provides an important conducting medium for heat transfer. Later it will become evident that differences in the insulating properties of tissues such as fat, skin, and muscle essentially reflect the water content of these tissues.

Interestingly, water in its pure state is not a particularly good conductor of charges; in practice, though, body water always contains ionized solutes, and electrical conductivity is therefore relatively high. This will be found to be particularly cogent when consideration is given

to the propagation of bioelectrical signals in the next chapter.

Surface Properties

The surface of a container of water exhibits characteristic properties resulting from the colligative phenomena described earlier. Individual molecules are continually entering and leaving the vapor phase above the surface; the highly ordered molecular packing suggested by Figure 2–11 is a gross oversimplification. However, intermolecular associations are considerable within the liquid phase and somewhat different at the interface. There is a net tendency for interfacial molecules to be more strongly attracted downward into the bulk volume than laterally across the surface. This asymmetry of forces leads to formation of a meniscus, as seen in a water-filled tube (Figure 2–12).

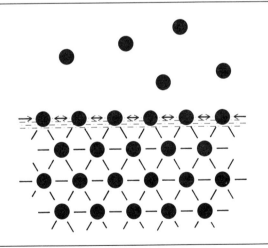

Figure 2–11. Liquid and vapor phases of water. This simple diagram shows the highly ordered nature of water in its liquid form (lower), the interface with the atmosphere (center), and the lesser density of molecules in the vapor phase (above). Interfacial molecules are strongly attracted downwards into the bulk volume of the liquid phase.

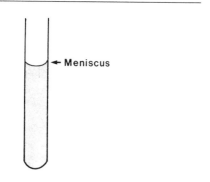

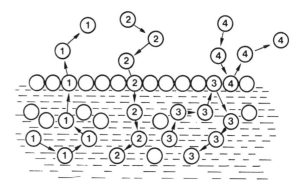

Figure 2–12. Surface tension: the meniscus. The attraction of interfacial molecules to each other and to the liquid below the surface generates the characteristic meniscus that is seen in a water-filled glass tube.

Similarly, the surface properties require energy to be expended so that a given molecule can break free and enter the atmosphere as a vapor phase molecule (Figure 2–13). This requirement is part of the latent heat of vaporization noted above. In the normal situation, molecules are continuously in motion, striking one another in random fashion described as Brownian. The collisions result in release of much of the energy; and the movements increase in intensity when external energy is supplied, for example when water is heated. With sufficient *momentum*, which is the product of mass and velocity, some molecules may strike the interface with enough vigor that they exceed the cohesive threshold of the surface and pass into the vapor phase. In reverse fashion, vapor phase molecules are also randomly striking the interface, and if their momentum falls below the cohesive threshold of the surface, they are absorbed and retained to be incorporated into the liquid phase, rather than bounced back off into the atmosphere. The net movement between the

Figure 2–13. Liquid–vapor exchanges. Water molecules are in continuous motion within both the liquid and vapor phases. At equilibrium, water leaving the liquid phase is balanced by water leaving the vapor phase and returning to the liquid. Molecule #1 from the liquid phase reaches the surface with enough momentum to "break through" and enter the vapor phase. Molecule #2 reaches the surface from the vapor phase with little momentum and is incorporated into the liquid phase through the process of condensation. Molecules #3 and #4 reach the interface from the liquid and vapor phases, respectively, but #3 has insufficient momentum to overcome surface tension and is retained, while #4 hits the surface with enough momentum to bounce back into the atmosphere.

phases is described by the terms *vaporization,* or volatilization, and *condensation,* and these exchanges reflect the interplay of numerous factors, including temperature, vapor pressure, surface area, and so on. These variables will feature extensively when consideration is given later to some aspects of thermoregulation and respiration. The concept of surface tension usually causes students some difficulty. An expanded and more formal treatment of the topic is given in Box 2–1.

Box 2–1   Surface Tension

This discussion is provided for completeness of the description of the most important properties of water. It is a conceptually difficult topic for many students. The reader is encouraged to study this material because it explains a number of phenomena referred to in the text.

Surface tension is the term used to describe the force operating perpendicularly to a unit length of the surface. Surface tension may be considered as the force required to expand the area of the surface, or the force underlying the tendency for the area of a surface to be reduced to the minimum possible. This is illustrated by the effect of surface tension underlying an everyday phenomenon—the formation of a near-spherical drop of water by pinching off to minimize the ratio of area to volume (Figure 2–14). The sphere is the optimal body in this regard. Surface tension is quantified in terms of force per unit length, or newtons per meter. Pure water, under standardized conditions of temperature and pressure, exhibits a surface tension of 7 N/m. By comparison, a solution of a mild detergent may have a surface tension of 3 to 4 N/m; blood plasma, a surface tension of approximately 3.5 to 4 N/m; and the surface tension of a lung extract may be as low as 0.1 to 0.5 N/m. The surface tension–low-

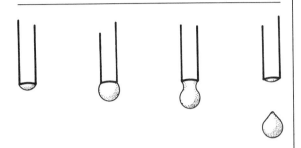

Figure 2–14. Surface tension in action. A hanging drop of water generally assumes a near spherical shape, minimizing its surface area relative to its volume. In doing so, the weight of the droplet causes it to pinch off and fall. For the same reasons, if a hydrophobic surface is misted with water, nearly perfect spherical droplets form.

ering effect of detergents and proteins results from the *amphipathic* properties of these molecules: that is, the regionally distinct polar and apolar domains. The charged or hydrophilic portions intersperse between the water molecules, and at the surface the hydrophobic regions are held out into the atmospheric phase. This is crudely illustrated in Figure 2–15. The effect of these substances at the liquid-vapor interface is to reduce water-water cohesion and so reduce surface tension.

Protein solutions and detergents read-

Figure 2–15. Surface-active molecules. Amphipathic molecules (such as many detergents) reduce surface cohesiveness or tension. The polar portions of the molecules (shaded circles) intersperse between the water molecules of the surface (empty circles) while their apolar portions stand out into the atmospheric phase.

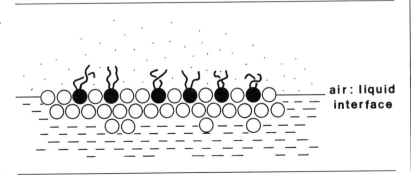

air : liquid interface

ily foam, and quite stable "bubbles" may result. An air-filled bubble is an excellent example of the role of surface-active substances (surfactants) and also exposes the relationship between pressure and volume described by Laplace's law (Figure 2–16).

In any homogeneous space bounded by a "wall" or enclosing membrane, there exists an outwardly directed force that is constant in all directions. It is pressure, expressed in units of force/area (N/m²), or pascals (Pa). Pressure, acting radially outward, is opposed by surface tension in the wall or membrane. Surface tension is the

tendency for the surface area to collapse to the minimum possible.

Acting over the whole spherical surface, surface tension in effect becomes a net inwardly directed force that balances pressure. The relationship between pressure and tension is described by Laplace's law:

$$P = \frac{2\omega \, T}{r} \qquad (1)$$

where T is surface tension in N/m, P is pressure in N/m², r is radius in meters, and ω is a unitless coefficient descriptive of the wall or membrane film.

Laplace's law can be rewritten in the following ways:

$$r = \frac{2\omega T}{P}$$

or

$$T = \frac{P \times r}{2\omega}$$

From equation 1, given in its various forms, it is apparent that, at a given pressure, tension is directly proportional to radius: the greater the radius, the greater the tendency for collapse to minimize the area. Similarly, for a given tension, pressure varies inversely with radius. This may be readily visualized with the aid of Figures 2–17 and 2–18.

Suppose that a large bubble forms in a soapy solution. As noted earlier, the size of the bubble reflects the outward, or distending, influence of pressure and the inward, or collapsing, tendency of surface tension. Any reduction in surface area resulting from surface tension necessarily reduces the volume of the spherical bubble. Because the number of gas molecules inside the bubble is constant, any reduction in the volume in which they are dispersed must increase the pressure exerted by the

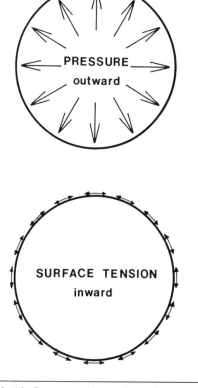

Figure 2–16. Pressure–volume relationships. Pressure is an outwardly-directed force that tends to "stretch" the wall. It is opposed by surface tension, which acts to reduce the stretch on the wall and, over the whole surface, serves as a net inwardly-directed force.

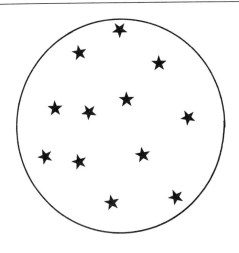

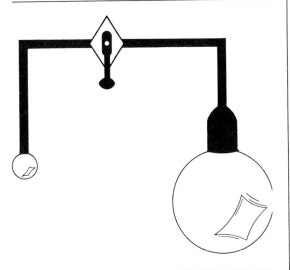

Figure 2–18. The paradox of the bubbles. The greater pressure in the small bubble (see Figure 2–17) will cause it to empty into the larger bubble when the two are interconnected.

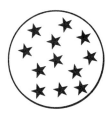

Figure 2–17. Pressure–volume relationships. Molecules exert a far greater outward pressure in bubbles of small radius or volume (in which they are compressed) than in bubbles of larger radius or volume.

gas in a net outward direction (see Figure 2–17):

$$\textbf{Pressure} \times \textbf{Volume} = \textbf{constant} \quad (2)$$

If two bubbles of different radii were formed from the same soap solution, then interconnected, the smaller bubble with higher pressure $[P = (2\omega T)/r]$ would collapse into the larger, lower pressure bubble (see Figure 2–18).

The aforementioned principle is of relevance in numerous physiologic situations in which spaces are subject to distension, with resultant *pressure-volume-tension* rela-

tionships. The terminal air spaces of the lung, the alveoli, are of various sizes or volumes, depending on the particular stage of the inspiratory-expiratory cycle. If the alveoli were moistened only with water, or even a simple physiologic salt solution, surface tension would cause the smaller alveoli to collapse completely whenever expiration occurred. This does not happen because the alveoli contain a lining layer of a highly specialized surfactant. This material, a mixture of proteins and dipalmityl lecithin, a specific phospholipid whose structure is shown in Figure 2–19, exhibits surface tension–lowering properties. The ability to act as surfactant varies with the effective concentration of the molecule. This characteristic is in contrast to the properties of water, for in water the surface tension remains constant even when the surface is expanded or compressed. Pulmonary surfactant is most effective in lowering surface tension when it is present at high concentration; it is relatively ineffective when present at low concentration. Because the

Figure 2–19. The lecithins: dipalmitylphosphoryl-choline. This member of the lecithin class of phospholipids (described in detail later in this chapter) has two palmityl ($C_{16:0}$) side-chains, which makes it somewhat unusual. Most lecithins contain at least one unsaturated fatty acid. The lecithin shown is an important constituent of surfactant in the fluid lining the alveoli of the lungs. Note the charged choline moiety within the polar portion of the molecule.

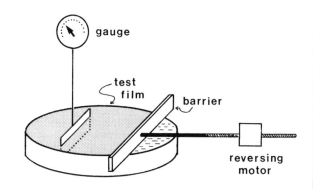

lecithin molecules are organized in the manner shown in Figure 2–15, as the diameter of the alveolus decreases during expiration, a given number of surfactant molecules become more tightly packed at the liquid-air interface. Pulmonary surfactant is most effective under precisely these conditions.

The effectiveness of any surfactant can be assessed by the technique depicted in Figure 2–20. If a washing of lung fluid or a simple lung tissue extract were applied

Figure 2–20. Surface tension measurements. In the upper diagram, a force-measuring gauge, or transducer, is monitoring the surface tension by means of the suspended plate sensor while a barrier is moved to increase or decrease the area of the film making up the test surface. In the lower figure, a washing of lung fluid exhibits a marked reduction in surface tension during compression and an increase in tension towards that of water as the compression is removed. The barrier has no effect on the surface tension measured when the apparatus contains pure water.

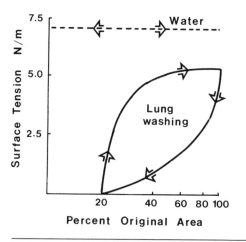

as a film on a surface of water, and the film area were stretched out, the opposing surface tension would bear a complex relationship to the change in area. Tension would increase quite rapidly from the very low (<0.5 N/m) initial value, with relatively little change in area. However, with further expansion, surface tension would change only slightly, then not at all. In all states, its value is substantially lower than the surface tension value of pure water. During compression of the film of surfactant, surface tension decreases quite rapidly to very low values. This marked decrease in surface tension as the surfactant molecules are compressed together is the sole reason why the alveoli do not collapse during expiration. In the description of pulmonary mechanics in Chapter 5, it will become obvious that this effect of surfactant markedly reduces the inspiratory effort required to expand the alveoli for re-aeration. In Chapter 10 we will see that the first appearance of surfactant in the lung, just before birth, is a critical event in the preparation of the fetus for extrauterine life.

2.3 • An Introduction to Cell Biology

Cells are functional masses of *protoplasm*, or living matter, that contain or have previously contained a nucleus and are limited peripherally by a membrane. The surface membrane, or *plasmalemma*, protects the interior from the immediate external environment of the cell and provides a measure of structural support, because many internal parts of the cell are anchored to this membrane by the cytoskeleton. The plasmalemma plays such an important role in the everyday business of the cell that some effort should be devoted to understanding its structure and composition. The next section of this chapter details the nature and properties of membranes. Typically, the surface membrane is a mere 70 to 100 angstroms (Å) thick (0.000007 to 0.00001 mm) and has very little tensile strength. Perhaps the usual small size of cells (10 to 100 μ, or 0.01 to 0.1 mm in diameter) is necessitated by the fragile nature of this limiting membrane.

Within the cell and suspended in the cytoplasm, or the amorphous fluid portion, is a wide array of subcellular structures called *organelles*. In most cells the *nucleus* is the most obvious organelle. The role of the nucleus in directing synthetic activities of the cell, and specific consideration of mechanisms of nuclear and cell division, will be described in Chapter 8. The specialized nuclear membrane has characteristic pores and is continuous with an internal, tortuously folded membrane system called the *endoplasmic reticulum*. The endoplasmic reticulum may be smooth or may appear to be rough surfaced because of the presence of *ribosomes*, structures that are intimately involved in the assembly of amino acids into proteins.

Mitochondria (Figure 2–21) are probably the most highly specialized organelles, both in terms of structure and function. Mitochondria are responsible for the major energy transformations in the cell. The process of oxidative phosphorylation enables energy harvested from controlled hydrolytic reactions to be incorporated

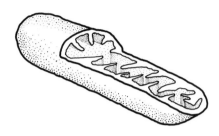

Figure 2–21. Mitochondrion. This simplified diagram shows part of the internal structure of the mitochondrion. The internal membrane is thrown into a series of folds, called cristae.

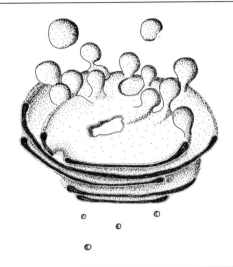

Figure 2–22. The Golgi apparatus. The Golgi is a series of interconnected laminar membranes. Newly synthesized proteins are gathered into the lowermost portion. They may be modified, especially by the addition of sugar residues, then they are packaged into membrane-enclosed granules and released off the upper surface. The membrane wrapping will become incorporated into the plasmalemma of the cell when the contents of the granule are released during secretion.

into the highly labile and energy-rich phosphorylated compound called *adenosine triphosphate* (ATP). Oxygen is consumed in order to produce ATP, and water is produced as a byproduct.

Another organelle with characteristic form is the *Golgi apparatus* (Figure 2–22), a specialized membrane system located near the nucleus. The Golgi apparatus is particularly evident in cells engaged in secretory, or export, function, and its membranes contain enzymes capable of modifying newly synthesized proteins from the ribosomes before the proteins are packaged into secretory units and moved to the cell surface.

A variety of membrane-bounded vesicles can be discerned in most cells. Some of these have characteristic properties associated with degradational activity and have been called *lysosomes.* Lysosomal enzymes usually have pH optima less than 6 and they seem to be responsible for autodigestion of damaged cells: a type of scavenger role. Additionally, complex molecules and particles can be engulfed by some cells in a process called endocytosis, and the vesicles so formed fuse with lysosomes so that digestion can occur before the products gain access to the true cytoplasmic phase of the cells.

Recent studies indicate that this amazing array of intracellular organelles is organized on an internal latticework of filaments referred to as the *cytoskeleton.* Highly specialized proteins, including tubulin, become polymerized and provide a three-dimensional scaffolding upon which the organelles are attached (Figure 2–23). The

cytoskeleton is dynamic and can break down then reform, as would be required in a cell capable of changing its shape in order to perform its function. This is exemplified by the phagocyte, a cell that in effect wraps itself around a particle in order to engulf it for internal digestion. These cells are important in defense mechanisms, as will be described in Chapter 9.

Specialized cells, of course, have additional internal features, such as the contractile apparatus of muscle cells and the enormous fat droplets that dominate the interior of an adipocyte. Additionally, secretory cells seem to be packed with membrane-bounded granules awaiting release from the cell.

The cytoplasm, or fluid remainder of the cell, can only be described in a very general way as a mixture of *colloid* and solution. The key elements of the mix include proteins, lipids, carbohydrates, salts, and water, though the com-

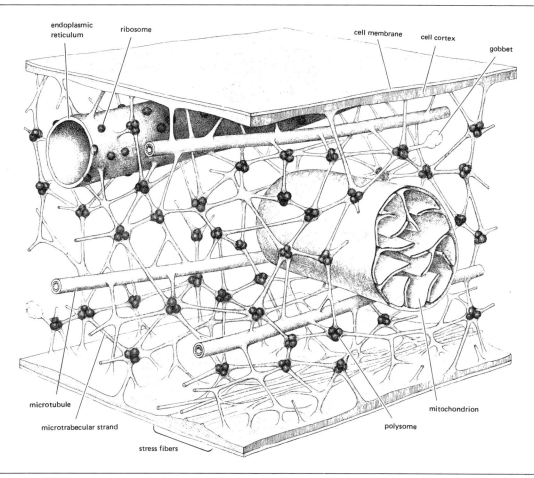

endoplasmic reticulum ribosome cell membrane cell cortex gobbet microtubule microtrabecular strand stress fibers mitochondrion polysome

Figure 2–23. The cytoskeleton. This diagram has been synthesized from hundreds of images obtained from a powerful, high-voltage electron microscope. This instrument can produce images of internal three-dimensional structure from relatively thick specimens. The various organelles are suspended on a latticework formed from tubulin and microtrabeculae. (Reproduced by permission of the publisher. From Porter, K.R. and Tucker, J.B.: "The Ground Substance of the Living Cell," *Scientific American,* March 1981, p. 59. Copyright © 1981, Scientific American, Inc. All rights reserved.)

binations that occur, such as lipoproteins, glycolipids, metalloproteins, and so on, make an orderly classification very difficult. Perhaps the most important characteristic to grasp is that these constituents exist more as colloids than as true solutions. Colloids are heterogeneous solid-liquid mixtures that exist in various physical forms. Some appear very liquid, such as milk (a *sol*), while others appear quite solid, such as Jello

(a *gel*). Using milk as an example of a colloid, we can continue with some definitions: micelles, or aggregates, of casein and other proteins are dispersed in a watery medium. This gives milk its characteristic opacity. The micelles are not in solution and yet are not so large that they settle out, except when milk is centrifuged or clotted, as in cheese making. The fat in milk may behave the same way, because in the milk of some species, creaming or the floating of fat droplets to the surface does not normally occur; instead, the fat remains colloidally dispersed.

It should be obvious from the foregoing that cells represent collections of "compartments" separated one from another by *membranes*. Usually the cells in a tissue are not really independent but rather act and interact with some harmony. For this to occur, communication between the cells, or the transfer of information, is important in the same way that transfer of materials such as fuels and wastes is important.

Much of the next two chapters of this text is concerned with information transfer, while a sizable portion of the later chapters will address materials transfer. To appreciate the mechanisms and consequences of such transfers, the following section examines the nature of membranes in some detail. Aspects of materials transfer across such membranes are described in section 2.5.

2.4 • Structure and Properties of Membranes

Biologic membranes delimit compartments of various sizes in the body. Of greatest importance here is the plasma membrane, or the limiting membrane that separates cytoplasm from interstitium. Naked cytoplasm does not exist. There is a long history of various models proposed to account for the functional, biochemical, and structural properties of these membranes. The most useful model, and currently the most generally acceptable, is Singer's fluid mosaic (Figure 2–24), which provides for proteins and lipids coexisting in a dynamic structure. Lipids, including a high proportion of distinctly polar molecules, are oriented into hydrophilic surfaces with a hydrophobic interior. Interspersed in this lipid matrix are various proteins, as shown in Figure 2–24. Some of the proteins are peripheral and exposed on either the external or internal faces. Others traverse the lipid matrix and, in the special case of channel proteins, or pores, provide hydrophilic domains through the essentially hydrophobic inner region of the membrane.

The proteins and lipids interact extensively and dynamically, providing an ordered structure while at the same time enabling channel proteins to open and close their lumina, and allowing others to move radially in and out through the thickness of the membrane. Additionally, some proteins are able to move laterally within the plane of the membrane, sometimes transiently forming clusters of similar proteins at particular loci.

The basis of *lipoprotein* interaction stems from the ordered polar-apolar orientation of the membrane lipids (Figure 2–25), and the ability of proteins to alter their higher order structure. These conformational changes alter the distribution and charge density of hydrophilic and hydrophobic domains on the proteins. The important membrane lipids responsible for these interactions are described below.

The fluidity of the lipoprotein mosaic varies with temperature. In part this is a reflection of the fatty acid composition of the lipids intrinsic to the membrane. The physical state of lipids

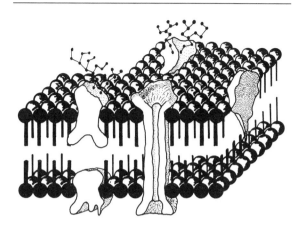

Figure 2–24. Membrane structure: the fluid mosaic. In this illustration of the membrane bilayer, proteins float in a sea of lipid. Note the presence of the channel protein, providing a hydrophilic "pore" through the thickness of the membrane. Other proteins are shown exposed on the external face (upper) and on the internal face (lower). Two of the externally exposed proteins are decorated with chains of carbohydrate residues; these are glycoproteins. The carbohydrate makes up the glycocalyx, an external coat over the cell. The membrane lipids are shown with polar heads on the surfaces and apolar tails extending into the inner matrix, or core.

varies from crystalline at low temperatures to fluid at a critical "melting" temperature. This is much the same as the phenomenon whereby butter melts into oil at a warm temperature. The critical temperature for such a phase change is quite low (approximately 20 C) because much of the hydrocarbon in the polar lipids of membranes is unsaturated, possessing an abundance of double bonds. Appendix B explains what is meant by unsaturated and gives examples of such fatty acids. Only at temperatures below 20 C can the high degree of molecular packing required for solidification, or crystallization, be achieved. Some of the strategies used by cold-blooded animals to maintain membrane fluidity at temperatures less than 20 C are noted in Box 2–2.

The plasma membrane of the erythrocyte is the best-studied mammalian membrane. The extent to which the erythrocyte plasma membrane is typical of membranes in general is uncertain,

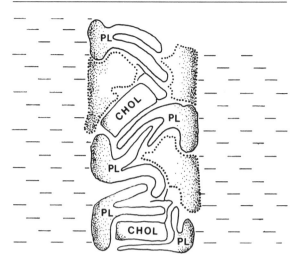

Figure 2–25. Polar–apolar organization in membranes. Phospholipids (PL), cholesterol (CHOL), and proteins (dotted outline) coexist with their more polar regions (shaded) in proximity to the surface, while the less polar portions are retained within the thickness of the membrane. All of these molecules are amphipathic because they have regionally distinct polar and apolar portions.

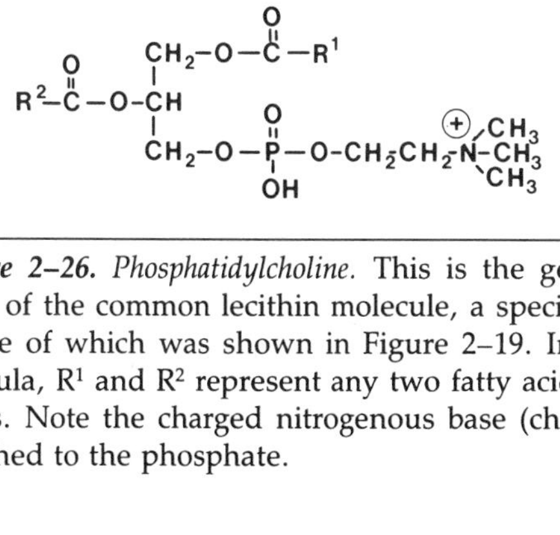

$$R^2 - \overset{\overset{\displaystyle O}{\|}}{C} - O - \underset{\underset{\displaystyle CH_2 - O - \overset{\overset{\displaystyle O}{\|}}{\underset{\underset{\displaystyle OH}{|}}{P}} - O - CH_2 CH_2 \overset{(+)}{N} \begin{smallmatrix} CH_3 \\ -CH_3 \\ CH_3 \end{smallmatrix}}{|}}{CH} \quad \begin{smallmatrix} CH_2 - O - \overset{\overset{\displaystyle O}{\|}}{C} - R^1 \end{smallmatrix}$$

Figure 2–26. Phosphatidylcholine. This is the generic form of the common lecithin molecule, a special example of which was shown in Figure 2–19. In this formula, R^1 and R^2 represent any two fatty acid residues. Note the charged nitrogenous base (choline) attached to the phosphate.

but many properties of this model appear to be similar to those of the plasmalemmas of more complex cells. Both the lipids and proteins of this membrane have been extensively characterized.

Of the lipids the *lecithins,* a family of *phosphatidylcholines* (Figure 2–26), are of particular importance. The fatty acid esterified in position 2 is most often a polyunsaturated 18-carbon acid, the acid in position 1 is generally saturated and so has no double bonds, and the phosphoric acid attached to position 3 is coupled to choline, a charged nitrogenous base. The *cephalins,* or the family of *phosphatidylserines,* are similar except for the presence of the amino acid serine on the phosphate (Figure 2–27). The carboxyl (−COOH) and amino (−NH$_2$) groups readily assume charges depending on pH in the immediate environment (see Figure 2–27). The charged region is spatially separate from the noncharged or apo-

lar fatty acid chains. This is the basis for what is termed the amphipathic nature of the phospholipids, illustrated in Figure 2–28.

Also in the family of cephalins are the *phosphatidylethanolamines* in which a weak base, ethanolamine, is coupled to the phosphate group (Figure 2–29). The quantitatively minor lipids include *cholesterol* (Figure 2–30) and complex lipids such as *cerebrosides, sphingomyelins,* and *gangliosides.* The latter are shown in Figure 2–31 simply to illustrate the structural diversity and complexity of the very polar lipids. The reader should not try to memorize these structures.

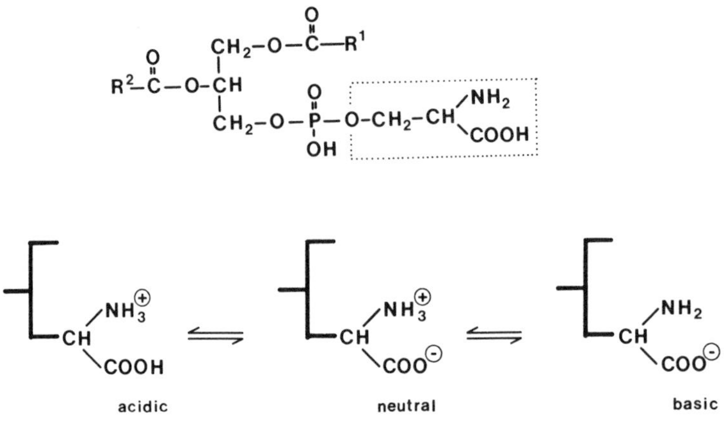

Figure 2–27. Phosphatidylserine and its charges. Phosphatidylserine contains a serine residue (dotted) linked to the phosphate group. The −NH$_2$ and −COOH groups of the serine assume charges (−NH$_3^+$ and −COO$^-$), depending on the pH of the environment. As a result, this phospholipid is particularly polar.

acidic   neutral   basic

<hr>

Box 2–2   Membrane Specializations

Mammals and birds, being homeotherms with core temperatures far above the critical temperature, do not depend on the special devices used by lower animals to protect the integrity of their membranes. For example, the critical temperature could be lowered further by a higher content of branched chain and polyunsaturated fatty acids and incorporation into the membranes of additional complex lipids. These

serve to decrease the stability of the lipoprotein matrix as it approaches a phase change at very low temperatures. Fish use this adaptation so that their membranes remain fluid despite low environmental and body core temperatures. The fatty acids of the lipids of fish are particularly enriched in polyunsaturated fatty acids (see Appendix B).

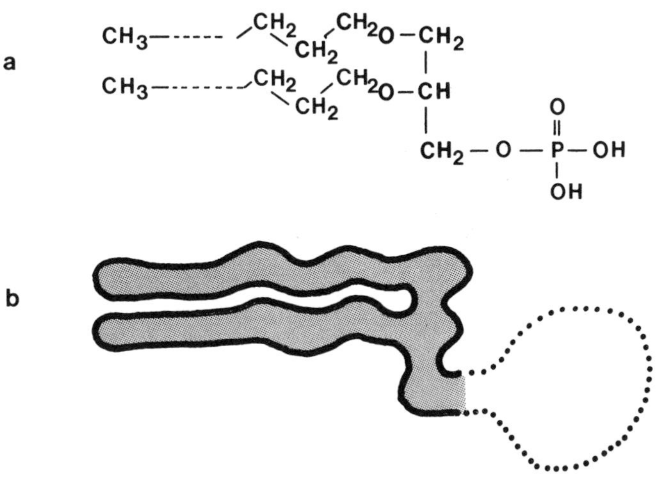

Figure 2–28. *Amphipathic nature of phospholipids.* In *a*, the chemical structure of the phospholipid parent structure, phosphatidic acid, is shown in a form slightly modified from that used elsewhere in this chapter. Note the two hydrocarbon chains connected to two of the three carbons of glycerol, which is drawn vertically. The third hydroxyl group of the glycerol is involved in the linkage with the phosphate group. Usually, the phosphate is in turn connected to additional charged groups, as shown in Figures 2–26, 2–27, and 2–29. In *b*, the hydrocarbon "tails" are shaded and the polar portion is shown as a "head".

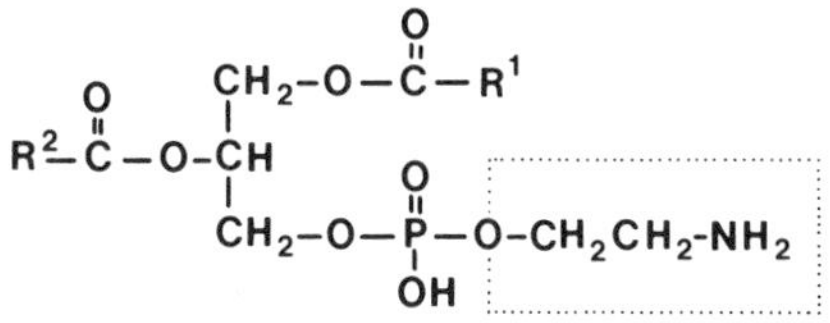

Figure 2–29. *Phosphatidylethanolamine.* Another member of the cephalin class of phospholipids is shown with the phosphate group connected to a weak nitrogenous base, ethanolamine (dotted). The $-NH_2$ residue can become positively charged ($-NH_3^+$) by taking up a H^+ ion when the pH is less than neutral.

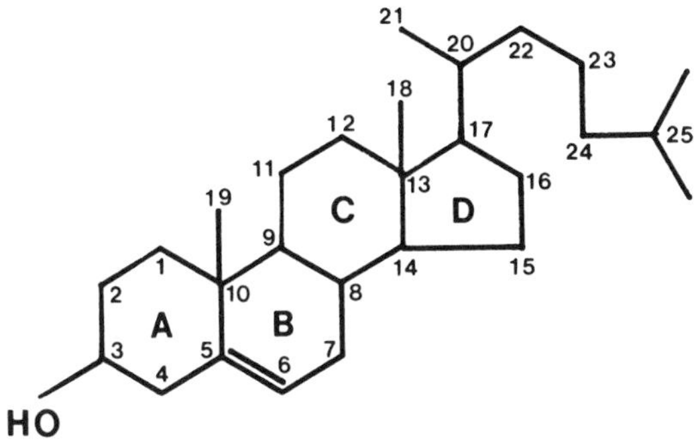

What is important in relation to membrane structure and function is the following:

> the polar heads of the phospholipids align to form hydrophilic surfaces, as was indicated in Figure 2–15, when surface-active molecules were described. In cells, the more hydrophobic chains, or tails, associate with each other within the thickness of the membrane while the polar heads align on the internal and external surfaces (see Figure 2–25).

The precise structural relationships among

Figure 2–30. *Cholesterol.* The cholesterol molecule is shown with ring assignments (A through D) and each carbon is numbered. Later, when describing steroid hormones, which are derivatives of cholesterol, these numbers will be used to locate a variety of substitutions on the parent structure. For now, you should be able to identify the four rings and be able to recognize positions 3, 11 and 17.

the lipid components are best understood in the compound membrane of the myelin sheath. The sheath is a coiled bilayer (see Figure 1–19) of virtually pure plasmalemma formed by processes of Schwann cells, tightly wrapped in spiral fashion around the axon. Sufficient myelin can be obtained in its native state for physico-

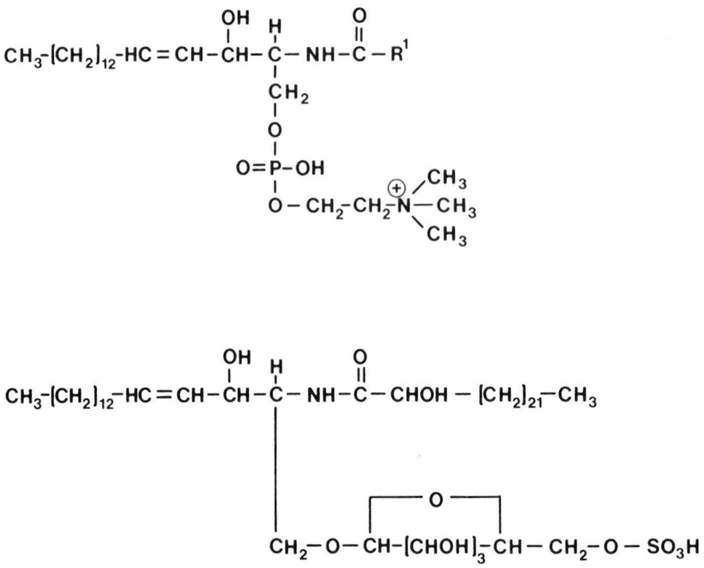

Figure 2–31. Complex polar lipids. The great diversity in the structure of the polar lipids is illustrated by these two examples: sphingomyelin (top) and a cerebroside (bottom). Note that the cerebroside has a sulfuric acid residue, capable of serving as a strong acid, as its most polar group. Sphingomyelin contains a choline moiety attached to the phosphate group, as in lecithin (see Figure 2–26).

chemical analyses, including x-ray diffraction examination, to be performed. A wide array of physical methods can be applied to study isolated fragments of plasmalemma and, in selected examples, while the intact membrane still surrounds a cell. These methods, used in physical biochemistry and biophysics, are beyond the scope of the present discussion.

2.5 • Materials Transfer across Membranes

There is much traffic of materials (water, gases, solutes) across membranes. Because of the wide array of physicochemical properties of these substances, and the need to regulate what can and cannot traverse the membrane, several mechanisms exist. Membranes are best thought of as being *selectively permeable* to molecules: they allow certain substances to pass with ease and exclude others. The lipoprotein nature of the membrane, and its orderly arrangement into hydrophilic and hydrophobic domains, determines most of these permeability characteristics. For example, lipid-soluble molecules such as carotene, the orange pigment of many plants, pass from the interstitial fluid through the lipid domains in the cell membrane by simply dissolving in the membrane, establishing a concentration gradient from outside to inside, then flowing from regions of high concentration to regions of low concentration.

The simplest form of bulk flow is *filtration,* a term usually applied to the movement of solutions across barriers when hydrostatic pressure is the driving force. Chapter 5 describes the role of filtration from the pressurized cardiovascular system into the extravascular tissue spaces. In the kidney, similar filtration causes enormous bulk flow of a plasma filtrate into the nephron, or renal tubule. Filtration direction is purely the result of a *pressure gradient:* fluid flows from high-pressure regions to those of lower pressure in an attempt to equalize pressure on either side of the barrier. The fluid consists of solvent, usually water, and dissolved solute. The barrier can be thought of as a rather coarse filter (Figure 2–32). There is only limited opportunity to retard the passage of solute, although very large molecules (e.g., proteins and lipoproteins) may be held back; and in most cases free cells such as blood cells are unable to traverse filtration barriers.

Another major mixing process that contributes to movement of materials across barriers is *diffusion.* Diffusion is a consequence of the intrinsic Brownian motion (Figure 2–33) of molecules, which randomly bounce off other molecules in a fluid, either liquid or gas, until a relatively homogeneous mixture results (Figure 2–34). If solute molecules are taken up by a membrane, as in the case of carotene, the remaining molecules in solution will redistribute to remove concentration gradients in the bulk phase of the solution. Processes such as this ensure that polar molecules and ions have some chance of coming close to more specialized regions on the membrane that may facilitate their passage through the otherwise hydrophobic barrier.

A well-known transfer phenomenon that occurs across semipermeable membranes is called *osmosis.* In osmosis, water moves to equalize solute concentration on either side of the membrane. Water moves from the more dilute side to the more concentrated side (Figure 2–35). Solute molecules such as large proteins that are unable to easily cross membranes contribute to the development of *osmotic pressure,* a drawing force that attracts water. In Chapter 5 it will be-

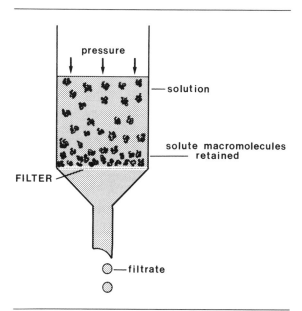

Figure 2–32. Filtration. This diagram shows a solution of a macromolecule in a reservoir on a filter. The solvent passes through, but the large molecules are retained and concentrate in the vicinity of the filter. The "column" of solution above the filter provides a hydrostatic driving force for the passage of solvent.

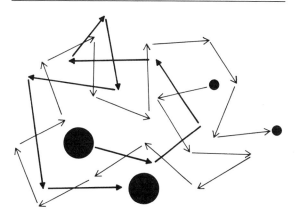

Figure 2–33. Brownian motion. Molecules are intrinsically mobile; the paths they follow in a confined space are quite random because of chance collisions with other molecules. These movements give rise to mixing and provide the basis for diffusion.

Figure 2–34. Diffusion. Diffusion is the consequence of random motion, as illustrated by molecules in chambers. Assume that space B is initially a vacuum and the dots in space A represent gas molecules. When the two chambers are connected the concentration of the gas in A reduces as the concentration in B increases. These changes in concentration with time are shown in the graph. Eventually, the concentration will be equal in A and B, when the distribution of the gas molecules has become homogeneous.

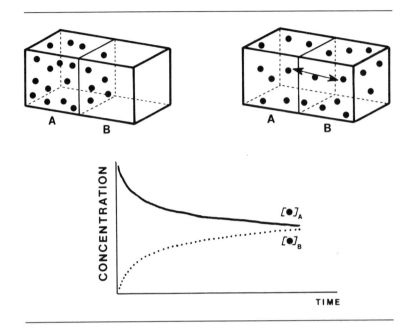

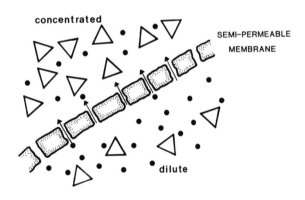

Figure 2–35. Dialysis and osmosis. In this semipermeable membrane, the "pores" permit solvent (dots) to pass while preventing solute molecules (triangles) from redistributing across the membrane. The higher concentration of solute above the membrane is drawing solvent from the more dilute side. Provided there is sufficient room for expansion in the space above the membrane, this osmotic drag will continue until the concentration of solute is identical on either side. It will be shown later that this process can cause cells to expand to the point of rupture.

come obvious that a major role of plasma proteins is to provide an osmotic driving force that acts in part to oppose water movement out of the blood vessels. This is an example of two mechanisms—one filtration, the other osmotic drag—that act against each other. In severe protein malnutrition, the concentration of plasma proteins is reduced and colloid osmotic pressure is less than normal. The effect is excessive extravascular accumulation of fluids, a phenomenon called *edema.*

Somewhat similar to osmosis, though depending on the nature of the membrane and solute involved, is *dialysis.* In this case a permeant solute rather than the solvent redistributes itself across a membrane in an attempt to achieve molecular balance on both sides. Usually osmosis and dialysis will occur together, with solute and solvent moving in opposite directions. If excessive solvent moves into a restricted space, there is a real risk of swelling and possible rupture of that space. In Chapter 5, when the effects of salt solutions on cells are considered, the damaging effects of dilute solutions and of pure water on cells will be noted. These insults result in an osmotic drag of water into cells proceeding to the extent that the resulting cell swelling causes *lysis,* or rupture, of the cell. This is well known for blood cells that are transferred into pure water, whereupon swelling and rupture are easily detected by the release of hemoglobin from the cells, a process called *hemolysis.*

In addition to the processes described above, in which simple physicochemical forces account for materials movement, mechanisms exist for energy-consuming selective movement that can overcome chemical or concentration gradients across membranes. Energy, usually obtained by controlled hydrolysis of ATP, is used to ''pump'' substances against concentration gradients. In some cases the energy is used to provide the driving force for a *carrier molecule,* or pump, in the membrane to move substances from one side to the other. These pumps may be extremely selective for a given ion or molecule, or they may be capable of handling a whole class of closely related substances. In some instances they serve to exchange one or more ions moving into a cell for one or more distinct ions moving out. The Na^+-K^+–ATPase of the plasmalemma uses ATP-derived energy to pump Na^+ ions out in exchange for K^+ ions being brought in. In the next chapter this pump will be shown to be a key factor in the behavior of excitable tissues, because it regulates in part the balance of charges across the membrane.

2.6 • An Introduction to Homeostasis

The preceding sections of this chapter have provided an overview of the chemical makeup of the body as a whole, the variety of compartments used for convenience in description, and the specific nature of cells. Although the details provided are sometimes the result of research performed very recently, it has long been recognized that living creatures exhibit some features that are truly distinct from inanimate objects.

About 100 years ago the French physiologist Claude Bernard was the first to formally distinguish between the *milieu interieur,* or the internal environment of animals, and the *milieu exterieur,* or the world at large. In Bernard's analysis, importance was placed on the notion that living beings expended effort to preserve the internal environment, quite distinct from that prevailing outside.

For 50 years physiologists explored the mechanisms that served in this protective role and reinterpreted older discoveries, most of which had been made in the preceding 300 years. Finally, about 50 years ago, an American physiologist, Walter B. Cannon, assembled this great body of knowledge into the most important conceptual dictum of this discipline. Cannon hypothesized that the central purpose of physiologic mechanisms was to provide *constancy* of the internal environment. The internal *milieu* is potentially subjected to external influences that threaten its stability; physiologic mechanisms continually operate to oppose and offset these changes. Cannon's recognition of the relative stability of virtually all physiologic parameters such as body temperature in homeotherms, blood glucose concentrations, blood gas levels, and the like has dominated all subsequent developments in physiology.

The terms *steady state* and *homeostasis* are widely used to describe relative constancy, and mechanisms providing for this stability are called homeostatic. The concept of homeostasis is exceedingly valuable in trying to understand the minute-by-minute adjustments that occur in almost all physiologic quantities. In simplified terms, any factor that tends to disturb a variable, such as body temperature, away from its steady-state value will be opposed by homeostatic mechanisms that attempt to reestablish the normal value.

As shown in Figure 2–36, a *perturbation*, or disturbance, of the steady state triggers compensatory reactions that serve to restore the steady state. For example, an animal suddenly subjected to excessive ambient temperatures may experience an increase in body temperature, but this is promptly offset by the activation of heat-losing mechanisms. The phenomenon of some disturbance leading to one or more reactions is the basis for living tissues being described as *irritable*: a *stimulus* or *action* can be expected to provoke one or more *reactions*.

The steady-state value represented by the solid horizontal line in Figure 2–36 is somewhat contrived. In reality, the steady state is rather imperfect and is better represented by a range of values that encompasses a *comfort range*. Within the comfort range, small changes in the actual value are of no great consequence and may provoke no reaction. Disturbances that shift the variable beyond the comfort range, however, do activate *compensatory* mechanisms to bring the value back into the range (Figure 2–37). The comfort range of values may be very narrow, as in the case of a variable that is very closely regulated. Alternatively, if a sizable variation can be tolerated, close regulation may be unnecessary, and the comfort range may be quite wide. In Chapter 9 the notion of comfort ranges is used to construct a working definition of stress as any influence that forces a physiologic variable far beyond the limits of the comfort range. It will also be shown that long-term physiologic adjustments may actually include shifting the comfort range to new values. For example, in fever, body temperatures are still regulated by a series of compensatory mechanisms, but all take place at temperatures greater than normal.

The compensatory changes that are activated when a variable shifts from the comfort range can be in either direction. If the disturbance increases some quantity, the reaction is likely to cause a decrease, and vice versa. This is analogous to the behavior of a mass, suspended from a spring, that is disturbed from its

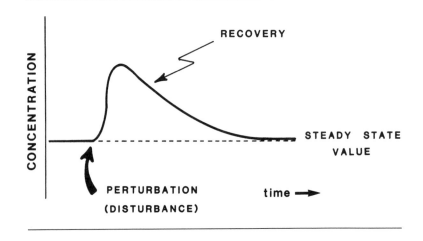

Figure 2–36. Physiological adjustments. The dotted horizontal line represents a steady-state quantity of any physiological parameter; it could be a concentration of some constituent in the blood—glucose, for example. When the steady-state concentration is disturbed for some reason, a compensatory reaction brings about recovery and the concentration returns to the resting value. This graph depicts changes in concentration (ordinate) against time (abscissa).

Figure 2–37. The comfort range.
This figure shows a quantity
undergoing small changes
within the comfort zone, followed by a major disturbance
that drives the value beyond
the lower limit. The marked
disturbance provokes compensatory reactions that restore the
quantity back into the comfort
zone. Changes within the limits
of the comfort range are incon-
sequential and they represent
normal variation that requires
no special compensation. The
types of variation and changes
shown here are physiologically
more realistic than the simple
pattern shown in Figure 2–36.

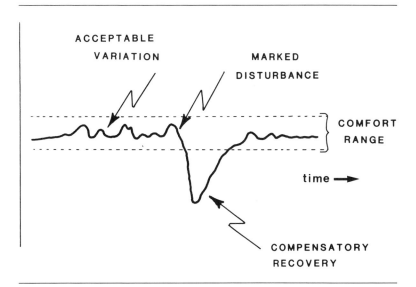

resting position. Any upward disturbance will
be opposed by gravity working downward while
a downward disturbance will be opposed by the
recoil of the spring working upward. Of course,
these reactions do not occur instantaneously, and
they do combine with each other: if the mass is
pulled down then released, a characteristic pattern of up-and-down movements will follow until the movements become imperceptibly small
and the resting position is regained. If the movements of the mass were recorded on a moving
chart, a tracing such as that shown in Figure 2–
38 would result. Position is shown on the ordinate and time on the abscissa; the pattern
shown is that of a *damped oscillation*. When the
reaction process carries the variable beyond the
resting value, the term *overshoot* is applied; the
overshoot in turn provokes a reaction in the opposite direction.

Physiologic homeostasis usually employs a
combination of opposing mechanisms. Often,
several complementary devices operate in each
direction. The various mechanisms have characteristic *lag times* and *response times:* some come
into play very promptly (short lag time after
stimulus) but may be short-lived (short response
time), while others may be sluggish in onset
(long lag time) but may be persistent (long re-

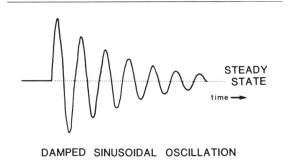

Figure 2–38. Damped oscillation. This figure represents
the vertical movements of a mass, suspended on a
spring, that has been disturbed and bounces up and
down until coming to rest at some later time. The
figure shows changes in a quantity—vertical location
in this case—against time. Note that the initial compensatory reactions overshoot the resting, or steady-
state, value. With time, the reaction becomes progressively less; hence the oscillation is considered
damped.

sponse time). This added complexity makes
analysis difficult but it provides living systems
with great flexibility in control.

The formal study of these actions and reactions is called *control theory*, and in physiology
it is called *cybernetics.* In its simplest form, cy-

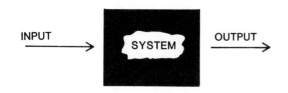

Figure 2–39. The essential elements of a control system. This primitive control diagram shows the input feeding into a system and resulting in an output from that system. By simple analogy, this diagram could represent electric current as the input, an electric motor as the system, and some form of work as the output. It is possible to mathematically relate the output to the input, without having to understand how the motor actually functions.

bernetics is concerned with examining the relationships that exist between an input and an output from some system (Figure 2–39). In most cases, little is known with certainty about the system, and the image of a *black box* is appropriately used. Physiologists study the relationships between inputs and outputs and sometimes generate equations that adequately describe what happens to an output for a given change in input. These analyses are usually not very profound. They must be heavily qualified, and exceptions abound.

Most homeostatic reactions are compensatory and act to oppose the original disturbance. In control theory, this is called a *negative feedback,* and it is the dominant characteristic of most physiologic controls. An input is sensed as a disturbance to the steady state, and the output from this sensor serves to feed back and counteract the original disturbance (Figure 2–40). With reference to Figure 2–37 and the concept of comfort ranges, the *sensor* is the component of the system capable of detecting when the variable has been disturbed to the outer limit of the comfort range. This limit value represents a threshold value, or *setpoint,* for the system. The sensor triggers the output or reaction from the system

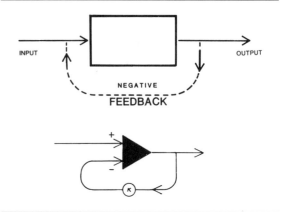

Figure 2–40. Closed-loop negative feedback. Most control systems include a provision for the output to feed back and modify the input; the most stable systems involve negative feedback. For example, a furnace in a house delivers heat when called to do so by the thermostat, the sensor for this system. The heat so provided is sensed at the thermostat and eventually causes the furnace to be shut off. The output (heat) serves as a negative feedback on the input (room temperature).

and so is a key part of the black box. Physiologic sensors are called *receptors,* and much will be said about them in the next two chapters.

At this stage the reader should be comfortable with the concepts that the internal milieu is maintained distinct from the external milieu, that homeostatic mechanisms tend to stabilize the internal environment, that most physiologic reactions are compensatory, and that physiologic controls can be modeled and expressed in terms of an input, a system, and an output. Variables of critical importance are usually closely regulated within narrow limits, while others may be controlled less strictly.

The remainder of this text uses this framework to explore the nature of the array of mechanisms that have evolved to protect the integrity of living animals.

2.7 • Exercises

1. Select the most appropriate item from the alphabetic list to match with each of the prompt terms. Each item should be used once. Be sure that you understand why you make the selections.

plasma proteins	cybernetics
apolar	filtration
hydrophobic	comfort zone
latent heat	surface tension
amphipathic	receptors

a. Polar lipids _____

b. Pressure gradient _____

c. Stable foam _____

d. Biologic sensors _____

e. *Kybernetes* (Greek for "helmsman") _____

f. Colloid osmotic pressure _____

g. Nonionizable _____

h. Homeostasis _____

i. Nonwetting _____

j. Evaporation _____

2. Draw a simple control diagram for a system that assures maintenance of the state of hydration of the body. Identify one factor that could lead to dehydration, then note two obvious "reactions" that might be invoked to offset this dehydration.

3. Provide concise definitions for the following terms:

Active transport _____

Extracellular space _____

Dialysis and osmosis _____

Organelle _____

Membrane fluidity _____

4. The pH of urine, about 5.4, is less than that of blood, about 7.4. Which of the following statements is/are correct?

a. Plasma contains twice ($7.4 - 5.4 = 2$) as many H^+ ions as urine.

b. Urine is less basic than plasma.

c. Urine contains 100 times more H^+ ions than blood.

d. Urine contains 1,000 times more H^+ ions than blood.

e. Urine contains twice the H^+ ions contained in blood.

The Excitable Tissues: Nerve and Muscle

3

3.1 • Electrophysiology

Some aspects of selective ion transport across membranes will be described in this section. In Chapter 2 it was noted that the intracellular and extracellular fluids are quite different in composition. This discussion will be mainly concerned with the two cations of sodium (Na^+) and potassium (K^+).

Part of the movement of ions across membranes is due to the "leakiness" of the lipoprotein barrier, which allows ions to flow down concentration gradients. Even though the ionic radius of K^+ exceeds that of Na^+, differences in the degree of hydration make the hydrated K^+ ion, $K^+ \cdot (H_2O)_x$, smaller than the hydrated Na^+ ion. The Na^+ ion attracts water dipoles more strongly than does the K^+ ion. Under physiologic conditions the effective particle radius is that of the hydrated ion. As a result of these hydration differences, K^+ is some 50 to 75 times more mobile than Na^+.

A major factor acting to maintain ionic gradients across the excitable membrane is the Na^+-K^+–sensitive adenosine triphosphatase (ATPase) located in the membrane itself. This enzyme uses hydrolysis energy from adenosine triphosphate (ATP) to pump Na^+ out and K^+ in across the cell membrane (Figure 3–1). Because of the unequal distribution of ions inside and outside the cell, there is a resting potential or voltage of about 60 millivolts across the membrane. Because the voltage is expressed inside relative to outside, the membrane in its resting state has a negative potential. The membrane is said to be *polarized*.

The membrane behaves as a dielectric, because it serves to separate charges on either side.

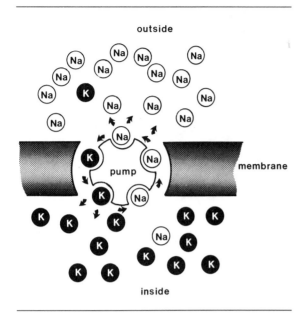

outside

pump

membrane

inside

Figure 3–1. Sodium, *potassium-adenosine triphosphatase.* This membrane enzyme pumps Na⁺ ions out of cells in exchange for K⁺ ions being brought in. ATP is hydrolyzed to furnish the energy needed for the operation of this ion pump, called the Na⁺-K⁺-ATPase. Note the relative abundance of Na⁺ and K⁺ in the extracellular and intracellular compartments.

The term dielectric was introduced in Chapter 2, and a simplified description of the meaning of the electrochemical terms is provided in Box 3–1. The reader should be comfortable with the use of these terms before proceeding with the remainder of this chapter.

The membrane is an imperfect dielectric because some leakiness of ions is quite normal and metabolic energy is expended by the pump to sustain the ion distribution. A sizable proportion of the total energy cost of keeping an animal alive is expended in driving the Na⁺-K⁺–ATPase pump. In addition, specific proteins embedded in the rather hydrophobic lipid matrix serve as ion channels (Figure 3–2). The channels provide a means for rapid transit of ions across the membrane under certain controlled conditions, depending on whether the channel is open or closed. The channels can be opened by chemicals such as *neurotransmitters,* or by *voltage field effects.* Both mechanisms are of importance. Consider an action potential or impulse suddenly impinging on a portion of the membrane that is at rest. For the moment, it will suffice to consider an action potential to be simply a large voltage, with a polarity that is the reverse of the normal membrane potential. A transient increase in sodium conductance occurs because the field that exists in concentrated form, immediately ahead of the action potential, opens the sodium channels. This phenomenon is termed voltage gating, and Na⁺ ions pour down their concentration gradient into the cell. The result is to render the inside temporarily and focally positive with respect to the outside. At the moment when total charge density is the same on either side of the membrane, a state of depolarization exists, although for convenience the whole process, extending until the charge is completely reversed (that is, the outside rather than inside becomes negative), is termed *depolarization.* Within milliseconds, Na⁺ starts to be pumped back out because of the action of the Na⁺-K⁺–ATPase pump. K⁺ is also permitted to flow out, the driving force being simply the concentration gradient of K⁺ from inside to outside. Together, these processes redistribute the ions to repolarize the membrane. Because these ions are charged, their flow is equivalent to "currents" in an electronic sense. They have been studied most extensively in experimentally provoked stimulus situations in the giant axons of squids. A more detailed treatment of these events is provided in Box 3–2.

The brief period of Na⁺ *conductance,* when Na⁺ pours into the cell, is very important, as is the drop-off phase, when Na⁺ influx slows, then ceases. The channel can be opened by fields, as in the case of the applied stimuli described in Box 3–2. The channels can also be opened by specific chemical signals received on the outer face of the membrane, as will be described in the next section. The channel can also be closed, or inactivated, by very high concentrations of Na⁺ in the vicinity of the intracellular opening of the channel. This mechanism limits the extent of Na⁺ influx at a given location. As the channel opens, Na⁺ pours in and high concentrations of this ion accumulate in the immediate vicinity of the internal opening (Figure 3–4). This high concentration then acts to close the channel. It is

Box 3–1   Terms Used with Bioelectrical Events

Some familiarity with simple physics or electronics is required in order to understand the electrochemical basis for events occurring across cell membranes. Because ions are *charged,* they carry *current* when they redistribute across membranes. The terms used in electrophysiology are quite simple but have precise meanings. However, unless the reader has been exposed to an introductory treatment of electronics, the words may have little meaning.

The following analogy between fluid flow and important aspects of current flow will give the reader an everyday idea of the meaning of key variables used in this field. Be certain that you understand what the terms mean before continuing with this chapter.

Mechanical analogues of electromotive forces and variables: Fluids flow from regions of high pressure to those of low pressure. The rate of flow is constrained by *resistance* from the walls of the conducting system on the moving fluid within.

The driving force, equivalent to pressure differential, for the movement of charges is *voltage* or *potential difference.* The rate of flow of charges per unit time is *current.* Flow is opposed by *resistance.* The variables voltage, current, and resistance are related by *Ohm's law:*

Potential = Current × Resistance

In units:

Volts = Amperes × Ohms

$$V = I \times R \qquad (1)$$

Therefore:

$$I = \frac{V}{R} \text{ and } R = \frac{V}{I}$$

Power is the product of voltage and current, or the magnitude of current flow times the pressure drop through which it flows:

Power = Volts × Amps

Substituting from equation 1:

Power = Amps × Amps × Ohms

$$P = I^2 R \qquad (2)$$

If charges are separated by a nonconducting barrier, a potential exists across the barrier. If the barrier then becomes conducting, current flows in an attempt to reduce the potential to zero. The term *resistivity,* and its reciprocal, *conductivity,* describe the effectiveness of this barrier to flow. The amount of charge that can accumulate on one side of the barrier is referred to as *capacitance.*

Imagine yourself standing under a canvas awning supported on four sides and rapidly filling with rain. The canvas serves as a barrier, the resistivity of which depends on its quality. Water accumulates up to a given capacity before pouring over the edge. If the canvas starts to leak when it becomes grossly distended, this represents a change in conductivity. The water falls because gravity provides a potential difference between the awning and the ground.

Figure 3–2. Ion channel proteins. Certain membrane proteins (see Figure 2–24) provide hydrophilic domains across the thickness of the membrane. The channels can be selectively opened (top) to permit the influx of ions from the interstitium, or they may remain closed (bottom). The opened–closed status reflects conformational (or shape) changes in the protein brought about by voltage fields (voltage gating) or by chemicals such as neurotransmitters (chemical gating).

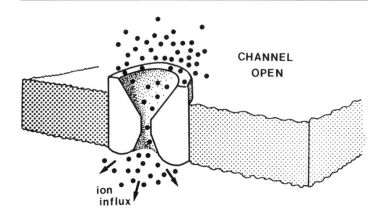

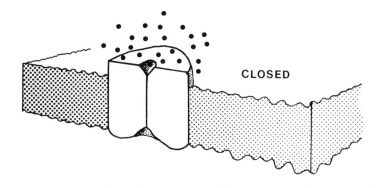

Box 3–2   Generation of Action Potentials

In Figure 3–3 a step voltage stimulus is applied across the membrane of a large axon, between an electrode placed inside the axon and one placed outside. In part a, the current due to *sodium influx* increases very quickly, peaks, then falls off. Potassium current, which is outwardly directed, builds up more slowly but is sustained for many milliseconds. This *efflux* of K^+ is most important for repolarization of the membrane. In part b, the net or overall current flow across the membrane is shown, with directionality. The initial blip is due to discharge of the capacitance, or charge storage, of the membrane and can be ignored here. The rising phase of an action potential is produced by Na^+ influx, which is shown here as a downward current. Finally, the combination of K^+ efflux and Na^+ pumping, by the Na^+-K^+–ATPase pump, gives rise to the sustained current that eventually restores the potential to its resting state. This is called the recovery phase of an action potential.

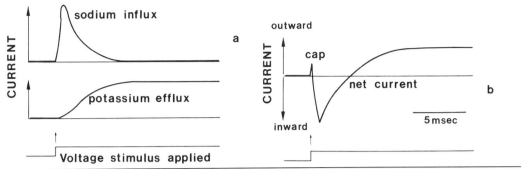

Figure 3–3. *Ion currents resulting from voltage gating.* These two figures illustrate the way in which currents made up of the flow of Na⁺ and K⁺ ions across the membrane relate to each other during depolarization. *a:* The upper trace shows the inward current due to Na⁺ when a voltage stimulus is applied across the membrane. The current increases rapidly, then falls off. The K⁺ efflux current is slower in onset; it builds up slowly as the Na⁺ current is decreasing, but it is sustained. *b:* The two currents are totaled to provide the net current across the membrane. A downward signal is a net inward current flow while the upward signal is a net outward current flow. The small "blip" is due to the discharge of capacitance of the membrane, and can be ignored for the present. The time–scale bar indicates the rapidity of these events.

signaled by the Na⁺ ion itself, so it is termed *sodium inactivation.* Following closure of the channel by this mechanism, another period of sodium conductance cannot occur unless there is at least a brief period of repolarization. This is the basis for action potentials having a finite duration and also for the separation of action potentials. Since the interval between action potentials can be varied down to a finite minimum, information can be coded by *frequency modulation.* This type of coding is analogous to that used for FM radio transmission.

The phase when another applied threshold stimulus fails to elicit an action potential is termed the *refractory period.* In reality there are two forms: The *absolute refractory period* occurs during generation of the action potential and prevails during most of the sodium inactivation phase. No matter how powerful the next applied stimulus is, no new sodium influx can occur during the absolute refractory period. The *relative refractory period* prevails during the final phases of repolarization, or recovery to the resting potential. During the relative refractory period a second stimulus, much larger than that normally required, may be able to elicit another action potential.

What is meant by the term *threshold?* It is the strength of a stimulus causing sufficient change in Na⁺ conductance to the degree that it becomes self-sustaining and self-amplifying within limits set by its all-or-none character. The initial influx sets up the voltage fields that open additional channels to allow still more Na⁺ ions to flow into the cell. This accounts for self-amplification. Sodium inactivation eventually limits the extent of voltage reversal and so accounts for the essentially invariant magnitude of the action potential. Depolarization either occurs or it does not; it is an *all-or-none* phenomenon.

The movement of Na⁺ shifts the transmembrane potential from the resting value toward zero. The transmembrane potential becomes less negative, inside relative to outside. In Figure 3–5a, a very weak stimulus causes a very minor potential change, because some ions have moved into the cell, but the change is self-correcting and fades out. In Figure 3–5b and c, the changes have the same overall characteristics because stimulus strength, although increasing, still fails to reach threshold. Finally, in Figure 3–5d, a threshold stimulus has triggered the self-sustaining action potential by the mechanisms noted above. It does not matter if the stimulus exceeds

Figure 3–4. Depolarization. This figure depicts the distribution of charges in the vicinity of a single sodium channel at a site of depolarization. In the resting state (top), the channel is closed and the membrane is polarized. The inside bears a negative voltage with respect to the outside. When an adequate stimulus (see Figure 3–2) impinges on the channel (right), the channel opens and sodium ions pour into the cell, eventually leading to an accumulation of excess positive charges on the inner face and a deficit of positive charges (or net negativity) focally on the external face. Polarization of charges has been reversed from that of the resting state; the membrane is said to be depolarized. Sufficient accumulation of Na⁺ ions in the vicinity of the inner opening of the channel (left) causes Na⁺-inactivation or closure of the channel. Finally, the distribution of ions is restored to normal by the operation of the Na⁺-K⁺-ATPase.

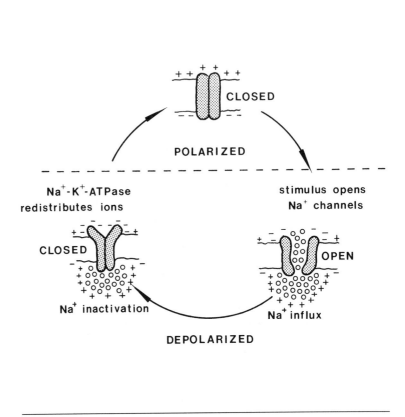

threshold; the depolarization will be of the same magnitude. Hence the all-or-none description applies to the spike phase of the change in potential.

Because there is little or no control over the magnitude of the action potential, there is no provision for coding information by *amplitude modulation.* Amplitude and frequency modulation are depicted in Figure 3–6.

Summary of Selective Ion Transport across Membranes

- In neurons, Na⁺ is the major ion that carries charge inward. Sodium channels are gated chemically or by electric fields.

- With appropriate applied fields, Na⁺ influx begins and can become self-accelerating, then finally self-limiting.

- Ionic movements are of sufficient magnitude to reverse charge polarity across the membrane.

- Recovery to the resting state, or repolarization, requires pumping of Na⁺ to the outside in exchange for K⁺. During this phase, the absolute refractory period and then the relative refractory period ensure that no new depolarization can occur.

- The magnitude of the voltage change occurring beyond threshold is essentially invariant, so coding of information is possible only by varying, up to a maximum limit, the frequency of action potential discharges.

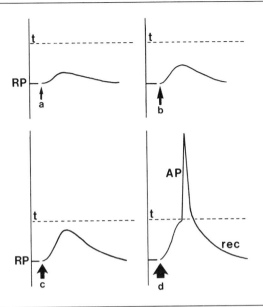

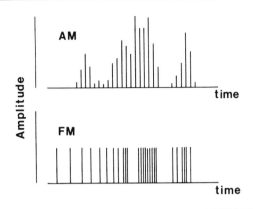

Figure 3–6. Amplitude and frequency modulation. Amplitude modulation (AM), depicted in the upper figure, shows signals of different sizes (actually voltages) occurring at a constant frequency. Information could be coded by varying the amplitude of a given signal. In the lower figure, depicting frequency modulation (FM), the amplitude is quite constant and the only variable is the number of signals per unit time. Frequency modulation is achieved in neural processing by varying the number of action potentials in a unit of time.

Figure 3–5. The threshold stimulus. These figures show potential changes, or voltages, measured across the membrane in four situations. The horizontal broken line (t) represents a particular voltage called threshold. The resting potential (RP) is negative inside relative to outside and is approximately −60 millivolts. A very small applied stimulus (a) causes only a transient change in potential. The change is a little greater in magnitude with a larger stimulus (b), but is still short-lived. The voltage change almost reaches threshold with a larger but still subeffective stimulus (c), but again it declines to the resting state. In these cases, some Na^+ influx has occurred but it has been offset by the action of the Na^+-K^+-ATPase pump, which has restored the ion distribution to the resting state. A large, effective stimulus (d) provokes sufficient Na^+ influx for the potential to reach threshold, whereupon field effects open still more Na^+ channels and the massive influx of ions results in the action potential (AP). The voltages measured here are all the result of currents from ions redistributing across the membrane. After the "upswing" phase of the action potential, reflecting depolarization, a recovery phase (rec) then restores membrane potential to its resting value.

The ability of the membranes of certain cells, notably neurons and muscle cells, to discharge action potentials in the manner described above is the basis for their being called *excitable cells.*

3.2 • Propagation of Nerve Impulses

In order for nerves to transmit coded information around the body, directionality is needed. In part directionality is achieved anatomically, by the network of sensory and motor nerves, and in part it is achieved by the properties of the junctions, or synapses, between neurons. Synapses employ chemical transmitters, produced by the *afferent* (incoming) neuron and recognizable by the *efferent* (outgoing) neuron. The mechanism of synaptic transmission will be described in the next section. For now, simply assume that the neurotransmitter is able to initiate action potentials in the efferent cell. Reverse information transfer through the synapse is not possible, which makes this structure equivalent to a *diode* in an electronic circuit. This property of the synapse provides the basis for unidirectional communication within a specific neural circuit.

Also needed is a basis for movement of the focal area of depolarization along the axon of the neuron. Details of this mechanism are given here, and C. F. Stevens's article "The Neuron" in *Scientific American* (241(3):55–65;1979) provides a most lucid account of propagation.

The distribution of charges (+ and −) on each side of the membrane around a focus of depolarization is shown in Figure 3–7. Assume that initial directionality was provided by synaptic initiation of the action potential. A complex series of local charge fields surrounds the site of depolarization, but when simplified as shown, current flows into the neuron at the active region, down the *axoplasm* in the cell interior in both directions, from positive to negative, back out through the membrane, then along the extracellular solution of electrolytes bathing the axon (again from positive to negative). Note the charge reversal at the active region, with + on the inside, and also that charge density on the membrane is weakened immediately ahead of the active region when compared to more distant portions of the membrane.

At any cross-sectional point, net longitudinal current is zero because the current inside flows in an opposite direction to the current outside. However, the density of longitudinal current is not the same, because the cross-sectional area of the axon is quite limited, whereas outside currents can be dispersed through the large extracellular space. The strictly limited cross-sectional area of the axon is important in concentrating longitudinal current flow in the axoplasm. It is part of the reason why transmembrane current is also concentrated right at the depolarized site.

The density of current flow through the membrane is greatest in the depolarized region and weakens with distance along the axon in either direction. The dense current flow exerts *field effects* that in turn open new sodium channels immediately ahead of the depolarized region. This allows influx of Na^+ and so causes the region of depolarization to advance. Directionality of propagation is possible because Na^+ influx on the tailing side of the depolarized area cannot occur, even though current density may be just as high at that point. The reason is quite simple. Because the depolarization has already passed over this portion of the axon, it is in a time domain corresponding to the refractory period. Indeed, the absolute refractory period prevails immediately behind the new depolarization site where the field effect is greatest. Further back, the recovery events may be more complete and the relative refractory period will prevail. Much further back, the membrane is fully recovered and is ready for another depolarization.

These events of current flow provoking Na^+ influx and then complete depolarization are rapid but nevertheless require finite amounts of time. They permit only slow propagation of nerve impulses. For rapid neural transmission, another structural device called *myelination* has evolved to "insulate" the membrane for all of its length along the axon (see Figure 1–19), except at the *nodes of Ranvier* (Figure 3–8).

The naked membrane, or axolemma, is ex-

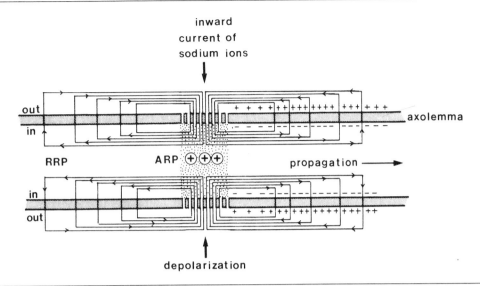

inward
current of
sodium ions

depolarization

Figure 3–7. Propagation of action potentials. This schematic shows the charge distribution on either side of the membrane (axolemma) around a locus of depolarization. The depolarized region is propagating to the right. The pattern of current flow (+ to −) is shown behind (to the left) and ahead (to the right) of the depolarized region. The density of current flow is greatest in close vicinity to the depolarized region. At this location, the inside of the neuron is positive relative to the outside because of the influx of Na⁺ ions. On the leading side, the high current density causes voltage gating of new Na⁺ channels; as a result, the depolarization locus moves to the right. On the tailing side, comparable fields are ineffective in opening Na⁺ channels because the membrane is in absolute refractory period (ARP). Farther back, the redistribution of ions will place the membrane in relative refractory period (RRP), or the membrane may return to its resting state.

Figure 3–8. Myelin sheath and Nodes of Ranvier. Cellular processes of the Schwann cell, which spirally-envelop the axon, make up the myelin sheath. The sheath is interrupted at nodes where the axolemma is exposed to the interstitium. Current flow across the membrane can only take place at the nodes, so action potentials are propagated very rapidly by skipping (saltatory conduction) from node to node. (Reproduced by permission of the publisher. From Leeson, C.R., Leeson, T.S., and Paparo, A.A.: *Textbook of Histology,* 5th edition, Philadelphia: W.B. Saunders Company, 1985.)

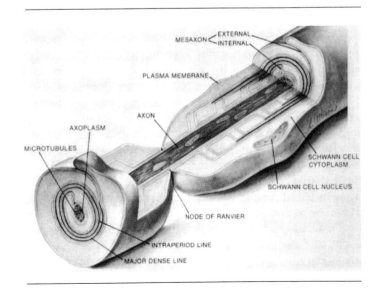

posed to the interstitial fluid only at these gaps in the myelin sheath, so they are the only places where transmembrane current flow can occur. The depolarized region then jumps from node to node, a process called *saltatory* conduction. All of the membrane events described above take place exclusively at these nodes. The delays that are inherent in each phase of action potential generation are minimized, thereby providing for very rapid propagation rates. Major myelinated nerves are capable of conducting action potentials at velocities as high as 120 meters per second (m/sec). In contrast, nonmyelinated neurons propagate only at about 2 m/sec.

3.3 • The Synapse

Nerves communicate with each other via cell-cell structures known as *synapses*. There may be thousands of such structures on the dendritic tree of a given neuron. In such a situation, the potential exists for thousands of input neurons to have the opportunity to influence the activity of a single output neuron. The former are called afferent neurons and the latter are called efferent neurons. At the terminal part of an axon, neurons are nonmyelinated and the axon is enlarged into what is called a *synaptic bouton* (Figure 3–9). The axolemma is therefore naked at this location and it is intimately associated with an exposed part of the dendrite of the efferent cell.

The membrane in the bouton region is slightly different from the remainder of the axolemma in that calcium ions (Ca^{2+}) rather than Na^+ serve as the inward *current carrier* for depolarization. These ions enter the cell through voltage-gated channels and flow down about a thousandfold concentration gradient from outside to inside. Within the bouton vast stores of neurotransmitter compounds are stored, packaged in membrane-bounded secretory granules. When an action potential passes along the axon and reaches the bouton region, there is influx of Ca^{2+}, and the intracellular concentration of this ion is rapidly increased. When intracellular concentrations of Ca^{2+} ($[Ca^{2+}]_i$) are sufficiently increased, the neurosecretory granules move to the surface and their membranes fuse with the axolemma, causing the neurotransmitter to be ejected (Figure 3–10).

The most common compound, and the one that will be considered here, is *acetylcholine*, a simple ester of *acetic acid* and *choline*, a nitrogenous base (Figure 3–11). The acetylcholine diffuses quickly across the narrow synaptic cleft, separating the efferent from the afferent cells. The distance traveled is less than a micron so only minimal time is required. A figure of 0.1 msec is considered typical for synaptic delay. Acetylcholine is taken up by *receptor* proteins concentrated in the membrane of the efferent cell in the vicinity of the synapse. This is referred to as the *postsynaptic membrane*.

The acetylcholine receptors, when occupied by acetylcholine, are capable of opening Na^+ channels and so they enable Na^+ influx to take place at the postsynaptic location. Enzymes capable of inactivating acetylcholine by splitting the ester bond between the acetic acid and the choline base (Figure 3–12) are located in close proximity to the receptor. The enzyme provides a means of promptly terminating the action of the transmitter soon after it has initiated the in-

Figure 3–9. *The synapse.* Synapses are communication and integration sites made up of a bouton (b)—the terminal non-myelinated portion of a naked afferent neuron (a) emerging from a myelinated axon (m)—and a closely adjacent receptor region, called the post-synaptic membrane (psm), on an efferent neuron (e). The bouton and receptor area are separated by the synaptic cleft (c), an extracellular space about 0.2 microns in width. Incoming action potentials are generated by Na^+ influx in the axon (triangles represent Na^+ channels); Ca^{2+} becomes the inward current carrier in the bouton (dots represent Ca^{2+} channels). Upon activation by Ca^{2+}, transmitter molecules, previously stored in the bouton in neurosecretory vesicles (n), are released from the pre-synaptic membrane into the cleft. They diffuse across, then bind to and activate receptors coupled to Na^+ channels (ch) in the post-synaptic membrane. With sufficient neurotransmitter traffic, excitatory or inhibitory post-synaptic potentials develop in the efferent neuron that may provoke or inhibit the development of action potentials.

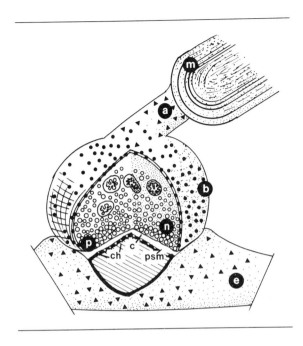

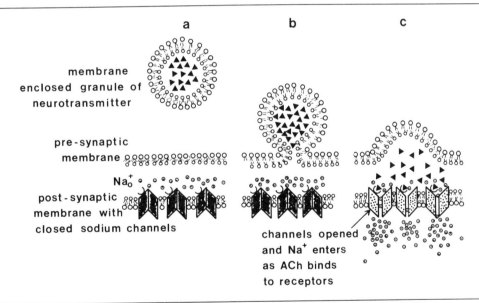

a

membrane enclosed granule of neurotransmitter

pre-synaptic membrane

Na_o^+

post-synaptic membrane with closed sodium channels

b

channels opened and Na^+ enters as ACh binds to receptors

c

Figure 3–10. *Neurotransmitters.* *a:* Neurotransmitters, such as acetylcholine, are packaged in secretory vesicles in close proximity to the pre-synaptic membrane. *b:* When action potentials reach the synaptic bouton, influx of extracellular Ca^{2+} ions triggers neurosecretion and the vesicles fuse to the pre-synaptic membrane. Until the vesicles release their contents into the cleft through exocytosis, the post-synaptic membrane is shown with unoccupied cholinergic receptors and closed sodium channels. *c:* The neurotransmitter is shown binding to receptors on the post-synaptic membrane. In many cases, the receptor serves as a chemically gated Na^+ channel so, upon occupancy by the neurotransmitter, Na^+ influx occurs, giving rise to an excitatory post-synaptic potential.

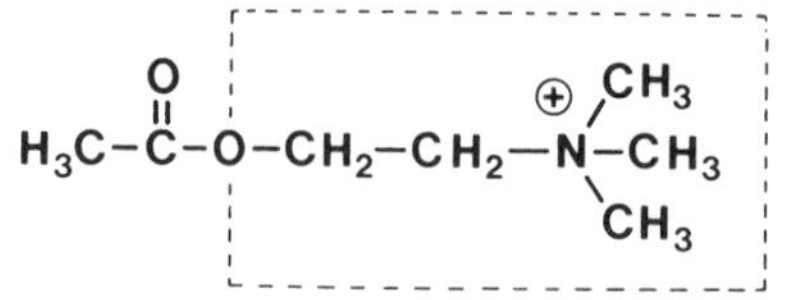

Figure 3–11. Acetylcholine. The most important neurotransmitter molecule is acetylcholine, a simple ester formed from acetic acid and choline (dotted box).

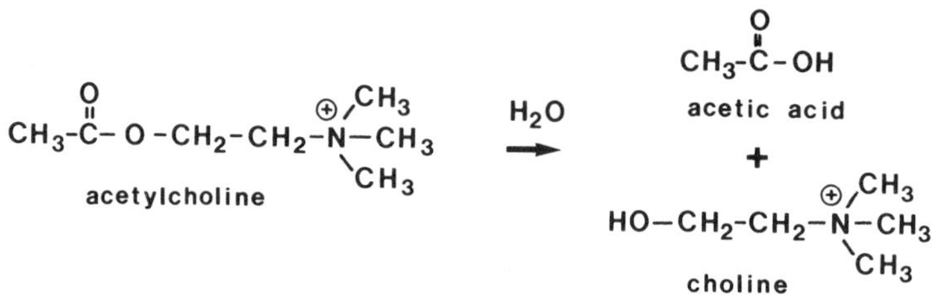

$$H_3C-\overset{\overset{\displaystyle O}{\|}}{C}-O-CH_2-CH_2-\overset{\oplus}{N}\overset{\nearrow CH_3}{\underset{\searrow CH_3}{-CH_3}}$$

Figure 3–12. Acetylcholinesterase. The enzyme acetylcholinesterase serves to hydrolyze the ester bond in acetylcholine to produce acetic acid and choline. Hydrolysis of the ester inactivates the neurotransmitter. The choline will be recycled back into the presynaptic bouton region to be resynthesized into new acetylcholine. Numerous drugs, capable of inhibiting the esterase or the re-uptake mechanism, make potent insecticides (see Table 3–2).

$$CH_3-\overset{\overset{\displaystyle O}{\|}}{C}-O-CH_2-CH_2-\overset{\oplus}{N}\overset{\nearrow CH_3}{\underset{\searrow CH_3}{-CH_3}}$$

acetylcholine

$$\xrightarrow{H_2O}$$

$$CH_3-\overset{\overset{\displaystyle O}{\|}}{C}-OH$$

acetic acid

+

$$HO-CH_2-CH_2-\overset{\oplus}{N}\overset{\nearrow CH_3}{\underset{\searrow CH_3}{-CH_3}}$$

choline

flux of Na^+. A single bolus of acetylcholine with its resultant effect in promoting Na^+ influx into the efferent cell is far too small to initiate an action potential in that cell. Only a large number—hundreds or thousands—of afferent neurons releasing acetylcholine at the synapses onto a given efferent neuron causes Na^+ influx of sufficient magnitude to trigger an action potential. The mechanism is outlined in Box 3–3.

Another mechanism enabling activation of the efferent neuron could consist of a series of action potentials, closely spaced one after another, reaching the presynaptic regions to cause a virtually continuous release of acetylcholine at relatively few synapses, sufficient to stimulate the efferent neuron to threshold. Much of the action potential traffic along neurons takes this form; it is called a *train* of action potentials (Figure 3–13).

It should be clear from this description that a single action potential reaching the presynaptic region from the axon of an afferent cell will be quite incapable, by itself, of initiating an ac-

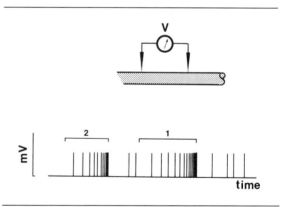

Figure 3–13. Trains of action potentials. Information is readily coded in neural and neuromuscular systems by groups of action potentials varying in number, frequency, and overall duration. Groups of action potentials encoding specific information, or some specific control signal, are called trains. The figure depicts a simple recording system for detecting voltage fluctuations on a nerve. The tracing shows two trains of action potentials with a few single "spike" signals. The trains shown here begin with a high frequency of action potentials, then the frequency decreases.

Box 3–3   Postsynaptic Potentials

The potential that results from the influx of Na$^+$ is called an *excitatory postsynaptic potential*. The excitatory postsynaptic potential is a *graded* potential, not an all-or-none phenomenon, that is proportional to the number of incoming action potentials. When it is of sufficient magnitude, the membrane potential reaches threshold and an action potential is fired.

Box 3–4   Inhibitory Postsynaptic Potentials

In addition to the excitatory synapses that use acetylcholine, there are other synapses that have an inhibitory effect on the potential of the efferent cell. An important inhibitory neurotransmitter is the compound, *γ-aminobutyric acid* (GABA) (Figure 3–14). GABA is released from synaptic boutons of inhibitory afferents and causes hyperpolarization of the efferent neuron. This means that the membrane potential is shifted further away from threshold. GABA gives rise to *inhibitory postsynaptic potentials*.

The mechanism involves selective control of chloride ion flux across the membrane. The net balance between excitatory and inhibitory transmitters—acetylcholine and GABA, for example—determines the relative dominance of excitatory versus inhibitory postsynaptic potentials and hence the resulting potential within the efferent neuron. Because excitatory and inhibitory postsynaptic potentials counteract each other, there is provision for yet another opportunity for integration via synapses.

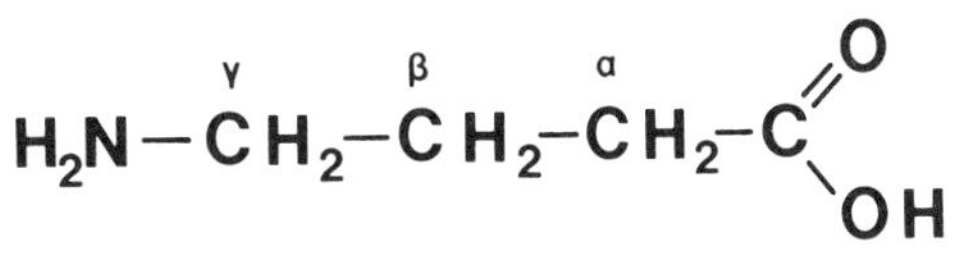

Figure 3–14. Gamma aminobutyric acid (GABA). GABA, the 4(or gamma)-amino derivative of butyric acid, is a common inhibitory neurotransmitter.

tion potential in the efferent cell. Because many afferent action potentials are needed for a single efferent action potential to be fired, there is a basis for *information processing*, or *integration*, at the synapse.

The term integration is used when the relationship of input to output is other than 1:1.

The synapse is ideally suited for an integrative role within the nervous system. This is particularly flexible because synapses can exert either excitatory or inhibitory influences on the efferent neuron. The basis for inhibitory synaptic transmission is described in Box 3–4.

3.4 • Skeletal Muscle Structure and Function

Muscle cells, or *myocytes,* are specialized contractile cells capable of performing mechanical work in response to excitatory events at their surface membrane. The prefix *sarco-* is used to specify muscle, so the excitable membrane can be termed the *sarcolemma.* All muscle types—skeletal, cardiac, and smooth—depend on excitatory events at the membrane to trigger the biochemical processes that bring about the mechanical response.

The linkage between action potential discharge and contraction of the myocyte is referred to as *excitation-contraction coupling.* The steps involved will be examined in some detail in this section.

It is convenient to begin with skeletal muscle, the most abundant type in the body. Adult-type myocytes are unusual in being *multinucleated.* This condition arises from the fusion of individual cells, or the donation of nuclei from specialized *satellite cells,* during muscle growth. The mature cells can be extremely large, both in length and diameter. These dimensions are important for excitation-contraction coupling. It is generally true that skeletal muscles are seldom fully relaxed, and because muscles are often arranged in *antagonistic pairs,* a balance usually exists between low-level activity in each of the members of the pair. This low-grade contractile activity is called *tone,* or *tonus.*

A typical muscle is shown dissected to progressively finer levels of detail in Figure 3–15. In skeletal muscle, the bulk of the myocyte is occupied by highly organized *myofibrils,* or longitudinal assemblies of *contractile filaments.* At the more gross myofibrilar level, characteristic striations or banding are evident and are due to the arrangement of the filaments. The interdigitation of thick filaments, made up of *myosin,* with thin filaments, which are mainly *actin,* is strictly controlled, with the thin filaments being anchored at the *Z-line.*

As shown in Figure 3–15, the *sarcomere* is the length of myofibril between two adjacent Z-lines. There is variation in the length of the sarcomere, depending on the state of relaxation (resting length) or contraction (shortened length). In certain situations, such as when the muscle is stretched, the sarcomere may be longer. However, there is both a minimum length, beyond which further shortening cannot occur, and a maximum length in stretched muscle, beyond which the sarcomere is torn or disrupted and the cell is damaged.

Contraction results from a fascinating series of interactions between the contractile filaments, the unraveling of which was a major biologic discovery that brought into play biochemistry, biophysics, electron microscopy, and crystallography.

As shown in Figure 3–16, each thin filament is surrounded by three thick filaments, while each thick filament is in turn surrounded by six thin filaments. The filaments have a distinct surface configuration, depicted in Figure 3–17 and more elaborately in Figure 3–18, that enables the actin and myosin molecules to interact with each other in a ratchet-like fashion.

For completeness of the description, a more detailed treatment of the proteins of the filaments and the contractile mechanism is provided in Box 3–5.

Excitation-Contraction Coupling in Skeletal Muscle

In skeletal muscle as in neurons, the major inward current carrier causing depolarization of the sarcolemma is Na^+. It is again emphasized that skeletal myocytes are very large cells, so the center of the cell is far removed from the surface membrane. A specialization exists in skeletal

Figure 3–15. Structural organization of muscle. The progressively finer breakdown of the structure of a muscle covers the full spectrum—from the intact organ down to the molecular level. In this figure, myocytes are identified as muscle fibers. Note that the sarcomere is the length of myofibril between two Z-lines. Different forms of thick and thin filaments are shown. The thin filament is made up of two helical strands of actin polymers with overlying strands of tropomyosin (dark), while the thick filament consists of arrays of myosin with protruding "heads" of heavy meromyosin. (Reproduced by permission of the publisher. From Hainsworth, F.R.: *Animal Physiology: Adaptations in Function,* Reading, MA: Addison-Wesley Publishing Company, 1981.)

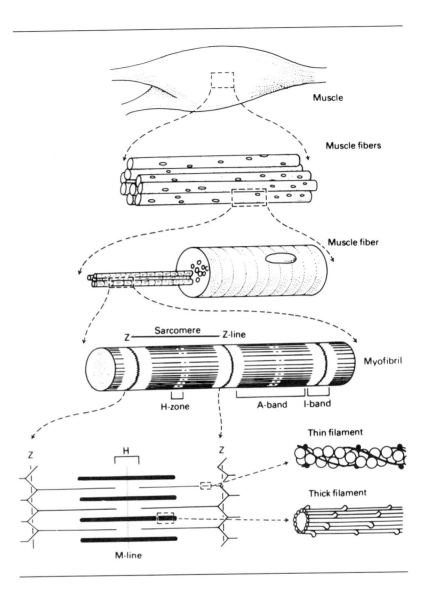

muscle by which the sarcolemma forms a series of extensive invaginations that extend the surface membrane deep into the interior of the cell, in among the myofibrils. These *transverse tubules* correspond roughly to the Z-lines on the fibrils. Action potentials evoked at the periphery sweep across the sarcolemma and down the transverse tubules.

In between the transverse tubules and in close proximity to the myofibrils (Figure 3–20) is an extensive intracellular membrane system called the *sarcoplasmic reticulum.* This structure is a highly specialized Ca^{2+} storage organelle and it responds to action potentials in the nearby transverse tubules by releasing a flood of Ca^{2+} ions into the cytoplasm. The cytoplasmic concentration of Ca^{2+} rapidly increases from about $10^{-7}M$ to about $10^{-5}M$, thereby reaching the critical concentration needed to trigger the biomechanical events that cause the ratchet mechanism to operate and shorten the cell. Almost immediately after releasing Ca^{2+}, the sarco-

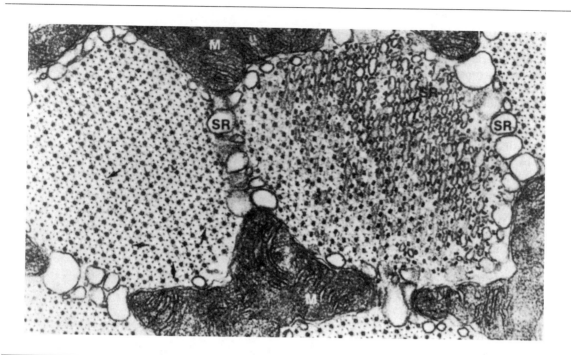

Figure 3–16. The sarcomere. An electron micrograph of a transverse section of skeletal muscle clearly shows the relationship between the thick and thin filaments in two my-ofibrils. Each thick filament may be surrounded by six thin filaments; each thin filament is surrounded by three thick filaments. The arrows indicate apparent connections between the thick and thin filaments and are likely to be the heavy meromyosin "heads" that are depicted in Figure 3–17. The fibril at right is sectioned in the H-zone (see Figure 3–15) and hence is relatively devoid of thin filaments. Sarcoplasmic reticulum (SR) and mitochondria (M) are evident. ($\times$ 83,000. Reproduced by permission of the publisher. From Kessel, R.G. and Kardon, R.H.: *Tissues and Organs: A Text-Atlas of Scanning Electron Microscopy,* San Francisco; W.H. Freeman and Company, 1979.)

plasmic reticulum proceeds to sequester it again, using energy from ATP hydrolysis to pump the Ca^{2+} against a considerable concentration gradient.

The foregoing is a description of the events resulting from a single depolarization in which the mechanical response is very short-lived, lasting less than 1 sec, and is known as a single *twitch.* When a sustained contraction is required, it is achieved by repeated depolarizations. As in the case of neurons, action potentials in muscles are also followed by refractory periods during which the membrane potential recovers to its resting state. Repeated depolarizations may occur with a frequency up to the limit set by the refractory period. The refractory period is brief relative to the time required to pump Ca^{2+} back down to resting concentrations, so it is possible to have an almost continuous release of Ca^{2+}, and sustained elevated concentrations can be maintained in the cytoplasm of myocytes.

Figure 3–17. Organization of the filaments. The thick filament is made up of myosin molecules packed as shown with the light meromyosin (LMM) forming parallel arays and the heavy meromyosin (HMM) "heads" extending out from the surface. The lower portions show the assembly of G-actin units into the helical polymer (called F-actin). Along with the tropomyosin and troponins, they comprise the thin filaments. (Reproduced by permission of the publisher. From Hainsworth, F.R.: *Animal Physiology: Adaptations in Function,* Reading, MA: Addison-Wesley Publishing Company, 1981.)

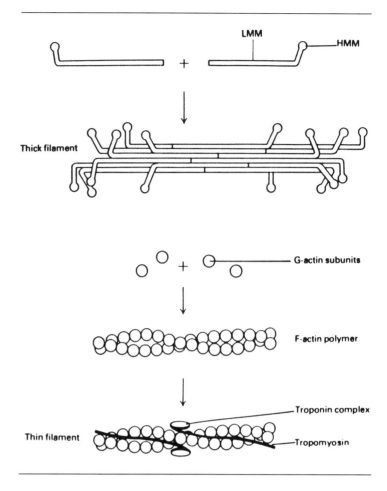

Figure 3–18. Exposure of cross-bridge binding sites. The upper figure depicts a thin filament in resting muscle where concentration of Ca^{2+} in the sarcoplasm is very low ($<10^{-6}M$), and Ca^{2+} binding sites on troponin are unoccupied. The cross-bridge binding sites on the actin (small black dots) are obscured by tropomyosin. In the activated muscle (lower), sarcoplasmic concentrations of Ca^{2+} have increased about 100-fold, the ion has bound to troponin, and the Ca^{2+}-troponin complex has rolled the tropomyosin away to expose the cross-bridge binding sites. Actin can now bind with the heavy meromyosin "heads" of adjacent thick filaments to form an actomyosin complex (see part *b* in Figure 3–19). (Adapted by permission of the publisher. From Vander, A.J., Sherman, J.H., and Luciano, D.S.: *Human Physiology: The Mechanisms of Body Function,* 3rd edition, New York: McGraw-Hill Book Company, 1980.)

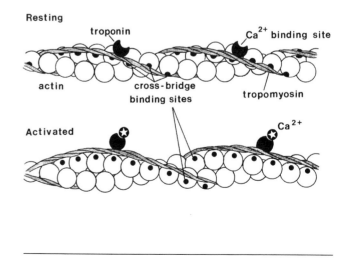

Box 3–5   Myofilaments and Contraction

The thick filament is made up of myosin molecules that comprise two portions, or *meromyosins* (Figure 3–17). *Light meromyosin* is a rodlike portion, several of which constitute the body of the filament. Each light meromyosin is associated with a more specialized head region called *heavy meromyosin*. The head region contains enzymatic capability for hydrolyzing ATP to furnish energy. The head can be considered to be mobile and capable of swiveling, perhaps through 35° to 60° with respect to the light meromyosin. The head also has the ability to form complexes with specific regions on the thin filaments. This complex is called *actomyosin* and results from the formation of *cross-bridges* between heavy meromyosin and actin (Figures 3–18 and 3–19).

Actin exists in various forms, but interest can be focused on the filamentous, polymeric form made up from two chains of actin monomers (G-actin) wound together as a helix. In addition, long filaments of *tropomyosin* are wrapped around the actin polymers and serve to mask cross-bridge binding sites in the muscle at rest (see Figure 3–18). During activation, the tropomyosin is rolled away so that the cross-bridge sites become exposed, enabling the actomyosin complex to form.

The movement of the tropomyosin is controlled by regulatory proteins called *troponins*, one of which, troponin C, is a spe-cific binder of calcium ions (Ca^{2+}). In the presence of a critical concentration of Ca^{2+}, the troponins are activated, tropomyosin is moved, the cross-bridge sites are exposed, and the filaments can interact with each other. This is shown in stylized fashion in Figure 3–19. The central regulatory role is played by Ca^{2+} ions. In Figure 3–19, the heavy meromyosin is shown in its resting state charged with a bound molecule of ATP (no enzyme hydrolysis at this stage) and the heavy meromyosin is blocked from forming a cross-bridge by tropomyosin. With a suitable increase in Ca^{2+} concentration, not only are the cross-bridge sites on actin exposed, but the Ca^{2+} destabilizes the heavy meromyosin. This enables cross-bridges to form; at the same time, the enzymic function of the ATPase is activated:

$$ATP \rightarrow ADP + P_i + energy$$

As ATP is hydrolyzed to adenosine diphosphate (ADP) and inorganic phosphate (P_i), energy is released, which provides the power stroke as the heavy meromyosin swivels and the thin filament is moved relative to the thick filament. Another Ca^{2+} action now takes place as ADP is released. This enables another ATP molecule to be bound, so that the *ratchet movements* can continue.

Activation of Skeletal Muscle

Skeletal muscle is activated physiologically by specific and precise *motor* neural signals. The various forms of *neuromuscular* interactions will be outlined later in this chapter, and the present treatment is very simple. Skeletal muscle can be actively excited, but not inhibited, at the level of the muscle cell itself. The cells are therefore passively relaxed (noncontracted) or are actively

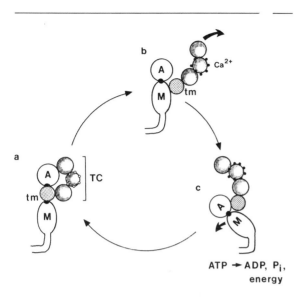

Figure 3–19. *The ratchet mechanism.* The troponin complex (TC), consisting of a series of molecules, is shown in relation to actin (A), the heavy meromyosin "head" of myosin (M), and tropomyosin (tm). In resting muscle *(a)*, tropomyosin interposes between the actin and myosin, thereby preventing cross-bridge formation. When the muscle is activated *(b)*, Ca^{2+} and troponin C interact (small dots), and the troponin complex displaces the tropomyosin, so actin and heavy meromyosin form an actomyosin complex. This also activates the ATPase to release energy from ATP, as shown in *c*. The head swivels and causes the actin filament to be moved. The cross-bridges then break and the head returns to its original orientation on the thick filament. So long as both Ca^{2+} and ATP are present, the swiveling is repeated in a ratchet-like fashion. If the muscle is no longer activated (sarcoplasmic Ca^{2+} concentrations returned to resting levels), tropomyosin rolls back to prevent cross-bridge formation *(a)*.

excited. Skeletal muscles are innervated with motor nerves and a single myocyte has but one axon supplying it. The contact area of the nerve terminal with the sarcolemma is usually located in the central region of the cell surface and it is called a *motor end-plate*.

Action potentials that reach the axon terminus provoke release of acetylcholine as the neuromuscular transmitter; the acetylcholine diffuses across a very narrow extracellular space to cholinergic receptors in the motor end-plate (Figure 3–21). Chemically gated sodium influx follows, causing focal depolarization which then propagates in all directions over the sarcolemma and into the transverse tubules. The acetylcholine is normally subjected to rapid deactivation by acetylcholinesterase, a constituent protein in the motor end-plate. The depolarization at the motor end-plate is therefore short-lived. The motor end-plate is specialized to provide a 1:1 coupling of action potentials in the motor nerve with action potentials in the myocyte. This high-fidelity coupling is quite different from what was described in the previous section for synaptic coupling.

As the action potential sweeps away across the sarcolemma, a process of depolarization similar to that described for the axon occurs and the myocyte is readied for yet another depolarization, once the membrane comes out of the refractory period.

From the foregoing, it should be obvious that without the delivery of nerve impulses, there is no source of excitation. Without muscle action potentials, the sarcoplasmic reticulum firmly binds up Ca^{2+} and the troponin system is unable to maneuver the tropomyosin, so no cross-bridges can form. Of course, in the absence of ATP, the sarcoplasmic reticulum is unable to maintain very low cytoplasmic concentrations of Ca^{2+} because the Ca^{2+}-ATPase pump stops working. Cross-bridges can and do form and give rise to a partial contraction whenever Ca^{2+} concentrations in the sarcoplasm rise above the resting level. In the case of postmortem *rigor*, brought about by the mechanism just described, this contraction will persist for hours or days. Rigor eventually ends when *autolysis* begins to break down the muscle cell filaments.

Muscle Energetics and Fuels

The ultimate *energy carrier* in all muscles is ATP, with its labile high-energy bond at the terminal

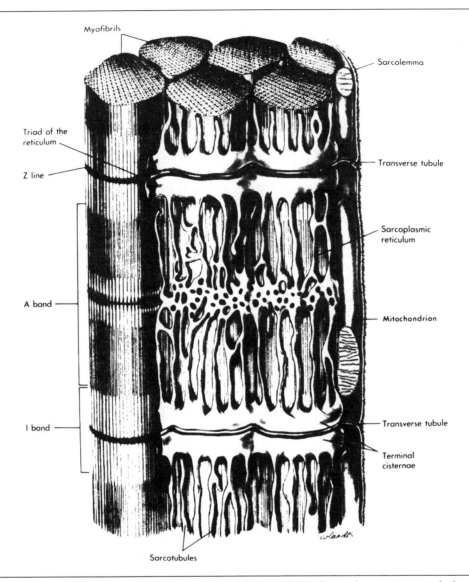

Figure 3–20. *The membranes of skeletal muscle.* This construct shows the transverse tubules extending from the surface as processes of the sarcolemma, deep in among the contractile myofibrils. In close proximity, an extensive sarcoplasmic reticulum serves as the principal intracellular depot for Ca^{2+} ions. When action potentials pass down the transverse tubules, the sarcoplasmic reticulum releases Ca^{2+} into the sarcoplasm as a key component of excitation-contraction coupling. A Ca^{2+}-pump is then activated to cause re-uptake of the Ca^{2+} ions by the sarcoplasmic reticulum. The decrease in Ca^{2+} concentration in the sarcoplasm then brings about relaxation. (Reproduced by permission of the publisher. From Bloom, W. and Fawcett, D.W.: *A Textbook of Histology,* 9th edition, Philadelphia: W.B. Saunders Company, 1968.)

Figure 3–21. The motor end-plate. The motor neuron terminal is closely associated with a discrete receptive region of the sarcolemma called the motor end-plate (MEP). In the terminal, non-myelinated portion of the motor neuron, Na^+ serves as the inward current carrier, but this function is assumed by Ca^{2+} ions in the bulbous structure packed with vesicles of neuromuscular transmitter. Influx of Ca^{2+} upon arrival of an action potential causes acetylcholine to be released from the neuron into the neuromuscular junction. It diffuses to the MEP, binds to cholinergic receptors that are coupled to Na^+ channels, and causes depolarization. The action potential then propagates away from the MEP in all directions across the sarcolemma and down the t–tubules. Note that Na^+ again serves as the inward current-carrying ion. Acetylcholine is promptly inactivated by acetylcholine esterase, as noted before in Figure 3–12.

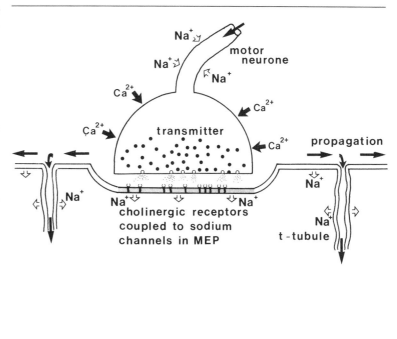

phosphate group. The quantity of ATP available at any one time is very limited and could sustain a mere few twitches. Muscles store additional energy in creatine phosphate (Figure 3–22), a form that can be easily used to replenish the supply of ATP. Creatine phosphate is formed from ATP during times of ATP excess by the reversible reaction:

$$ATP + creatine \rightleftharpoons creatine\ phosphate + ADP$$

It is believed that the enzyme involved in this phosphoryl transfer, creatine kinase, may be specifically located within the region of the heavy meromyosin, as well as on the outer mitochondrial membrane, where it may assist in transferring energy out to the cytoplasm.

Despite the reserve of creatine phosphate, the total amount of high-energy phosphate is probably still only sufficient for a few seconds of contractile activity. Skeletal muscle, and particularly red skeletal muscle, quickly replenishes the energy stores by aerobic or oxygen-depen-

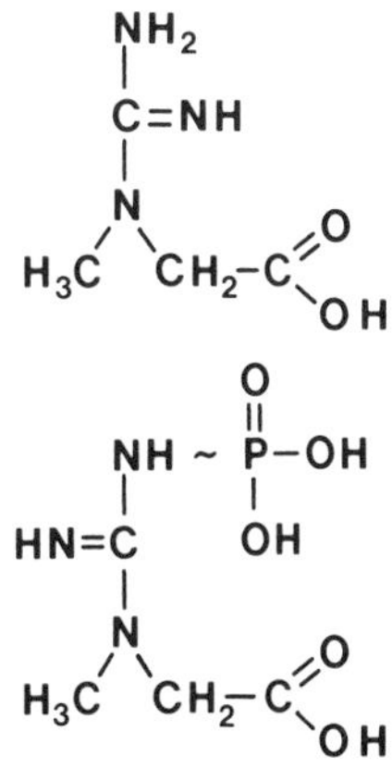

Figure 3–22. Creatine and creatine phosphate. Creatine phosphate serves as a reserve of labile high energy to buffer the amount of ATP in certain cells, notably muscle. The high energy is contained within the bond to the phosphate (see the ∼ bond in the lower figure) and is readily transferred to and from ATP by the action of creatine kinase. The non-phosphorylated form, creatine, is shown above.

dent catabolism of stored fuels. The major reserve is glycogen, a storage polymer of glucose, and it is rapidly broken down to monomers, and then to acetyl coenzyme A (CoA) for further degradation to CO_2, H_2O, and the transfer of energy into newly synthesized ATP. The steps involved in liberating the energy from the fuel molecules will be described in detail in Chapter 7. It is now apparent that the enzymes promoting glycogen breakdown can be activated by Ca^{2+}, at the concentrations that prevail during excitation-contraction coupling.

The mechanism described above requires oxygen if it is to proceed to completion. Red skeletal muscle in particular has high concentrations of *myoglobin*, which is an intracellular oxygen carrier somewhat like the hemoglobin in red blood cells. Myoglobin buffers the muscle cell against oxygen deficiency, or *hypoxia*, which could otherwise occur very quickly whenever oxygen consumption outstripped oxygen delivery from the blood. There is a compensatory increase in blood flow to active tissues, such as contracting muscle, but sustained muscular activity still usually results in hypoxia. Under such conditions, another adaptation becomes operative by which the carbohydrate fuels are only partly degraded, so the need for oxygen is minimized. Lactic acid is produced by this *anaerobic* process. It may accumulate in the muscle, giving the sensation of muscular pain, but most of it diffuses into the blood and is carried away. A mechanism called the *Cori cycle* recycles the lactate back to the muscle as glucose (see Chapter 7).

Anaerobic glycolysis as described yields a mere fraction (1/18) of the ATP available from glucose if it were completely oxidized by aerobic mechanisms. If ATP is consumed at a faster rate than it can be generated, a state of *fatigue* prevails.

The Work Performance of Muscle

When a muscle contracts and is allowed to shorten, the contraction is described as *isotonic*, implying that the tension on the muscle is relatively constant. Alternatively, if the muscle is prevented from shortening, a contraction results in an increase in *tension* development. Contractions of the latter type are called *isometric* to indicate that length does not change. Muscle contractions in the body are neither purely isotonic nor purely isometric, because although most muscles do actually shorten, they do so against the elastic resistance of antagonistic muscles or of connective tissues such as tendons and ligaments.

The nature of simple contractions can be best examined using an isolated frog muscle, the gastrocnemius, with its insertion via the Achilles tendon. This isolated preparation has minimal requirements to perform reliably. The muscle can be mounted isometrically, or at a fixed length, on a transducer that converts tension into a signal that can be written onto rapidly moving chart

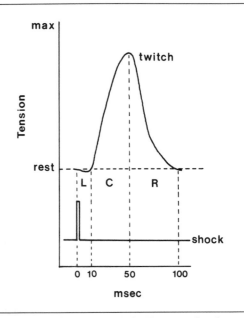

Figure 3–23. The simple twitch. Tension development in the muscle is plotted against time after the delivery of a discrete electric shock as the stimulus. Note that a latency period of about 10 milliseconds (msecs) precedes the development of tension. Tension builds to a maximum during a period of about 40 msecs, then declines over about 50 msecs as the muscle relaxes.

paper. With appropriate electrical stimulation delivered into the body of the muscle, a single applied shock evokes a single isometric twitch. The response can be considered in three main phases (Figure 3–23): first, a *latent period* of about 10 msec after the shock is applied; second, a *contraction period* of some 40 msec; and third, a *relaxation period* of about 50 msec. If a stimulus of inadequate intensity is delivered, there is no response, and such stimuli are called subthreshold. As stimulus strength is increased, a minimal response is eventually obtained and the stimulus is now at threshold. Further increases in stimulus strength produce progressively larger responses, or graded responses, as more and more myocytes with slightly differing thresholds are activated. This phenomenon is called *spatial summation* of contraction. As the cells are arranged in a parallel fashion within the muscle, the effects of their individual contractions summate to provide the overall tension recorded. Eventually a stimulus strength is reached at which every cell is recruited into the response and maximal tension results. Further increases in stimulus strength cannot result in increased tension. Twitches, being single discrete contractile events, either occur maximally for an individual cell or they do not occur at all. The graded response obtained from whole muscles is due to spatial summation.

Over a reasonable period of time and with periodic moistening of the frog gastrocnemius muscle, twitches can be obtained for as long as stimuli are applied, provided sufficient time elapses between shocks for complete relaxation to occur before the next depolarization-contraction-repolarization-relaxation cycle is begun. Of course, the muscle preparation will eventually fatigue and deteriorate. When stimuli are delivered repeatedly, the result depends on the frequency, or the interval between successive depolarizations. The various responses are described in Box 3–6.

3.5 • Cardiac and Smooth Muscle

Myocardium: Specialized Muscle of the Heart

As briefly introduced in Chapter 1, the myofibrils of *myocardiocytes* are quite well organized and striations are apparent, just as in skeletal muscle. The cells are not exclusively arranged as a mass of parallel units because that is inappropriate for a hollow organ required to function as a pump. The cells are uninucleate and possess obliquely branching processes, the ends of which form intimate contacts with adjacent cells. These contact areas are the *intercalated disks*, and they function in *electrocoupling* of adjacent cells. Action potentials can therefore pass rapidly from cell to cell, enabling the bulk of cells to be excited almost simultaneously.

The cardiac cells are arranged around a matrix of connective tissue elements that fuse in selected locations as fibrous bands. There is no insertion onto any skeletal structure. Support is also obtained from the *pericardium*, a tough membrane that envelops the heart, which additionally serves in providing lubrication of the surface of the myocardium.

Myocardiocytes are spontaneously active, even when totally isolated from the body as dispersed cells. The cells have a wide range of intrinsic beating frequencies but because they are so tightly electrocoupled within the heart, pacing of excitation is dictated by the cells with highest intrinsic frequency. A group of cells called the *sinoatrial node* generally serves to control excitatory events in the rest of the heart (Figure 3–25). This constitutes the heart *pacemaker*. In Chapter 5 it will become evident that the SA node is subject to *inhibitory* motor innervation from the autonomic nervous system, in striking contrast to neural control over skeletal muscle, which is exclusively excitatory.

There is a population of highly specialized myocytes that serves as a *conducting system* within the ventricles of the heart. They are not nerves yet they seem to function solely in the rapid delivery of action potentials throughout the ventricular muscle. This conducting system is made up of the *His bundle,* located in the wall, or septum, separating the two ventricles, and the *Purkinje fibers,* distributed throughout the marginal ventricular walls (Figure 3–25).

Myocardium exhibits a number of properties that are somewhat intermediate to those of skeletal and smooth muscle (see below). Electrophysiologically, the initial event in depolarization seems to be the opening of a Na^+ channel, yet Ca^{2+} channels also contribute, and Ca^{2+} ions seem to carry most of the inward current. Whether this extracellular Ca^{2+} is directly responsible for excitation-contraction coupling or acts to trigger release of much large quantities of intracellular Ca^{2+} is not clear. The most obvious specialization of the myocardiocyte is the very slow (hundreds of milliseconds) recovery of the membrane potential after depolarization. This serves to prolong the refractory period to

---

Box 3–6   Temporal Summation

If a series of submaximal stimuli is delivered, with only a brief interval between the end of relaxation before the next shock, each successive contraction will become slightly greater than the last. This is called the *staircase effect* (Figure 3–24) and may reflect the additive effect of a new activation over a very small residual activation from the previous cycle. This is due to incomplete removal of Ca^{2+} back to the normal resting concentrations before the next release of Ca^{2+} occurs. When the interval between two shocks is reduced further, it is possible to re-excite the cells before relaxation from the previous activation has progressed very far. Thus a new contraction occurs with greater magnitude than that resulting from single shocks applied less frequently. This is called *temporal summation*, or summation related to time. If the frequency of repeated stimulation is too high, the sarcolemma may be in its refractory period when the next shock arrives and, as expected, the latter will be quite ineffective in causing depolarization or contraction. This would occur in the frog gastrocnemius if the shocks are delivered with only about 4 to 5 msec separation.

If a series of shocks is applied at, say, 10 to 15 per second, the contractions partially fuse and tension progressively increases, without much relaxation between the events. At higher frequencies, say 35 to 50 per second, complete *fusion* occurs with no sign of relaxation. This sustained tension development is called *tetanus.* If a prolonged tetanus is provoked, a state of fatigue eventually develops because energy sources become depleted and metabolic toxins accumulate. In fatigue, the tetanus decays despite continued stimulation. In isolated muscle preparations, irreversible damage will occur.

Figure 3-24. *Temporal summation.* The periodic delivery of maximally effective stimuli (dots) elicits isolated twitch responses from a muscle (top row). The magnitudes of these responses are essentially constant. Note that the ordinate for each figure is scaled in "twitch units." When the frequency of delivery of the stimuli is increased slightly, a progressive increase in evoked tension is elicited, but each contraction is still quite discrete, or separate, from the others. This is the "staircase" effect, or *treppe*. In the middle row, repeated stimulation at a higher frequency provokes contractions; each occurs before relaxation from the previous contraction is complete. The contractions therefore are partly fused. The degrees of fusion and magnitude of the contractile response (in "twitch units") are greater when the interval between the stimuli is further reduced (right). In the lower row, the frequency of stimulation is still higher and complete fusion of contraction occurs. This is a tetanus, or a sustained high level contraction, that persists with continued stimulation, until fatigue develops.

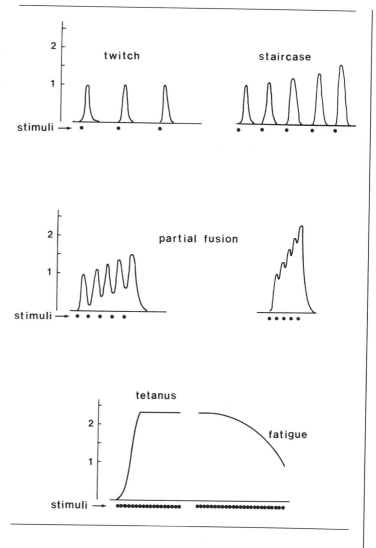

such an extent that temporal summation of contractions cannot occur, nor can a tetanus develop. From this, it follows that relaxation is an obligatory event between contractile episodes. Without complete relaxation, during which filling of the heart chambers occurs, the heart could not serve as a pump.

A discussion of factors influencing the rate and force of cardiac contractions will be deferred until Chapter 5.

Smooth Muscle

Many of the general principles underlying isometric and isotonic contractile function are common to all muscles, including smooth muscle. Very striking differences are also known, and they will be briefly summarized here. Throughout the rest of this text, various aspects of smooth

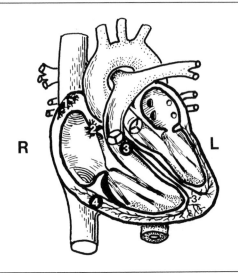

Figure 3–25. The conduction system of the heart. This cutaway view from the ventral side shows the specialized nodes, one of which—the sino-atrial note (1)—serves as the heart pacemaker. The atrio-ventricular node is shown located in the right atrium (2); it supplies the common His bundle (3). The bundle divides into two major branches (3') within the interventricular wall that pass toward the apex of the heart. Each branch then arborizes into Purkinje fibers (4) in the peripheral walls of the ventricles.

muscle function and regulation will be discussed, providing specific applications of the principles presented here.

Smooth muscle cells are fine, *spindle-shaped* units some 5 to 10 μ in diameter and 0.1 to 0.3 mm in length. They are uninucleate, and the nuclear region is the widest portion of the cell. The cells may be organized in bundles, but they exist in a framework of connective fibrils of collagen and elastin; sometimes these may be in the form of a ligament. There are no tendons and no mechanical attachments to the skeleton. Cells may also be found in isolation rather than in bundles or sheets. Smooth muscle cells are present in this isolated fashion in parts of many soft visceral organs such as the spleen.

The major occurrence of smooth muscle is in providing the wall or part of the wall of hollow structures such as blood vessels, the gut, the urinary duct system, and so forth. The muscle is usually organized in two distinct layers: an inner *circular layer* and an outer *longitudinal layer* (see Figure 1–17). The two are separated by a thin layer of connective tissue that may provide a route of access to the tissue for blood vessels and nerves.

At the light microscopic level smooth muscle exhibits no striations, and ultrastructural methods are required to show the presence of myofilaments. The actin and myosin filaments do exist but they are not so highly organized as in skeletal muscle, hence the absence of distinct banding or striations. Other major differences are also apparent at the fine level of organization. There is no transverse tubule system, the sarcoplasmic reticulum is sparse, there are relatively few mitochondria, and the sarcolemma is thrown into a series of very small pits or *caveolae*. There is a complete absence of organized neuromuscular junctions, so motor end-plates do not exist. In some smooth muscle systems, adjacent cells are very tightly joined by structures called *gap junctions*, membrane specializations that provide cell-to-cell continuity of the cytoplasm. The junctions vary in number in different smooth muscles. In some cases they seem to be very dynamic structures because they assemble and become functional under some conditions, yet disassemble and become nonfunctional under other conditions.

Because the myofilaments are less organized in smooth muscle than in striated muscle, there is no distinct sarcomere, or unit of length of the contractile apparatus. There are two main consequences. The mechanical response to a single depolarization is much less impressive than in skeletal muscle. Smooth muscle, however, can contract over a much wider range of lengths, as may be caused by *stretch*. These are important characteristics and need further analysis. Smooth muscle contractions differ from twitches in being slower in onset and longer in duration. The usual form of excitation at the membrane comes from trains of action potentials and the result is more like a tetanus than a twitch.

A slower, more sustained contraction is often

most appropriate for finely regulating the caliber of hollow tubular organs. Similarly, slow contractions are ideally suited for moving bulky contents, such as digesta, past an absorptive surface such as the intestinal mucosa. The importance of flexibility in the length at which contractions can occur relates to the extreme variability in the extent of distension of hollow organs at times when the muscle wall is called upon to contract. For more details, see Box 3–7.

As noted above, there are no moter endplates on the sarcolemma of smooth muscle cells. An alternative to end-plate potentials must therefore exist to initiate action potentials. Smooth muscle is classified functionally as being either *multiunit* or *single-unit*. Multiunit smooth muscle is subject to control by neuromuscular transmitters that are released from specializations of the terminal axons of the autonomic nervous system. A length of nonmyelinated axon lies reasonably close to a group of smooth muscle cells, but in place of the highly organized neuromuscular junction, a series of swellings termed *varicosities* is located along this terminal portion of the axon (Figure 3–26). The varicosities release transmitters that diffuse across the extracellular space to reach the sarcolemma of any myocyte in close proximity. A definite lag time is required for diffusion, and of course it is

purely a matter of chance which muscle cell is reached first. The 1:1 relationship of nerve action potential to muscle action potential noted for skeletal muscle is not applicable to smooth muscle.

Upon combining with receptors in the sarcolemma of smooth muscle cells, the transmitters bring about one of two effects. In contrast to skeletal muscle, smooth muscle may be *depolarized* or *hyperpolarized* by the transmitter. In the latter case, the resting potential is moved further away from threshold. Some smooth muscle can therefore be inhibited by neuromuscular transmitters, a situation quite different from what obtains in skeletal muscle.

The events occurring at the sarcolemma of smooth muscle cells are still poorly understood. Included are changes in chemically gated Na^+ *channels*, Ca^{2+} *channels*, regulation of *ion pumps*, and activation of the enzyme *adenylate kinase*. This enzyme causes ATP to be converted to *3'5'-cAMP* (Figure 3–27), an extremely important intracellular messenger that seems able to regulate the disposition of Ca^{2+} inside the cell. In contrast to skeletal muscle, where Na^+ movements are the basis for depolarization, the major inward current carrier during depolarization in smooth muscle is Ca^{2+}. This ion serves as the coupling agent to initiate contractions after com-

---

Box 3–7 Smooth Muscle Walls of Hollow Organs

As was noted for skeletal muscle, a combination of isotonic shortening and isometric tension development can result from smooth muscle activity. Isometric tension development is particularly important. A fluid-filled container exhibits an outwardly directed pressure that is counteracted by an inwardly acting force due to tension in the wall. Similarly, if tension builds up in the walls of a fluid-filled organ, the contents of the organ are put under pressure.

The tension is due to deformation of the collagen and elastin caused by the muscle cells as they attempt to shorten. In reverse fashion, as a hollow organ fills, it distends the wall and stretches the smooth muscle cells. Refer to Box 2–1 to review the relationship between pressure and wall tension. Stretch is a potent stimulus for smooth muscle excitability, or the tendency for cells to discharge action potentials and therefore to contract.

Figure 3–26. *Innervation of smooth muscle.* Terminal portions of autonomic neurons are nonmyelinated and are specialized by possessing varicosities in the axon. These structures are neurosecretory in function and, upon appropriate stimulation (arrival of action potentials), they release neurotransmitters into the surrounding interstitial space. The transmitter molecules reach the smooth muscle cells by diffusing over relatively long distances, then bind to receptors of various kinds in the sarcolemma. Note that there is no structural specialization like the motor end plate of skeletal muscle.

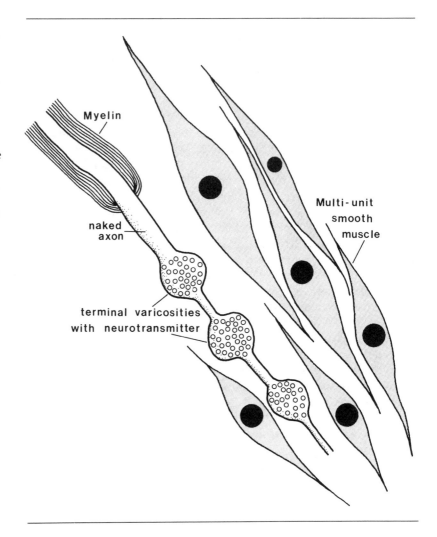

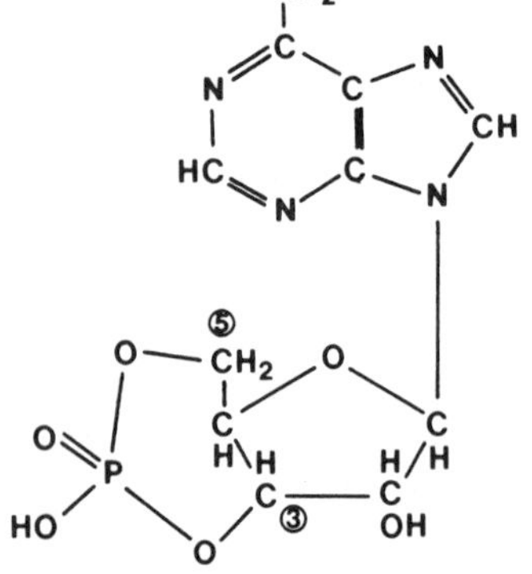

Figure 3–27. *3'5'-cyclic adenosine monophosphate (cAMP).* Cyclic AMP is a particularly important intracellular regulator. It consists of a cyclic phosphate moiety, involving carbons 3 and 5 of adenosine, generated from ATP by adenylate cyclase. Figure 7–3 illustrates other related adenosine derivatives. Figure 4–16 illustrates the involvement of cAMP in mediating hormone action.

bining with *calmodulin*, a small protein (see Box 3–8) that is remarkably similar to troponin C. Exactly how the Ca^{2+}-calmodulin complex activates the actin-myosin interaction is incompletely understood, but there is no doubt that Ca^{2+} triggers it. The device used by smooth muscle of employing the same ion to carry the current and to switch on the contractile machinery is effective only because of the small cross-sectional dimensions of the smooth muscle cell. Diffusion mechanisms that would be far too slow in the relatively enormous skeletal muscle cell are quite effective in cells that are just a few microns in diameter.

It is not certain how Ca^{2+} is removed back to resting concentrations so that relaxation can occur. Some sequestration of Ca^{2+} by organelles seems likely, along with an extrusion mechanism, possibly involving a *Ca^{2+} pump*, perhaps a Ca^{2+}-ATPase pump, located in the sarcolemma. A special feature of smooth muscles is the ability to initiate action potentials, apparently without the need for neural triggering. Some cells, particularly those in single-unit smooth muscle, exhibit *unstable resting potentials* that drift toward threshold, whereupon action potentials are discharged. A recovery phase follows, then the cycle is repeated of a slow depolarization to threshold followed by additional action potentials. This type of activity generates action potentials that are called *myogenic* and their excitation is propagated to adjacent cells via gap junctions. The phenomenon is termed *electrocoupling*. The cells responsible for the myogenic action potentials and capable of activating adjacent cells can be called pacemaker cells.

Another form of myogenic activity is commonly found in smooth muscle. The resting potential oscillates closer to and further from threshold with a periodicity of about 60 seconds; it is referred to as a *slow potential* (Figure 3–28). With suitable conditions, trains of action potentials may be released when the slow potential is closest to threshold. The discharge of action potentials is suppressed when the slow potential moves away from threshold. There is opportunity for extrinsic regulation to be applied over this background situation. For example, in myometrium (the muscle of the uterus), the sex steroid estrogen moves the slow potentials closer to threshold. Additional information about hormonal regulation of smooth muscle is provided in Box 3–9.

Stretch of the uterine wall has the same ef-

Box 3–8   Calmodulin

Calmodulin is a recently discovered regulatory protein that is present in a wide variety of cells in a diverse range of species. It is relatively small (molecular weight = 16,700 daltons) and quite acidic, as it has about 30% of its amino acids as aspartic acid or glutamic acid. At physiologic pH, these acidic residues provide *negatively charged* or *anionic* domains. (The relationship between the type of amino acid and the net charge on a protein was described in Chapter 2.) The anionic domains seem to be ideally suited for binding Ca^{2+} cations. The molecule is conformationally mobile, or capable of striking changes in shape, but it is most stable when occupied by four Ca^{2+} ions. In this Ca^{2+}-stabilized form, calmodulin is capable of regulating other proteins, activating some and inactivating others. The molecule can be regarded as both a *Ca^{2+} receptor* and a *Ca^{2+}-activated regulator* of other proteins.

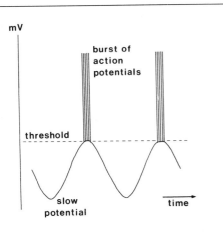

mV

burst of
action
potentials

threshold

slow
potential

time

Figure 3–28. Myogenic slow potentials. Slow potentials are low frequency oscillations of the "resting" potential of certain types of smooth muscle. The periodicity of the oscillation may be about 0.3 to 1.5 per minute. Whenever this potential reaches the threshold for the cell, a burst of action potentials is discharged. These are described as being *myogenic* because they are intrinsic to the muscle and require no external prompting. In some tissues, hormonal factors may suppress the occurrence or magnitude of slow potentials and so influence the activity state of the muscle.

Box 3–9 Humoral Regulation of Smooth Muscle

In addition to *neural control,* many smooth muscles are subject to regulation by *hormones.* Hormonal regulatory actions fall into two categories, based on the time course of action: *acute* and *chronic.* Acute regulation is not dissimilar to that afforded by neurotransmitters. Indeed, the action of norepinephrine is identical, irrespective of whether it is delivered from axon varicosities or from the adrenal medulla. Acute regulation is *rapid in onset* and of *strictly limited duration.* A number of hormones of the gastrointestinal tract are acute regulators of gut smooth muscle. Some peptides produced by enzymic cleavage of circulating plasma proteins exert potent contracting and relaxing actions on vascular smooth muscle. Oxytocin from the posterior pituitary is a well-known acute stimulant for myometrial contractions.

The second form of humoral regulation is much more complex because it is *slow in onset* and *persists for hours* rather than seconds, as is the case for the acute regulators. The muscles of the female reproductive tract are subject to chronic regulation by sex steroids. The effect of estrogens on the magnitude of slow potentials is an example of chronic regulation. Sex steroids regulate growth of the myometrium, influencing both the number and size of cells, the excitability of the cells, the nature of the connective fibrils responsible for the length-tension relationship noted earlier, and so on. Fascinating possibilities for regulation and control result from the chronic regulators determining if the tissue is reactive or refractory to the acute regulators, such as oxytocin. For example, in Chapters 4 and 10 the responsiveness of myometrium to oxytocin will be shown to depend on the ability of estrogen to increase the number of oxytocin receptors in the sarcolemma of the muscle. Finally, to indicate the breadth of these controls, the sex steroids determine if gap junctions are absent or present, if the cells can electropropagate, and therefore if the myometrium acts as a true single-unit muscle. Indeed, these chronic regulator hormones largely dictate whether or not the uterus will accommodate a conceptus during pregnancy, then initiate the events causing birth.

fect. Clearly, when a muscle has this intrinsic activity, there will be situations when it will be physiologically appropriate to suppress excitability. It is therefore no surprise that the nervous system is able to provide inhibitory influences on this type of muscle.

It is believed that myogenic activity is particularly suited for ensuring a tonic low level of activity. This sustained low-level activity is sometimes called tonus, but the terms *contracture* and *resting tension* are probably better.

3.6 • Organization of the Nervous System

The discussion so far has considered the general nature of animal tissues and the continued regulation of processes that maintain the integrity of living tissues. The key properties of excitable tissue, particularly neural and muscular tissues, have been examined and a basis established for their participation in regulation. This section addresses the organization of the nervous system and shows how stimuli are integrated to elicit particular responses. The description of regulatory mechanisms is expanded in Chapter 4 with a thorough treatment of hormonal communication and regulation. Important applications of this material will appear in the remaining chapters, so after this initial exposure, the reader should be certain to return and review the material whenever necessary.

The nervous system can be divided, both anatomically and functionally, into two major divisions: the *central nervous system* (CNS) and the *peripheral nervous system*. Operationally, neural mechanisms are best described as *voluntary* and *involuntary*. Many involuntary neural mechanisms occur in what is known as the *autonomic nervous system*. As illustrated in Figure 3–29, the autonomic nervous system is distributed over both central and peripheral nervous systems.

The CNS comprises the *brain* and *spinal cord*,

highly specialized structures located entirely within a protective bony cage made up of the skull and the vertebral column. The peripheral nervous system consists of 12 pairs of *cranial nerves*, a variable number of paired *spinal nerves*, and the complex of nerves making up the autonomic nervous system.

There is some overlap in any classification, and the one presented here is no exception. For example, cranial nerve X, the *vagus nerve*, is a very important component of the autonomic nervous system and will be encountered time and time again in subsequent material.

The autonomic nervous system is conveniently considered as comprising two major subdivisions: sympathetic and parasympathetic. The sympathetic nervous system is also called the thoracolumbar system and the parasympathetic nervous system may be called the craniosacral system. These alternative designations indicate the portions of the vertebral column from which the CNS gives rise to the major nerves of each division. Major nerves from the thoracic and lumbar vertebrae, from the shoulders to the pelvis (see Figure 1–25), carry sympathetic outflow from the CNS to the body, while nerves from the cranial and sacral vertebrae carry the parasympathetic outflow.

The basic cellular unit of the nervous system

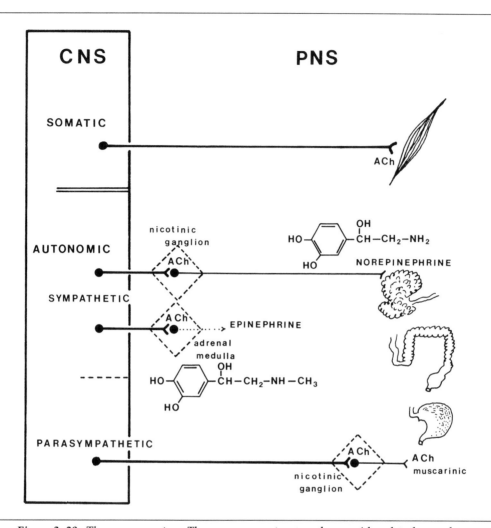

Figure 3–29. The nervous system. The nervous system can be considered to be made up of the central nervous system (CNS) and the peripheral nervous system (PNS). The CNS consists of the brain and spinal cord. The PNS includes both extensions of the voluntary, or somatic, and the involuntary, or autonomic, nervous systems. Note the synapses in efferent neurons in the autonomic nervous system (ANS). Clusters of synapses and cytons in major nerve trunks are ganglia. The adrenal medulla in the sympathetic nervous system releases epinephrine into the blood circulatory system and is an important neuroendocrine organ. Other sympathetic efferents release norepinephrine. In the ANS, the ganglia are classified on the basis of their differential sensitivity to drugs. For example, the cholinergic receptors at some synaptic loci are inhibited by nicotine (nicotinic receptors) while others are inhibited by muscarine (muscarinic receptors).

is the neuron. Neurons are highly specialized, and the body's full complement of neurons is probably present at birth. Nerves, made up of many neurons, can of course be repaired if tran-

sected, though it is not clear if cell division is part of the process. The various parts of the neuron—dendrites, cell body, axon, synaptic bouton, etc.—were described earlier. Outside of the

CNS, the cell bodies (cytons) of neurons form aggregates referred to as *ganglia*. Great masses of synapses are often found in close proximity to these cytons within the ganglia. The ganglia are important sites of *integration*, especially within the autonomic nervous system.

In addition to neurons, neural tissues in the CNS and ganglia contain glial cells that provide support and possibly nutritive assistance. The glial cells are of various types. Some seem to be involved in formation of the myelin sheath, while others make up the *blood-brain barrier*. Myelinated neurons make up the white matter of the brain and spinal cord while the gray matter comprises masses of unmyelinated neurons, or the dendritic portions of neurons.

Clusters of cytons are found within the CNS as well as within ganglia. These centers have well-defined roles and are usually anatomically discrete. In later chapters reference will be made to various *brain centers* that have integrative roles for many of the vital life-support systems.

The Brain

The brain is a highly specialized tissue comprised almost entirely of neural tissue. It is the major control center of the voluntary and many of the involuntary activities of the body. The brain is a hollow organ formed from the anterior portion of the embryonic neural tube. The central cavity is actually a combination of ducts and chambers, or ventricles, filled with *cerebrospinal fluid* (CSF). It is continuous with the fluid-filled central canal of the spinal cord. Surrounding the central cavity are concentrations of white matter made up from myelinated axons. Further out, the more peripheral portion of the brain is mainly gray matter. (This arrangement of gray and white matter is reversed in the spinal cord.) The CNS is surrounded by a multilayered membrane system, some details of which are provided in Box 3–10.

During brain development, constrictions in the neural tube define three primary segments: forebrain, midbrain, and hindbrain. The major parts of the brain and their relative locations, depicted in Figure 3–30, are important and are easily learned:

- The *cerebrum* is composed of the two largest structures of the brain, the right cerebral hemisphere and the left cerebral hemisphere. The outer layer of the cerebrum is called the *cerebral cortex.*

- The *cerebellum* is posterior to and sometimes slightly ventral to the cerebrum.

- The *midbrain* is located under the cerebrum and anterior to the cerebellum. The major part of the midbrain consists of cerebral peduncles, or the *cerebral stalk.*

Box 3–10   The Meninges

The soft tissues of the brain and spinal cord are surrounded by a triple-layered membrane system called the *meninges*. The membrane closest to the gray matter is the *pia mater*, the intermediate membrane is the *arachnoid*, and the most superficial membrane is the *dura mater*, the toughest of the three. Between the arachnoid and the pia mater lies a protective cushion of CSF. This fluid is similar to lymph or an ultrafiltrate of plasma. It is actively secreted by cells lining the specialized capillary beds in the ventricles of the brain.

Figure 3–30. The bovine brain. This lateral view of the bovine brain shows the major parts of the brainstem. The olfactory bulb (O) connects with the midbrain as does the cerebrum (C) with its highly contoured surface. The portion of the midbrain shown here is the cerebral peduncle (cp), or stalk, and the pons (P). The cerebellum (cb) lies posterior to the cerebrum and dorsal to the medulla oblongata (M). The latter communicates with the spinal cord. While not strictly part of the brain, the pituitary gland (pi) is shown, with its connecting stalk to the hypothalamus in the midbrain. For more detail, see Figure 3–31.

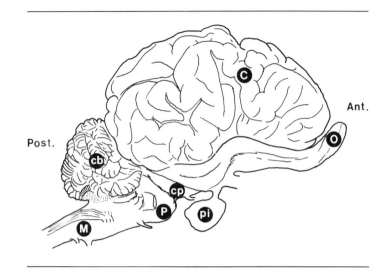

Figure 3–31. Equine brain. Two views are provided of the brain of the horse: the ventral surface (above) and a sagittal section (below). The ventral surface is labeled to show the cranial nerves (Roman numerals, described in Table 3–1). The sagittal section shows the general relationships between the structures of the midbrain and those of the hindbrain. (Reproduced by permission of the publisher. From Bone, J.F.: *Animal Anatomy and Physiology,* Reston, VA: Reston Publishing Company, 1979.)

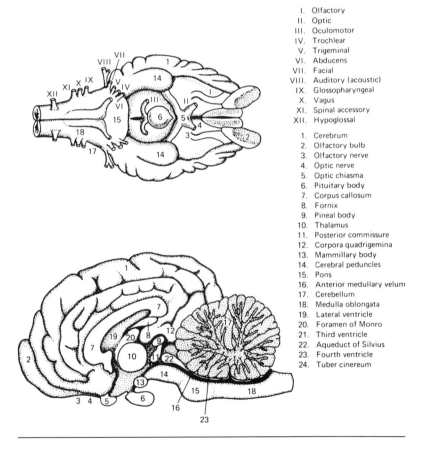

I.   Olfactory
II.   Optic
III.   Oculomotor
IV.   Trochlear
V.   Trigeminal
VI.   Abducens
VII.   Facial
VIII.   Auditory (acoustic)
IX.   Glossopharyngeal
X.   Vagus
XI.   Spinal accessory
XII.   Hypoglossal

1.   Cerebrum
2.   Olfactory bulb
3.   Olfactory nerve
4.   Optic nerve
5.   Optic chiasma
6.   Pituitary body
7.   Corpus callosum
8.   Fornix
9.   Pineal body
10.   Thalamus
11.   Posterior commissure
12.   Corpora quadrigemina
13.   Mammillary body
14.   Cerebral peduncles
15.   Pons
16.   Anterior medullary velum
17.   Cerebellum
18.   Medulla oblongata
19.   Lateral ventricle
20.   Foramen of Monro
21.   Third ventricle
22.   Aqueduct of Silvius
23.   Fourth ventricle
24.   Tuber cinereum

- The *pons* is located immediately posterior to the midbrain and anterior to the medulla oblongata.

- The *medulla oblongata* lies posterior to the pons and is the last part of the brain stem, making connection with the anterior portion of the spinal cord.

It is a little difficult to begin describing the major brain areas and their functions without excessive use of anatomic detail and the introduction of far more complexity than is necessary for most readers. It is sufficient to develop a general appreciation of the relative locations of the landmarks indicated on the median section shown in Figure 3–31. In addition, a ventral surface view of the horse brain is provided to show the location of the cranial nerves, indicated with Roman numerals. These nerves may carry *sensory* and or *motor* neurons, as indicated in Table 3–1.

The Spinal Cord

The spinal cord is an extension of the brain, or cranial portion of the CNS, into the vertebral portion. It is the means of communication between the brain and the body, provides communication pathways between portions of the cord itself, and provides sites of integration for various types of reflexes.

The organization of the spinal cord into white matter and gray matter is reversed from that of the brain, with white matter lying more peripheral to the gray matter. Because communication

Table 3–1. The Cranial Nerves

Name	Number	Origin	Termination	Function
Olfactory	I	Nasal epithelium	Olfactory bulb	Sensory
Optic	II	Retina	Optic chiasma	Sensory
Oculomotor	III	Cerebral peduncle	Muscles of the eye chamber	Motor
Trochlear	IV	Pons, anterior medulla oblongata	Muscles of the eye chamber	Motor
Trigeminal	V	Posterior pons	Face in general, buccal cavity	Mixed sensorimotor
Abducens	VI	Anterior medulla oblongata	Musculature of eye	Motor
Facial	VII	Medulla oblongata	Facial muscles, salivary glands	Mixed sensorimotor
Acoustic	VIII	Internal ear	Medulla oblongata, posterior to VII	Sensory
Glossopharyngeal	IX	Medulla oblongata	Buccal cavity	Mixed sensorimotor
Vagus	X	Medulla oblongata	Pharynx to lower abdomen	Mixed sensorimotor
Spinal Accessory	XI	Medulla oblongata	Neck and shoulders	Motor
Hypoglossal	XII	Medulla oblongata	Tongue	Motor

Box 3–11 The Spinal Cord

In cross-section (Figure 3–32) the cord appears to be almost completely divided into right and left portions by deep median folds of the pia mater. Dorsally, the fold is called the *dorsal septum*, while the other is the *ventral fissure*. The space overlying the pia mater and underlying the arachnoid is the subarachnoid space. Between the arachnoid and the dura mater is the subdural space, and between the dura and inner wall of the vertebra is the epidural space. There is no equivalent to the epidural space around the brain because the dura mater closely adheres to the cranium. A small central canal is a continuation of the ventricles of the brain and, like the subarachnoid space, is filled with CSF.

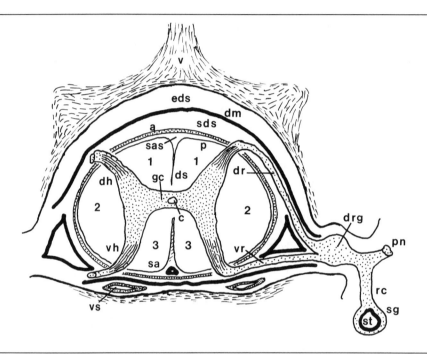

Figure 3–32. The spinal cord. A cross-section of the spinal cord shows the structures from the peripheral membranes to the central gray matter of the cord. Note the partial separation of the white matter into dorsal (1), lateral (2), and ventral (3) columns, and the relationship between the dorsal (dh) and ventral (vh) horns of the gray matter and the dorsal (dr) and ventral (vr) roots of the spinal nerves. The cord lies within the foramen, or canal, of the vertebrae (v) and is bounded by membranes and fluid-filled spaces: epidural space (eds); dura mater (dm); subdural space (sds); arachnoid (a); subarachnoid space (sas); and pia mater (p). The gray matter is organized into the horns on either side, connected by the gray commisure (gc) with the central spinal canal (c). The white matter is partly sectioned by the dorsal sinus (ds), and the ventral fissure which lies above the spinal artery (sa). Venous sinuses (vs) lie in the ventral portion of the epidural space. The dorsal and ventral nerve roots come together and exit via vertebral foramina and immediately form the dorsal root ganglia (drg), which supplies neurons forming peripheral nerves (pn). The ramus communicans (rc) connects to the sympathetic trunk (st), which runs parallel to the spinal cord between sympathetic ganglia (sg).

between the cord and the body tissues is via spinal nerves that are organized in close relation to individual vertebrae, it is convenient to regard the spinal cord as a longitudinal array of *segments*. The makeup of the cord is described in finer detail in Box 3–11.

The cross-section shows that the gray matter, consisting of cytons and unmyelinated fibers, extends into dorsal and ventral horns with a central connecting portion, the *gray commissure*. The white matter is divided into two *lateral columns*, a *ventral column* and a *dorsal column*. Each of these consists of myelinated nerves that tend to run up or down the length of the cord. There are well-defined *tracts* within these columns, and a neurologist can diagnose damage to specific portions of these tracts by testing the integrity of sensory or motor function reflexes that transit the columns.

It is sufficient that the reader recognize that the dorsal column is mainly concerned with sensory traffic, the ventral column with motor traffic, and that the lateral columns have mixed function. They are most important for communication along the spinal cord, from segment to segment, and to and from the brain.

The *horns of gray matter* communicate with the spinal nerves. Again, the dorsal portions or roots are sensory and the ventral roots carry motor nerve traffic. The cytons of the motor nerves are located in the ventral horns of the gray matter. Sensory nerves coming into the dorsal roots pass through dorsal root ganglia, aggregations of cytons of these neurons. The major roots fuse outside the spinal cord to form mixed peripheral nerves that carry both sensory and motor neurons and traffic. They also connect to a series of ganglia, one per vertebral segment, that together make up the sympathetic trunk of the autonomic nervous system (Figure 3–33). This connection is called the *ramus communicans*.

The nerve connections more peripheral to the site of fusion of the dorsal and ventral roots are really part of the peripheral nervous system. The peripheral nerve trunks divide as mixed function nerves and are broadly distributed to the body tissues. At their most peripheral locations, the sensory neurons originate at receptors for the generation of sensory information. More specific information about receptors is provided in Box 3–12. Motor neurons innervate effector organs by means of structures such as the neuromuscular junctions or the varicosities in smooth muscle, both of which were described earlier in this chapter.

The Autonomic Nervous System

A few additional remarks about the autonomic nervous system will complete this introduction to the organization of the nervous system.

Figure 3–33. The spinal cord and sympathetic trunk. This figure shows the organization of spinal nerves and the relationship between the series of sympathetic trunk ganglia and each of the spinal nerves. The illustrated structures are the dorsal horn of gray matter (a), ventral horn of gray matter (b), dorsolateral surface of the spinal cord (c), dorsal (sensory) nerve (d), dorsal root ganglion (e), ventral (motor) nerve (f), ramus communicans (g), sympathetic ganglion (h), spinal nerves (i), sympathetic nerves (j), and paravertebral sympathetic nerve trunk (k).

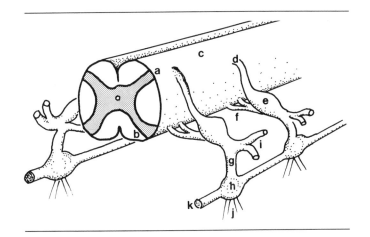

Box 3–12   Receptors

Receptors are specialized nerve endings that transduce various stimuli into frequency-modulated trains of action potentials for the sensory neuron. The receptors are complex in structure and take many forms. Differences in structure presumably underlie the *selectivity* of different types of receptors for stimuli of quite different physical or chemical forms.

Irrespective of variations in their precise nature, receptors are excitable structures capable of generating *receptor potentials* that increase in proportion to an applied stimulus. When the receptor potential

changes sufficiently, an action potential is generated and sent on its way along the sensory neuron. The receptor potential immediately decays; then, if the stimulus persists, it builds up again until another action potential is triggered.

It is not intended that the reader develop anything beyond this superficial understanding of the origin of these receptor-generated potentials. Note, however, that the receptor potential is not an all-or-none phenomenon as in the case of action potentials, but rather represents a *graded response* to a *graded input*.

In the earlier descriptions of neurons, the terms dendrites and axon were used to distinguish the afferent, or input, side from the efferent, or output, side of the cyton, or cell body. In descriptions of the peripheral nervous system, and particularly of the autonomic nervous system, it is more useful to distinguish between neuronal processes carrying impulses toward a ganglion *(preganglionic fibers)* and those carrying impulses away from the ganglion *(post-*

ganglionic fibers). In the autonomic nervous system the ganglia are also synaptic loci, so, from earlier remarks about multiple synaptic connections serving as a basis for integration, it can be expected that the ganglia are important in the integration of autonomic function. The role of the autonomic nervous system in regulation of visceral function will be described below, and then extensively in subsequent chapters.

3.7 • Synaptic Function in the CNS: Reflexes

Simple *reflexes* have some basic neuronal requirements and properties that are illustrated in Figure 3–34. The simple two-neuronal reflex arc, shown in Figure 3–34a, exhibits the following components:

a *receptor*, in this case a muscle spindle,

an *afferent neuron*,

an *afferent cell body*, in the dorsal root ganglion,

Figure 3–34. Components of simple reflex arcs. The components of the simple monosynaptic reflex are shown in part *a*. Afferent traffic originates at a receptor (a), passes along an afferent neuron (b) with its cyton (c), and enters the dorsal horn of the cord in the gray matter. After synapsing at (d), motor traffic passes through the efferent neuron (e) to supply the effector termini at motor endplates (f). This could be the process underlying a simple system such as the knee jerk reflex. *b:* The afferent neuron (b) synapses on an internuncial neuron (g) and on an ascending neuron (h) at two synaptic loci (d). The reflexes are described in detail in the text.

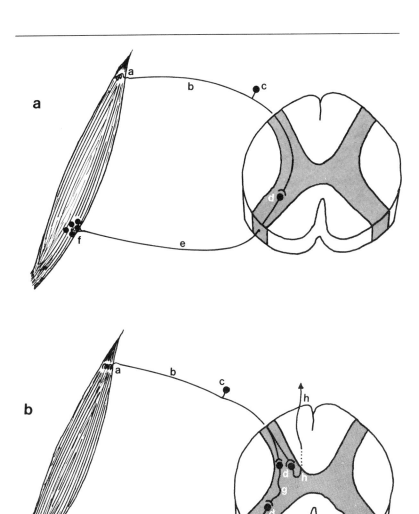

a *synapse,* in the spinal gray matter,

an *efferent neuron,* exiting from a ventral nerve root, and

a *neuromuscular junction,* innervating the target muscle.

Note that the cyton of the motor neuron lies close to the synapse within the ventral horn of the spinal gray matter. In this example, the receptive and motor components lie within the same tissue, a skeletal muscle, and the reflex could serve to protect the muscle from undue stretching. During stretching, activation of the reflex would elicit a reactive contraction, or shortening. The reaction could protect the myocytes or the tendons from being torn. The synapse is the simple site of integration, whereby sensory information from the afferent arm of the reflex leads to the effector response, being carried in the efferent neuron.

The second example, shown in Figure 3–34b, has a slight added complexity in that the basic reflex arc contains three neurons and is *bisynaptic*. The two synapses integral to this reflex circuit are separated by an *internuncial* or connecting neuron. Because the opportunity for integration at synapses is doubled, more subtle fine-tuning of the motor response is possible. An added feature is the branch on the axon of the afferent neuron that synapses in the dorsal horn of the spinal gray matter to provide input to an *ascending neuron*. This enables longitudinal integration within the spinal cord by passing sensory information to other spinal regions, as would be needed for more complex *multilevel reactions*. The same feature could allow transmission of sensory information to higher regions of the CNS, such as the cerebellum, where coordination of motor activity may be appropriate. This information would pass along tracts in the dorsal or lateral columns, as described before.

Increased complexity in the reflex can be achieved by *reciprocal control* over motor neurons innervating an *antagonistic pair* of muscles. Such an arrangement is described in Box 3–13.

The illustrations provided in Figures 3–34 and 3–35 are gross simplifications because the number of inputs may be several hundreds or thousands, while in the figures they are represented by single synapses. Similarly, the coordination of even simple spinal reflexes may involve reciprocal motor regulation on either side of the spinal cord. Note that a muscle is either activated into contraction or it is not. Inhibitory control is achieved at dendrites of the motor nerve, not at the motor end-plate. A muscle that is not stimulated to contract is free to be lengthened passively. This was referred to earlier as relaxation.

Box 3–13   Multisynaptic Reflexes

As illustrated in Figure 3–35A, the sensory or afferent neuron synapses at two loci. One synapse integrates the activity of the motor neuron innervating one of a pair of muscles. The other synapse is onto an internuncial neuron, distinguished in the figure by shading. Although the afferent input to these two synapses is excitatory, the subsequent output from the internuncial neuron is inhibitory and would be mediated by the release of an inhibitory neurotransmitter such as GABA. Integration at the most distal of the synapses is therefore achieved by inhibiting firing of the second motor neuron, so that the muscle it innervates is held inactive.

In Figure 3–35B, the inhibitory internuncial neuron is involved in a more complex control of the motor neuron with which it synapses. Note that the balance between two excitatory inputs, interacting with the inhibitory input, will determine if the second motor neuron is activated or not. In this case the additional input neuron may be part of an ascending or descending pathway, as would be needed for intersegmental coordination. In many instances, the integration of multisynaptic reflexes involves reciprocal events on both sides of the spinal cord. Thus, activation of motor neurons might occur on the left, while comparable motor neurons on the right may be inhibited. Consider the makeup of an avoidance maneuver, for example prompted by a sting or burn on one foot. The likely reaction will consist of flexion, or withdrawal, of the affected limb, combined with extension of the contralateral limb. The latter may be required to enable the noninjured limb to become load-bearing.

Figure 3–35. Components of more complex reflexes. These multisynaptic reflexes provide for reciprocal control over more than one effector organ (for example, a flexor and extensor muscle pair). *A:* The afferent neuron (a) synapses at b with a motor neuron (f) and an inhibitory internuncial neuron (c). The motor neuron to the flexor (f) is activated, while the motor neuron to the extensor (g) is inhibited. Note that the inhibition occurs centrally, at synapse (e), and is achieved by a GABA-releasing, inhibitory internuncial neuron (c). Relaxation of the extensor is achieved simply because there is no traffic of action potentials in the motor neuron (g). *B:* Multiple inputs, synapsing at (e) (see exploded view below) with the efferent neuron (g), arise from an excitatory descending neuron (h), an excitatory afferent (a), and an inhibitory neuron (d) crossing from the other side. A collateral (c) of one motor neuron (f) activates the inhibitory neuron. In this example, the two motor neurons (f and g) control muscles on either side. The balance of excitatory and inhibitory inputs to the motor neuron (g) determines if it is activated or not.

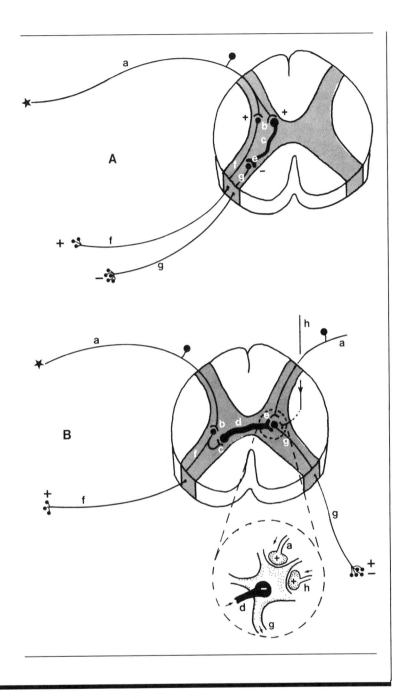

3.8 • Autonomic Motor Innervation of Visceral Organs

The autonomic nervous system has two major divisions, the sympathetic or thoracolumbar division and the parasympathetic or craniosacral division. The sympathetic nervous system forms a nerve trunk running along the spinal column, and outflows (for example from T-1 to T-4, T-5 to T-12, L-1 to L-5) are brought together in ganglia, as indicated in Figure 3–36. Then very long postganglionic fibers are dispersed to various visceral organs. In contrast, craniosacral outflow of the parasympathetic nervous system is by means of very long preganglionic fibers from

cranial nerves III, VII, IX, and X, or from ventral nerve roots at S-1 to S-4 or S-5. By far the most important of these is the vagus nerve, or cranial nerve X. Note that parasympathetic nerves synapse at ganglia that are located close to the effector organ; postganglionic fibers are therefore quite short. In both divisions of the autonomic nervous system, preganglionic fibers release acetylcholine for ganglionic synaptic transmission. They are described as being cholinergic. The acetylcholine receptors are not all the same; some distinctions are provided in Box 3–14.

Figure 3–36. The autonomic nervous system (ANS). The major parasympathetic (craniosacral) nerves are shown at left and the sympathetic (thoracolumbar) nerves are at right in this highly schematic (and somewhat fanciful) illustration. The viscera usually receive innervation from both divisions of the ANS. From top to bottom, the viscera depicted are lung (lu); heart (h); liver (li); stomach (s); intestines (i); kidney (k); bladder (b); and a unisex reproductive tract (r). In addition to cranial nerves, the parasympathetic outflow is from sacral segments of the spinal cord (depicted S–1 to S–4). Note the long preganglionic neurons and very short postsynaptic neurons. For sympathetic outflow between the first thoracic segment (T–1) and the last lumbar segment (L–5), short preganglionic neurons pass to major plexuses (stars) then innervate target structures by means of long post-synaptic neurons (dotted).

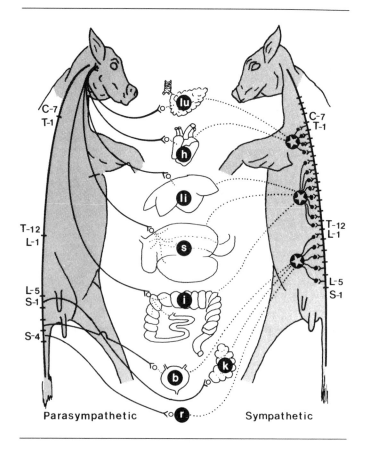

Box 3–14   Cholinergic Receptors

The acetylcholine receptors on the postganglionic neurons can be activated pharmacologically by the alkaloid *nicotine* and hence are termed *nicotinic*. Acetylcholine receptors in the effector organs innervated by parasympathetic neurons are not stimulated by nicotine but are activated pharmacologically by *muscarine*, an alkaloid from mushrooms, and so are termed *muscarinic*. A number of drugs and compounds having pharmacologic actions on excitable tissues are listed in Table 3–2. The differences in sensitivity of sympathetic and parasympathetic neurons to some of these agents are illustrated in adequate detail in Figure 3–29.

Table 3–2. A Selection of Neuro- and Neuromuscular-Active Agents

The agents listed below suggest the range of actions of various compounds that man has used in medicines, poisons, drugs of habituation, and so forth. The reader need not memorize this material.

Cholinomimetics are substances able to occupy and activate the cholinergic receptor (examples: acetylcholine, succinylcholine, carbacol).

Blockers of acetylcholine synthesis (include hemicholinium, which inhibits uptake by the axon of choline, produced after acetylcholinesterase has broken down acetylcholine in the postsynaptic membrane).

Blockers of acetylcholine release (include procain and the botulinum toxin).

CNS stimulants (include caffeine, which inhibits phosphodiesterase, the enzyme that normally inactivates 3'5'-cAMP, causing increased metabolic activity in the CNS; and strychnine, a poison that selectively blocks inhibitory pathways, thereby causing uncontrolled, convulsive activity in the CNS).

CNS and local anesthetics (include procaine and cocaine, both of which block sodium conductance and so prevent the generation of action potentials).

Cholinergic blockers (include atropine, which competes for acetylcholine binding sites on the postsynaptic membrane and at motor end-plates).

Ganglionic stimulators (include nicotine, which is initially stimulatory because it causes depolarization, but then becomes a blocking agent because it sustains the depolarization).

Neuromuscular blockers (include curare and bungarotoxin, which attach to motor end-plates, causing paralysis of muscle).

Acetylcholinesterase inhibitors, which block the enzymatic degradation of acetylcholine and so prolong all forms of cholinergic stimulation (include a wide range of agents—eserine, diisopropyl phosphofluoridate (DFP), various insecticides, nerve gases, etc.).

Inhibitors of action potentials in muscle (include quinine, an alkaloid that lengthens the refractory period and is used as a defibrillator, suppressor of shivering, and hence is antipyretic, the basis for its use in malaria, and in gin and tonic).

The final transmitter substance released to the effector organ by postsynaptic neurons differs between the two divisions of the autonomic nervous system. Sympathetic postganglionic fibers use norepinephrine and their effector organs have *adrenergic receptors*. Parasympathetic postganglionic fibers release acetylcholine and so are *cholinergic*. With just a few exceptions, dual innervation of an effector organ by the sympathetic and parasympathetic nervous systems provides for antagonistic control. Thus, motor neurons from one division may stimulate a given function, while neurons from the other division would suppress that function.

3.9 • Central Neural Integration

The preceding examples of reflex control of motor events have all used muscles as the effector organs. Similar principles apply when control of secretory activity is the end point of reflex control. For the present example, the neural integration of the control of salivary secretion is introduced. The applied aspects of this topic fit, of course, into a discussion of digestive mechanisms, so some of this will be noted again in Chapter 6.

The salivary glands are specialized for the production of a variety of secretions and their delivery, through ducts, into the proximal portion of the lumen of the digestive tract. The important components of the salivary secretory system are depicted in Figure 3–37.

On the afferent side of these reflexes there are several *receptive fields* within the buccal cavity that respond to chemical or physical stimuli. These include the taste and texture of feedstuffs. Afferent or sensory neurons pass through cranial nerve IX, also known as the glossopharyngeal nerve, to a group of cytons in the medulla oblongata. This area is called the *salivary center*. In addition, the medullary center receives inputs from the cerebral cortex and other ''higher centers'' of the brain that provide a means of bypassing the primary receptive field in the buccal cavity. The senses of sight, sound, and smell, with appropriate prior experience, memory, and conditioning, are all quite able to elicit active and copious salivation. The classic work of Pavlov, the Russian physiologist, on *conditioned reflexes* exposed the variety of cues that could be used to initiate salivary secretion, among a variety of autonomic responses, in highly trained dogs.

The salivary center communicates with the paired salivary glands via motor nerves. Cranial nerves VII, IX, and X, all mixed-function nerves that carry both sensory and motor information, are important in controlling the salivary glands. As noted earlier, these nerves form part of the cranial division of the parasympathetic nervous system. The preganglionic neurons are long and lead to ganglia located close to the salivary glands. Acetylcholine is released as the synaptic neurotransmitter and activates quite short postganglionic neurons that innervate the glands. These neurons also use acetylcholine as their transmitter and can reasonably be called secretomotor nerves. Acetylcholine provokes an altered distribution of ions across the membrane of the secretory cells that then causes an increased flux of water across the cells and into the lumen of the salivary acini. Some of the glands secrete a dilute solution of sodium bi-

Figure 3–37. Regulation of salivation. Afferent nerves from the buccal cavity, and higher brain inputs are integrated in the medullary salivary center. Secretomotor nerve traffic passes through cranial nerves VII, IX, and X to pairs of salivary glands [mandibular (m), parotid (p), submaxillary (s), and zygomatic (z)]. The efferent traffic is carried by cholinergic parasympathetic neurons in these mixed-function nerves. Notice the short post-ganglionic fibers into the mass of each gland.

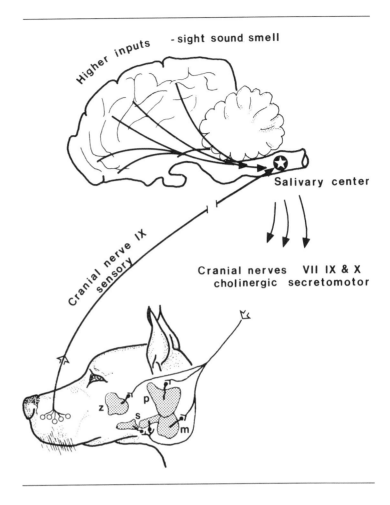

carbonate ($NaHCO_3$), others secrete heavily glycosylated molecules called mucus.

The increased secretion is due to acetylcholine occupying cholinergic receptors. The cholinergic receptors can be blocked with the drug atropine (see Table 3–2). A common medical use of atropine is to reduce salivation during oral surgery and as an adjunctive medication in general anesthesia when copious salivation is undesirable.

The reflex control of secretory events is quite equivalent to the control over skeletal muscles, described earlier. In both situations the reflexes have receptors, afferents, sites of integration, efferents, and effector targets.

3.10 • Exercises

---

1. True or false:

_____ The gray matter of the CNS lies peripheral to the more central white matter.

_____ Excitation and contraction are coupled by Ca^{2+} ions in all muscles through exactly the same mechanisms.

_____ Norepinephrine is the major neurotransmitter of the postganglionic sympathetic neurons.

_____ A single action potential arriving at a presynaptic bouton is transmitted chemically and initiates an action potential in the postsynaptic neuron with 1:1 fidelity.

_____ A persistent low level of contractile activity in a muscle or muscles can be called tonus.

_____ The dorsal portions of the spinal cord are mainly concerned with sensory traffic of nerve impulses.

_____ Acetylcholine is the neuromuscular transmitter at motor end-plates.

_____ In neurology, the term _ascending_ is generally synonymous with _cephalad_, meaning directed toward the brain, or _craniad_, meaning directed toward the head.

_____ The conducting system of the heart employs highly specialized neurons that form the His bundle and the Purkinje fibers.

_____ Internuncial neurons are included in the circuitry of polysynaptic reflex arcs. They may be either excitatory or inhibitory on efferent neurons.

2. The following is a control flow chart summarizing the events leading to a twitch contraction then relaxation in skeletal muscle. A number of important steps have been omitted. Use similarly brief one-line statements to complete the sequence, then use the chart for review purposes.

Action potential reaches terminal of motor nerve.

↓

↓

Action potential fires in the sarcolemma at the motor end-plate.

↓

It propagates across the surface of the myocyte.

↓

↓

Sarcoplasmic reticulum releases Ca^{2+} ions.

↓

↓

Cross-bridges form and filaments slide.

→ ATP is hydrolyzed and the bridges separate.

Another ATP molecule is bound by heavy meromyosin.

_or_

↓

Sarcoplasmic reticulum Ca^{2+}–pump operates.

↓

Tropomyosin moves to block actin-binding sites.

↓

Chemical Communication

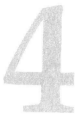

4.1 • Introduction to Endocrinology

Endocrinology, the study of the hormonal controls of bodily function, is one of the newer disciplines within physiology. This description attempts to convey the principles of endocrinology and to expose the reader to some of the exciting developments presently occurring in this field. It has to be balanced, however, with a need to avoid excessive biochemical complexity for beginning students. This requirement presents a dilemma because hormones are chemicals and their properties depend totally on the physicochemical makeup of the diverse array of molecules that behave as hormones. The material is exceedingly important for the reader who is trying to understand how animals function.

To help simplify portions of the description, much of the detail that is needed for completeness but that may detract the reader from easily obtaining an overview has been separated from the main text.

Chemically mediated controls of physiologic function are extremely diverse. Specific chemicals mediate critical processes in nervous function such as synaptic transmission, which involves the triggered release of neurotransmitters responsible for initiating action potentials in the postsynaptic neuron. Neuromuscular transmission is mediated by acetylcholine or by norepinephrine, depending on the division of the nervous system involved. In both cases specific molecules carry *information* from one cell to another. The responses to these transmitters are rather simple compared to those of other chemical mediators, but the communication principles involved are quite similar.

Somewhat related to the foregoing is the local exchange of information from one cell to others in close proximity in tissues other than in the nervous system. Such chemical mediators are called *paracrines,* or local hormones. *Autocrines* are chemical mediators that appear to have controlling actions on the very cells that produce them. Although autocrines and paracrines do not exhibit all of the characteristics of *endocrines,* the principles of information transfer again seem to apply. The release of histamine from specialized cells with resultant local vasodilation or "reddening" in adjacent tissues is an example of this mechanism. This is part of the reaction to local tissue damage such as that caused by the sting of an insect. Similarly, exercising muscle produces adenosine, a breakdown product of adenosine triphosphate (ATP) and related molecules, which is responsible for increased blood flow in active muscle.

Absolute distinctions between these groups of chemical mediators serve little purpose. For example, it matters little whether norepinephrine is classed as a neurotransmitter or as an endocrine.

Diseases of the endocrine system may result in startling dysfunctions, and many of these abnormalities must have been recognized thousands of years ago. For example, the gross symptomatology of *diabetes mellitus* was described by Hippocrates. *Gigantism* and *dwarfism* have always provoked interest. It is likely that the severe thyroid dysfunctions such as *cretinism* in the young and *goiter* (thyroid enlargement) in adults were also recognized. Man made use of the behavior modification of animals (and even other humans!) that results from castration, long before the endocrine function of the testes was understood.

Modern experimental endocrinology began with the studies of Bayliss and Starling at the turn of the 20th century. Their simple studies demonstrating the ability of aqueous extracts of intestinal mucosa to stimulate flow of pancreatic juice when injected into dogs led to the coining of the word *hormone* (from the Greek for *to arouse* or *to excite*), and the naming of the active principle as secretin. Within a brief period, several phenomena were described as being hormone

mediated, and numerous glands and tissues in the body were called endocrine, or glands of internal secretion. The glands and other tissues with endocrine function are shown in Figure 4–1.

A number of requirements usually had to be satisfied before a substance was generally accepted as a hormone. Some of these criteria are not always realistic, and the modern endocrinologist has powerful investigative techniques that partially substitute for the classic requirements.

A Hormone: To Be or Not To Be

- Hormones are usually produced in specific cells in endocrine *glands*. They are transported in blood to act on distal tissues, called *targets*.

- Surgical removal or other destruction of the gland or cells of origin causes abnormalities, or altered physiologic states.

- Suitable extracts of the gland are capable of correcting the deficiency or abnormality resulting from ablation of the gland.

- As extracts of the tissue are purified, the active principle, or the component that is responsible for the activity described above, becomes more active, or potent, when expressed on a weight basis.

- It is often possible to demonstrate higher activity in the blood draining an endocrine gland than in the blood supplying the gland.

While these guidelines were of major importance in the unfolding of knowledge of endocrine regulation, there were particular problems. In some cases, particularly for the specialized hormones of the hypothalamus, the site of action, the pituitary gland, is not distant from the origin: the pituitary is located just a few millimeters from the hypothalamus. Some tissues simply cannot be surgically ablated without

Figure 4–1. The endocrine glands. These organs and glands have known endocrine functions and comprise the bulk of the classic endocrine system: pineal (1); hypothalamus (2); pituitary (3); thyroid (4); parathyroid (5); stomach (abomasum in the case of ruminants) (6); duodenum (7); pancreas (8); adrenal (9); kidney (10); and ovary (testis in males) (11). Additional tissues function transiently as endocrine organs; the placenta in pregnant females is an example. Most tissues, such as the brain and liver, produce autocrines or paracrines, as described in the text. The role of this latter class of humoral regulators does not correspond exactly to that of classic hormones.

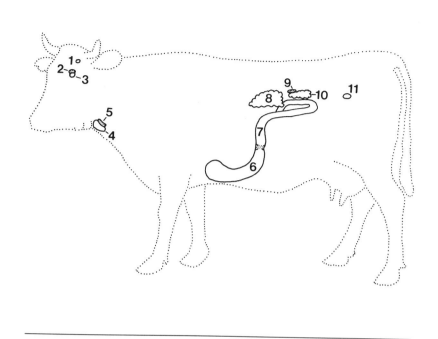

drastic consequences that have absolutely nothing to do with any hormone deficiency. For example, nephrectomy, or removal of the kidneys, usually causes death from uremia within a couple of days at most. It is quite obvious that the essential excretory function of the kidneys cannot be restored by injections of kidney extracts. The same difficulty applies to studies of the endocrine function of the brain or the liver. For similar reasons, studies of the placenta cannot use surgical ablation, if fetal survival is an end point of the investigation.

Another difficulty arises because the hormone in some cases is present in the gland only in particular physiologic states. Very recently the peptide oxytocin, which is normally considered to be a hypothalamic or posterior pituitary hormone, was discovered in many species in the corpus luteum, a temporary endocrine gland within the ovary. However, it is present only during cyclic stages or very early pregnancy, and disappears in advanced pregnancy. In contrast, another peptide called relaxin can be found in the corpus luteum of some species only during pregnancy, not during an estrous cycle. In a few species, such as the horse, relaxin is an endocrine product of the placenta, not the corpus luteum. From these observations it is obvious that the choice of tissue and the physiologic state during which tissues are obtained drastically influence the outcome. Additional problems in the identification of hormones are noted in Box 4–1.

What Do They Do?

As more and more molecules have become accepted as hormones, fairly comprehensive details of the range of activities of hormones have been established. The scope of hormonal action is amazingly broad and, for a given hormone, includes one or more of the following:

Box 4–1 Isolation of Hormones

Simple extracts may or may not contain the active principle, depending on the physicochemical nature of the hormone molecule. Very apolar *steroids* are virtually insoluble in aqueous solutions, so saline, for example, would not extract progesterone from the corpus luteum. In fact, the discovery of progesterone in 1929 depended in large part on the input of a student trained in organic chemistry who suggested to his professor to try an alcohol extraction in parallel with saline extraction of a mince of corpora lutea from pigs. Progesterone has high solubility in alcohol, and the student's ethanolic extract, but not the professor's aqueous extract, proved to contain the active principle that prevents abortion when injected into pregnant ovariectomized rabbits. There are many similar examples of difficulty in isolation and purification of hormones. Human prolactin is a good example of a case in which indirect physiologic evidence strongly suggested the existence of the hormone, but efforts to purify the protein took nearly 30 years before the goal was realized. Finally, because of the insensitivity of the biologic assays that were used almost exclusively before the last 10 to 15 years, it has only recently become a fairly simple matter to detect arteriovenous increases in concentration across a gland of secretion.

---

1. *Morphological changes:* Many gross changes in form, such as the differences in body shape between adult males and females or between intact and gonadectomized adults, are familiar examples.

2. *Cell division and differentiation:* Many hormones are specific mitogens for particular tissues—that is, the hormone stimulates accelerated rates of cell division. Differentiation is the process whereby daughter cells have different properties, such as cell structure or function, from the parent cell. In many cases the triggering signal is the presence of a particular hormone, or a group of hormones, just before the time of mitosis. Presumably, as a result, new genes are expressed or others are suppressed in the daughter cells.

3. *Protein synthesis:* There are numerous examples of increased synthesis of particular proteins being controlled by hormones, again presumably because new genes are exposed for expression. In addition, some hormones serve to stimulate protein synthesis in a more general manner. An example is the effect of some regulators in assembling ribosomes into polysome complexes to facilitate assembly of amino acids into proteins.

4. *Enzyme regulation:* This is an important end point in hormone action and may involve activation or inactivation of enzymes regulating anabolic or catabolic processes or more subtle enzyme adjustments. Some of these actions are direct, but many involve second messengers that mediate the action of the hormone within the cell.

5. *Stimulation of contractions:* Smooth muscle is, in many instances, subject to stimulatory control by hormonal agonists, or may be inhibited, or rendered quiescent, by hormonal antagonists. These actions may also be noted in muscle-like cells. For example, the myoepithelial cells of mammary tissue are stellate, contractile cells that surround the secretory units in mammary tissue. The hormone oxytocin is capable of provoking contraction of the myoepithelium to elicit milk ejection.

6. *Control of exocrine secretion:* First described for the control by secretin, a peptide hormone from the intestinal mucosa, of pancreatic secretions, this is a broad class of actions that is par-

ticularly important throughout the gastrointestinal tract.

7. *Control of endocrine secretions:* Several examples can be found of one hormone controlling the secretion of other hormones. This control may be either stimulatory or inhibitory. As a general phenomenon, it is especially important in the amplification processes characteristic of endocrine communication. It is also the mechanistic basis for feedback controls that can be expected in hormone systems.

8. *Regulation of ion movements across membranes:* Certain hormones act by chemically regulating ion channels in membranes and facilitating the redistribution of ions between the extracellular space and the inside of cells. Such actions at the cell membrane level probably underlie many of the actions already described, such as agonist or antagonist effects on motile cells.

9. *Control of permeability to water:* The flux of water between the urinary tubule and interstitial space within the kidney is in part controlled by antidiuretic hormone (ADH), also known as vasopressin. In the final stages of processing the contents of the kidney tubule into urine, water is recovered into the body, but only in the presence of ADH.

10. *Effects on behavior:* Some sex-related behavioral characteristics are quite clearly hormone-based though they are very complex. Long-term actions may be difficult to analyze because the critical event may involve the hormone having an effect during brain maturation, perhaps even before birth, but the consequences are noted much later. Hormones regulate maternal behaviors such as nesting activity, broodiness, protective activity, and the like. A new class of hormones has been recently discovered that seems responsible for pain tolerance.

How Do They Do It?

Hormone action is the most exciting area of investigative endocrinology and new discoveries have broad implications for the diagnosis and

management of disease, drug engineering, and for broadening our approach to understanding the very nature of chemical regulation of growth, differentiation, and control of function. Knowledge of this kind provides the rational basis for manipulation of animal performance.

In most cases, hormones act at specific target tissues and do so in a characteristic way. Some hormones have rather generalized targets but the response nevertheless is quite predictable. There is usually a well-defined relationship between the concentration of a hormone and the magnitude of the response. A similar pattern is also observed if the hormone is injected into test animals in different-sized doses. In both cases the phenomenon is called the *dose-response relationship* (Figure 4–2). The general characteristics of dose-response patterns provide clues about the mode of action. First, there is a *minimal dose* or concentration below which no response is discernible. Second, there is a *maximum dose* or con-

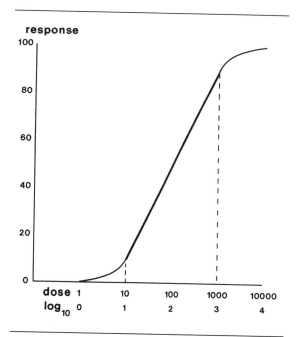

Figure 4–2. The dose-response relationship. This S-shaped, or sigmoidal, curve is typical of hormone responses when the dose of hormone is plotted on a logarithmic scale. The response, over a part of the range from minimal to maximal, bears a linear relationship to the $\log_{10}$ dose.

centration above which no further increase in response is obtained. Between the minimally effective dose and maximally effective dose is the *effective dose-response range*, and it usually spans about 1.5 to 2 orders of magnitude; a 35- to 100-fold range. The characteristics of the dose-response relationship provide the basis for bioassays, as described in Box 4–2.

Most of the characteristics of the dose-response relationship result from hormones acting only after combining with specific recognition sites, or *receptors*, in the target tissues. Receptors are analogous to locks. A key is only effective when used in the appropriate lock. A hormone is only effective when it can combine with the appropriate receptor. The receptor *transduces* the endocrine signal into the response system. Just as for other biologic transducers, hormone receptors serve to *filter* out the signal carried by the sole hormone of importance, then they initiate a very specific and predictable *response* to that signal.

Receptors will be considered in more detail later in this chapter. At this stage it is sufficient to note that if a particular tissue does not possess receptors to a given hormone, it cannot be a target tissue for that hormone. Conversely, if receptors can be identified in a tissue, there is every likelihood that the tissue is indeed a target for the given hormone.

Receptors are dynamic entities that may be present in some but not all physiologic states. The first appearance of receptors in tissues during development, or ontogeny, is an important regulatory event that may initiate new function in an organ or tissue, or may cause differentiation and the beginnings of a new organ or tissue.

Various systems of classification have been proposed to describe receptors and types of hormone action; all have shortcomings. It is most useful to classify hormones and their actions by the *chronobase*, or time course of their activity. Accordingly, hormones can be separated into *messengers* and *maintenance* types.

Primary or messenger hormones display a rapid onset of action, often within seconds. The action is of short duration, minutes at most. The response is obtained only while the hormone is present at the target; there is no carryover effect. Most primary or messenger hormones employ intracellular mediators, or *second messengers*, such as cyclic 3'5'-adenosine monophosphate (cAMP) (see Figure 3–27), or in some cases the action is mediated by calcium ions. Second messengers or mediators amplify the hormone signal and are subject to very precise control within the target cell.

The other major group is the secondary or maintenance hormones. Previously these were called trophic or growth-promoting hormones,

---

Box 4–2   Dose-Response Curves and Bioassays

For reasons that are incompletely understood, the response often relates linearly to the logarithm of the dose, so reference is often made to the *log-dose–response relationship*. For statistical reasons, the minimally effective dose and maximally effective dose cannot be measured with precision because beyond these limits, the responses are flat, or plateau values. Within the effective dose-response range, the slope of the line relating response to log-dose can be estimated accurately and statistical tests can be made to determine if a number of substances bring about the same response. The testing of unknowns for hormone activity initially depended totally on *biologic assays*, or *bioassays*, in which the biologic response observed in test animals served as the end point.

but not all of the actions can be described in this way. In contrast to messenger hormones, maintenance hormones exhibit a slow onset of action. The action is persistent and may continue long after the hormone has been degraded or left the tissue. Many of the maintenance hormones are *mitogens* for the target cells, or they may regulate gene expression in the synthesis of proteins. Finally, the action of these hormones seems not to depend on mediation by second messengers such as cAMP or Ca^{2+}.

4.2 • The Nature and Synthesis of Hormones

The hormones represent a diverse array of chemical classes of molecules, ranging in size from about 100 daltons to large proteins of more than 30,000 daltons. The size and other physicochemical properties of the molecules are important in relation to the methods of synthesis, secretion, transport, site of action, and method of elimination, all bearing on hormonal regulation.

The largest group of hormonally active molecules includes several chemical forms of a size between 100 and 1,000 daltons. They include *biogenic amines; peptides*, or small polymers of amino acids; *thyronines*, the iodine-containing hormones of the thyroid; *steroids;* and *prostanoids*, derivatives of long chain polyunsaturated fatty acids, especially arachidonic acid.

The Biogenic Amines

The simplest group of molecules are the *biogenic amines* (Figure 4–3), some of which are paracrines, some are neurotransmitters, and some are classic hormones. Paracrines are molecules that serve as local chemical mediators. Their actions share much with hormones in conveying information and in exerting control. They are 100

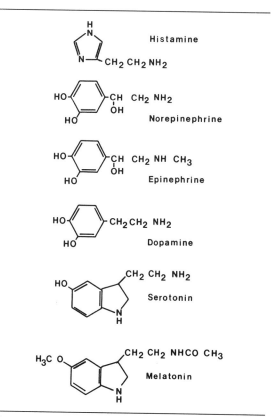

Figure 4–3. Biogenic amines. All the molecules shown serve as endocrines, paracrines, or neurotransmitters. They represent the simplest forms of information-carrying molecules in mammalian systems.

to 200 daltons in size and are distinguished from each other by the number, type, and location of *functional groups* on the molecule. Of this group, the catecholamines—dopamine, norepinephrine, and epinephrine—are derivatives of catechol, a dihydroxy-substituted benzene. The synthesis of epinephrine from norepinephrine is shown in Figure 4–4. This synthesis occurs predominantly in the medullary portion of the adrenal gland, a key part of the sympathetic nervous system. Interestingly, the ability to transform norepinephrine into epinephrine depends on an action of one of the steroid hormone products of the adrenal cortex.

The Peptides

Peptides are the smaller members of a wide range of polymers of amino acids that extend through to the massive proteins consisting of hundreds of amino acids. The smallest peptide hormone is thyrotropin-releasing hormone, an unusual tripeptide with just three amino acids that mediates hypothalamic control over the secretion of thyrotropin, or thyroid-stimulating hormone, from the pituitary. Thyrotropin may also contribute to the control of secretion of growth hormone and prolactin. The isolation and purification of thyrotropin-releasing hormones from hundreds of thousands of ovine hypothalamic fragments, then its subsequent structural analysis (Figure 4–5), enabling total chemical synthesis, was a major breakthrough in endocrinology in the late 1960s. The brain opiate peptides, including the enkephalins, are pentapeptides of 500 to 600 daltons.

An important pair of peptide hormones of about 1,000 daltons consists of oxytocin and ADH. They are structurally very similar, with only minor amino acid substitutions. Several very similar hormones sharing some of their biologic actions are found in more primitive vertebrates, which suggests that the evolutionary origin of these peptides is quite ancient. The examples in Figure 4–6 both possess a *disulfydryl* (S-S) linkage which creates a ring configuration. The integrity of rings such as these is critical for the biologic potency of many peptide and protein hormones. This is presumably because the receptor molecule requires the hormone to have a particular shape in order to bind it.

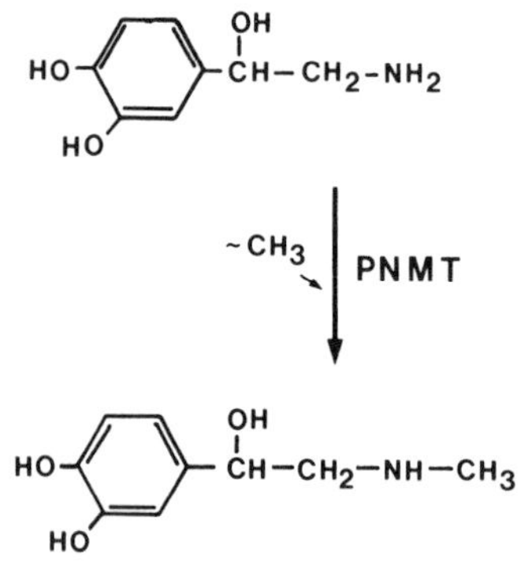

Figure 4–4. *Epinephrine synthesis.* Epinephrine is synthesized by the methylation of the primary amine group on norepinephrine. The enzyme responsible, phenylethanolamine-N-methyl transferase (PNMT), is found in highest concentrations in the adrenal medulla. The control of PNMT by cortisol, a steroid hormone of the adrenal cortex, will be described later as an example of one hormone controlling the synthesis of another.

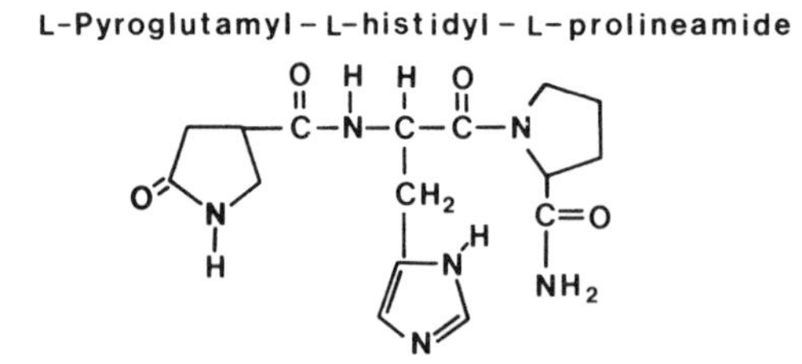

Figure 4–5. *Thyrotropin releasing factor/hormone (TRF).* This simple tripeptide structure is a hormone of the hypothalamus that regulates the synthesis and release of thyroid stimulating hormone from the pituitary gland. In addition, TRF may contribute to the control of secretion of growth hormone and prolactin. It was the first of the hypothalamic releasing factors to be analyzed structurally and to be prepared in mass quantities by chemical synthesis.

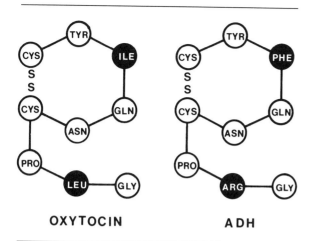

OXYTOCIN   A DH

Figure 4–6. Peptides of the posterior pituitary. Oxytocin and antidiuretic hormone (ADH), the most common examples of posterior pituitary peptides, are closely related structurally and exhibit some overlaps in function. Note that these two peptides differ in only two of their constituent amino acids.

Other peptides, ranging in size from 750 to 2,000 daltons, come from a variety of sources and evoke widely divergent actions. Some are additional examples of *releasing factors*, or hormones from the hypothalamus that seem to be solely concerned with the regulation of the secretory function of the anterior pituitary gland. The known members of this family will be described later in this chapter. Peptides of this size range can be readily synthesized once the amino acid sequence of the natural hormone is known. Peptide chemists can make a variety of changes in the sequence of amino acids to create synthetic analogues. These compounds are of great interest because some are extremely potent agonists while others may be potent antagonists to the natural hormone. Hormones engineered in this way are used in human medicine and have some potential as modifiers of animal performance.

Some peptides are derived from *precursor proteins* in the plasma, and they are cleaved off very specifically by regulator enzymes. These may not correspond to the classic definition of hormones, but they unquestionably carry information and elicit specific responses in target cells

by exactly the same mechanisms as those used by hormones generally. *Bradykinin* and *angiotensin* are examples of such peptides that influence the degree of constriction of small blood vessels, thereby influencing blood flow and contributing to the maintenance of arterial blood pressure.

Larger polypeptides and proteins, ranging upward from about 2,000 daltons, are described below.

The Thyronines

The thyronines are the major hormones of the thyroid gland (see Figure 1–8). Thyronines are substituted tyrosyl-tyrosines (Figure 4–7), having four iodines on thyroxine (T_4) and three iodines on triiodothyronine (T_3). Much of the T_3 is produced in peripheral tissues by enzymatic deiodination of T_4. The major form of thyroid hormone in the circulation is T_4, found in association with thyroxine-binding globulin. This is an example of a plasma-binding protein, or carrier, that transports the hormone and buffers, or stabilizes, the plasma concentrations of the free form. Being protein bound also protects the hormone from rapid elimination from the body; indeed, T_4 has one of the longest half-times of any of the hormones. The half-time is a measure of the kinetics of elimination of a molecule. It is the time required for reducing a given concentration by half. For the small ruminants, the half-time for clearance of T_4 is in excess of 24 hours. Thyroid hormones are maintenance hormones involved in regulating growth and other biosynthetic processes and in governing the efficiency of metabolic events, thereby influencing heat production.

The Steroid Hormones

Steroid hormones are all derivatives of cholesterol (Figure 2–30) and they exhibit a wide array

Figure 4–7. Thyroid hormones. The thyronines are derivatives of tyrosine, a phenolic amino acid (top). Thyroxine (T_4) is synthesized via diiodotyrosine within the thyroid gland. Triiodothyronine (T_3) is subsequently formed in peripheral tissues by selective removal of one of the iodines. The most important use of iodine (or iodide) in the body is in the synthesis of these hormones.

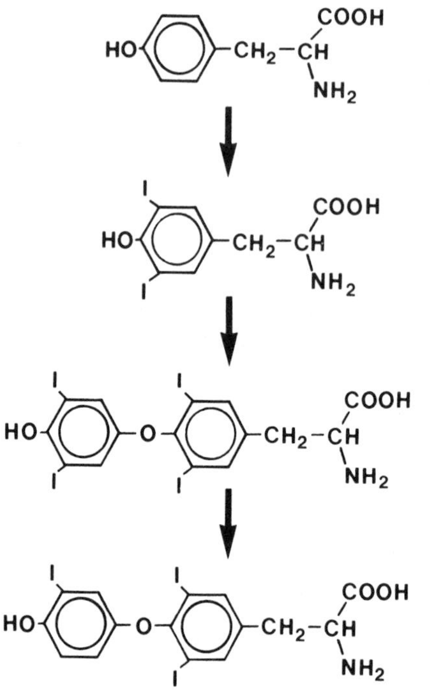

of substitutions that confer upon them their biologic activities. Families of similar molecules exist, and the steroids were first classified on the basis of their type of activity and the tissues of origin. Such a classification (Table 4–1) is still useful though distinct overlaps exist in both activity and sources in the body.

The Adrenal Steroids

Adrenal corticosteroids are produced in the outer or *cortical* region of the adrenal gland (Figure 4–8). Two major classes can be distinguished, with the glucocorticoids having effects on metabolism, differentiation, and an important stress-protection role, including anti-inflammatory actions. They play a critical integrating function in the fetus, coordinating a diverse series of maturational changes shortly before birth.

The mineralocorticoids are primarily concerned in the regulation of the ionic composition of the extracellular fluids because they contribute to the control of excretion of Na^+ and K^+

Table 4–1. The Steroid Hormones

Steroids of the adrenal cortex
    Glucocorticoids (e.g., cortisol)
    Mineralocorticoids (e.g., aldosterone)
Gonadal and placental steroids
    Androgens (e.g., testosterone)
    Estrogens (e.g., estradiol)
    Progestins (e.g., progesterone)

and, to a lesser extent, excretion of other ions in the kidney.

Of the wide array of steroids making up these two classes, *cortisol* is the most important glucocorticoid and *aldosterone* is the most important mineralocorticoid.

The Gonadal Steroids

The gonadal steroids are perhaps misnamed because they can be produced by the adrenal cortex

Figure 4–8. The adrenal gland. Adrenals are paired, bean-shaped glands located just cranial to the kidneys (see Figures 4–1 and 5–20) on the dorsal wall of the abdominal cavity. In most species, they are found close to the major trunk blood vessels. The gland is surrounded by a capsule (Cp$_L$, overlying the cortex (shown sectioned above and fractured below) and the inner medullary portion. The cortex is organized as zones. The zona glomerulosus (ZG), for example, is mainly concerned with synthesis of mineralocorticosteroids, and the zona fasicularis (ZF) is the source from which most glucocorticoids derive. The cells of the cortex form columns, adjacent to centripetally-draining sinusoids (SI). These vessels drain into the medulla, which is actually a specialized part of the sympathetic nervous system. In the lower figure, cells of the cortex appear to be extensively vacuolated as a result of the extraction of lipids (granules of steroids awaiting secretion); their close proximity to the capillaries (Ca) is apparent. (Reproduced by permission of the publisher. From Kessel, R.G. and Kardon, R.H.: *Tissues and Organs: A Text-Atlas of Scanning Electron Microscopy,* San Francisco: W.H. Freeman and Company, 1979.)

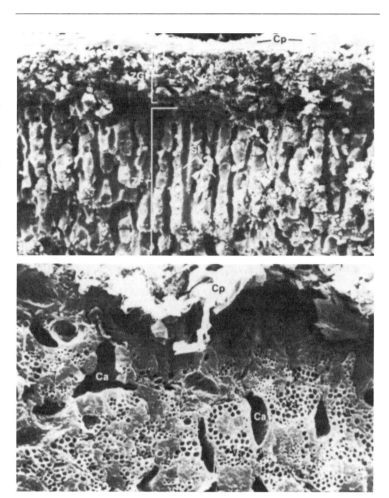

and the placenta of many species. As broad classes, androgens are male sex steroids, although females can and do produce them; estrogens are female sex steroids, though also present in males; and progestins are progestational, or pregnancy-protecting, steroids that can be present in males as well as females.

Steroid Synthesis

The overlaps implied by the preceding heavily qualified remarks result from the fact that steroid synthesis in vivo proceeds from class to class, and opportunity always exists for spill-out of the intermediate compounds at any stage. The steroids are manufactured from cholesterol by well-understood enzymic conversions. For present purposes an abbreviated outline will suffice. First, cholesterol is converted to the 21-carbon compound pregnenolone by cleaving off the side chain beyond C$_{20}$. Pregnenolone may be oxidized by giving up two hydrogen atoms at C$_3$ and rearranged to form progesterone (Figure 4–9). An alternate fate for pregnenolone is hydroxylation of C$_{17}$ by the enzyme 17-hydroxylase and, just as in the previous example, this enzyme is able to make similar modifications to other substrates, such as progesterone. These

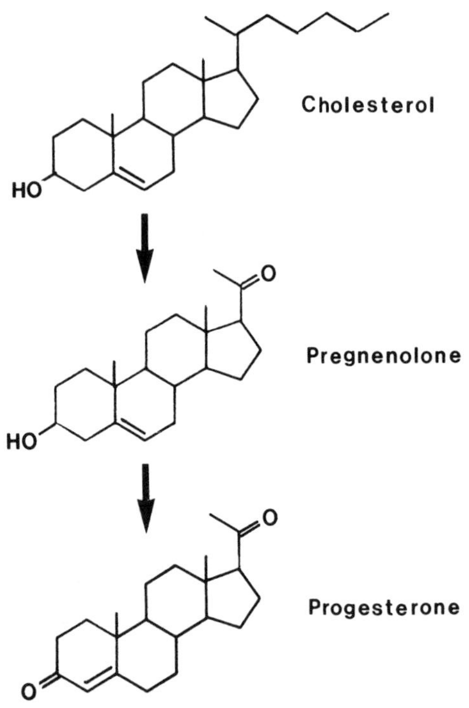

Figure 4–9. *Progesterone synthesis.* Acetate is the basic substrate used to construct cholesterol; however, the sterol is also taken in from the diet. Cholesterol is processed by removal of the side chain to yield pregnenolone. Oxidation at C_3 and relocation of the double bond from the B–ring to the A–ring produce progesterone.

initial transformations of the common precursor pregnenolone take place in all *steroidogenic* tissues at some time or other.

Further transformation of these progestins (progesterone, pregnenolone, and their 17-hydroxy derivatives) into corticosteroids occurs exclusively in the adrenal cortex. The steps involve additional hydroxylations and oxidations (Figure 4–10). Aldosterone is produced from corticosterone.

Androgens are produced from 17-hydroxy-progestins by conversion by a lyase, or C-C cleavage, reaction between C_{17} and C_{20}. The products are 19-carbon steroids that serve as androgens, or male sex steroids. The final important step in androgen synthesis is reduction of

the 17-ketone to a 17-hydroxy group, in either the β form to yield testosterone or in its relatively inactive 17α epimer called epitestosterone. Testosterone is the most potent naturally occurring androgen. The enzyme responsible for its formation is 17-hydroxysteroid dehydrogenase (Figure 4–11). Further interconversion is possible in some tissues with the formation of estrogens.

The A ring in estrogens has undergone a rearrangement called *aromatization*. The final structure, with a hydroxyl on C_3 and the unsaturated A ring (Figure 4–12), is like phenol, so the main estrogens are called *phenolic steroids*. As was the case for interconversions of androgens, estrone is interconvertible with estradiol-17β, or its very weak epimer estradiol-17α (see Figure 4–12). Estradiol-17β is the most potent naturally occurring estrogen.

Summary of Steroids

- All steroids are derived from cholesterol via the obligatory intermediate, pregnenolone.

- Pregnenolone is converted to progesterone and then to corticosteroids or androgens.

- Estrogens are formed by aromatization of androgens.

- There is considerable flexibility in substrates for particular enzymic conversions.

After a glance at the various structures of the steroidal hormones, it will be quite evident that hormones comprising a class with particular biologic activity, such as the progestins, the androgens, and the estrogens, have similarities in overall structure. The substitutions confer the basic physicochemical properties on these molecules, and relatively simple changes can rapidly inactivate the steroid (Figure 4–13). Such changes may also make them prone to further metabolic processing to facilitate excretion. For example, many steroids are *conjugated* with sulfuric acid or sugars in the liver, and the products are markedly more water soluble, in addition to being inactivated. As they become more polar, they no longer travel in the blood associated with

Figure 4–10. *Adrenal steroids.* Pregnenolone and progesterone are subjected to very extensive hydroxylation reactions in the adrenal cortex to give rise to the adrenal corticosteroids. In the example shown, progesterone (Prog) is hydroxylated at C_{21} to produce 11-deoxycorticosterone (11-DOC), and then hydroxylated at C_{11} to produce corticosterone (B). Hydroxylation at C_{17} produces cortisol (F), or rearrangement of C_{18} into an aldehyde produces aldosterone (Aldo). Some of the adrenal steroids are largely glucocorticoid in action (for example, B and F) while others are mainly mineralocorticoid (for example, Aldo and 11-DOC), as detailed in the text.

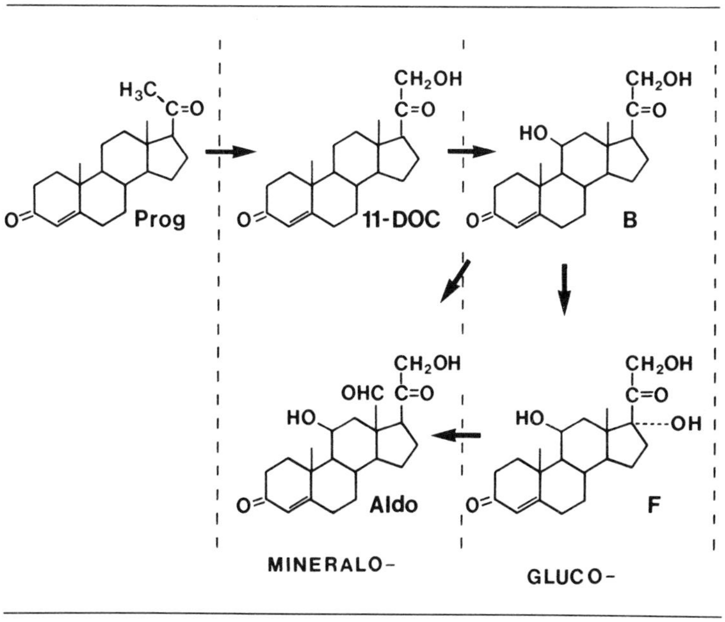

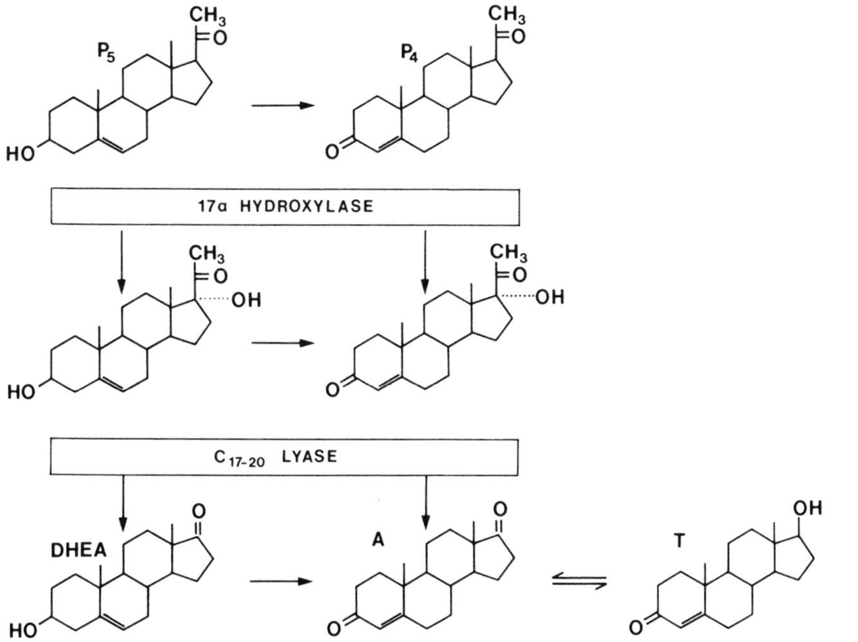

Figure 4–11. *Androgens.* The synthesis and interconversions of the male sex steroids involve hydroxylation of a progestin precursor at C_{17}, loss of the C_{19} and C_{20} sidechain, and oxidative or reductive events at C_3 and C_{17}. The Δ^5 pathway converts pregnenolone (P_5) to its 17α-hydroxy derivative and then to dehydroepiandrosterone (DHEA). The same enzymes can convert progesterone (P_4) to androstenedione (A) via the Δ^4 pathway. Androstenedione and testosterone (T) are interconverted readily by oxidoreduction at C_{17}.

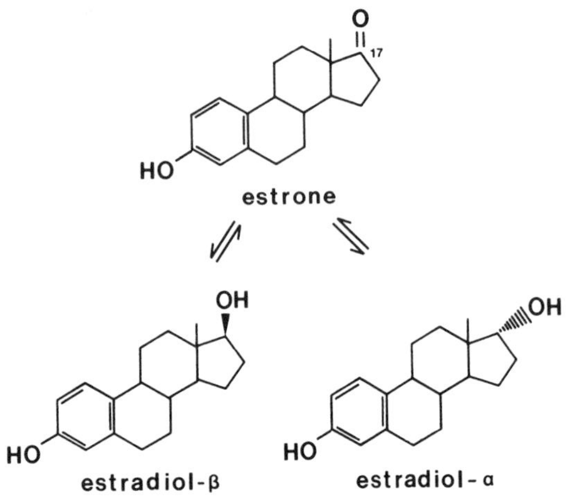

Figure 4–12. *Estrogen interconversions.* Estrone, the 17-keto compound, may be reduced to either estradiol-17α or to estradiol-17β, by addition of hydrogens at C_{17}. Note the rearrangement of the A–ring into a phenol-like structure in these naturally occurring estrogens. The hydroxyl group at C_{17} in estradiol may be standing out from the plane of the paper (the β form), or the reverse (the α form). Estradiol-17β is about 10 times more potent as an estrogen than is estrone, and about 100 times more potent than estradiol-17α.

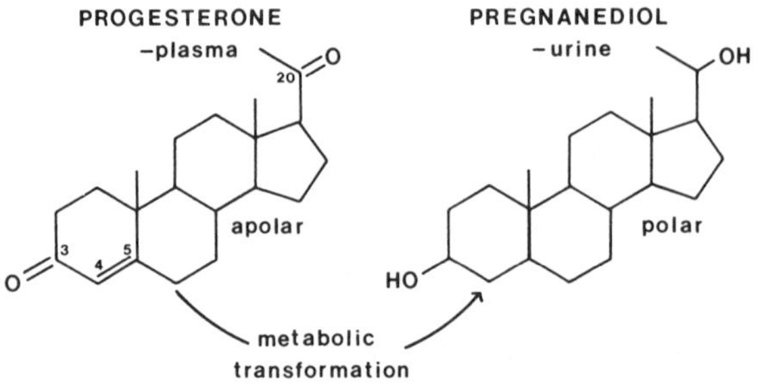

Figure 4–13. *Steroid metabolism.* Inactivation of progesterone involves reductions, or additions of hydrogens, at C_3 and C_{20}, and saturation of the double bond at C_4. The more polar product, pregnanediol, is markedly more water soluble, has little biological potency, and because it does not associate tightly with serum proteins, it is readily filtered by the kidney and excreted into the urine.

carrier proteins, and this makes them more readily filtered at the kidney. In their original active form, the steroids are relatively apolar and they associate in plasma with hydrophobic domains on serum albumin, or with specific binding sites on specific carrier globulins. In this bound form, the effective size of the steroid is in excess of 60,000 to 70,000 daltons, instead of 350 or so. The large complex cannot be filtered, but a molecule of 350 to 500 daltons—the size typical of steroid sulfates or glucuronic acid conjugates—is filtered very efficiently.

The Prostanoids

Another class of hormones, or paracrines, of special importance are the prostanoids. The original discoveries were made on materials extracted from accessory male sex glands, but in recent years many members of this family have been found in virtually every tissue in the body. They are highly specialized fatty acids derived ultimately from arachidonic acid, a constituent of many polar lipids, especially common in the 2 position of many lecithins. Arachidonic acid ($C_{20:4}$) is a derivative of arachidic acid ($C_{20:0}$), which has four olefinic bonds. The fatty acid esterified to position 2 in the polar lipids is hydrolyzed by phospholipase A_2, a Ca^{2+}-dependent enzyme often localized inside lysosomes. Under certain conditions, including those of cell deterioration, lysosomes release their enzyme content. The lecithin, of course, is mainly found in the plasmalemma or other membranes of the cell. Free arachidonic acid, made available by the action of the phospholipase, is very rapidly converted into one or another prostanoid (Figure 4–14).

One major pathway begins with conversion by an enzyme complex called a *cyclooxygenase,* which can be inactivated by simple drugs such as aspirin or by other drugs called *nonsteroidal anti-inflammatory agents.* During recent years, an alternate pathway of arachidonic acid metabolism called the *lipoxygenase* pathway has been

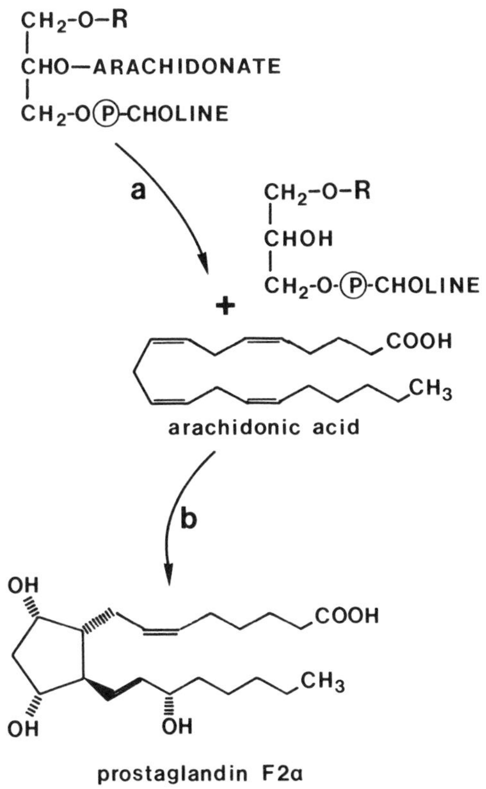

Figure 4–14. Prostanoid synthesis. The key steps in the synthesis of the family of prostaglandin-like molecules are shown here. Arachidonic acid is usually obtained by hydrolysis off a phospholipid, in this case a lecithin, by an appropriate phospholipase (reaction a). One important enzyme is Ca^{2+}-activated phospholipase A_2, which hydrolyzes lecithin into lysolecithin and a free fatty acid. The free arachidonate (shown folded for convenience) is subjected to a series of rearrangements and oxidations to form any of a variety of prostanoids (reaction b). Conversion of arachidonate to prostanoids is blocked by nonsteroidal anti-inflammatory drugs and antipyretic drugs such as aspirin. The product shown here, prostaglandin $F_{2\alpha}$, has important regulatory actions in reproduction (Chapter 10).

discovered. The products of arachidonic acid metabolism are varied and complex.

The prostanoids seem to be more active as local hormones, or paracrines, than as typical circulating hormones; and normal distribution to distant tissues via the circulation is problematic. This is because the lung is capable of rapidly deactivating many prostaglandins and only a small fraction of those entering the venous circulation after secretion from the tissues escape pulmonary destruction before they reach the arterial blood and have access to distal target tissues.

Polypeptide and Protein Hormones

Polypeptides range in size up to 10,000 to 15,000 daltons. There are too many to describe in detail at this time, but the group includes some hormones of the gastrointestinal tract, those of the pancreas, additional brain and pituitary hormones, and some from the thyroid and parathyroid glands. The parathyroids are usually located as a pair just beside the lobes of the thyroid. The various hormones and their functions will be described in later sections of this and other chapters.

Peptides of this size consist of up to 100 amino acids in strict sequence, and the opportunities for substitutions on the molecules, arrangements of polar and apolar domains, and special conformations that favor interaction with receptors are quite extensive. The same is true for the protein hormones or those with molecular sizes of 20,000 daltons or greater. These molecules may be single peptide chains or may consist of two *subunit* proteins. Many of them are heavily glycosylated, and so are called *glycoproteins*. They include the majority of the pituitary hormones and some placental proteins from certain species.

Polypeptide and protein hormones are best considered to form families of related molecules. For example, there is a group of hormones and hormone-like factors that are closely related, both structurally and functionally, to insulin (Figure 4–15). Included are insulin, relaxin, nerve growth factor, and the somatomedins, or insulin-like

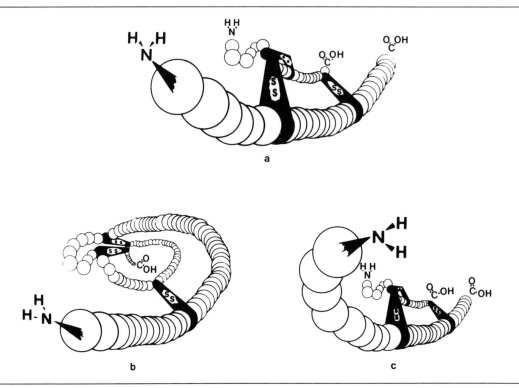

Figure 4–15. Insulin-like peptides. Three members of a family of similar molecules have some structural and activity characteristics in common. Insulin *(a)*, a well known hormone of the pancreas, is involved in metabolism through the regulation of substrate availability to cells. Nerve Growth Factor *(b)*, a regulatory factor, mainly influences hypertrophic expansion of neurons during nervous system development. Relaxin *(c)*, a hormone, or paracrine, of the reproductive tract, is predominately concerned with connective tissue turnover and regulation of reproductive smooth muscle. Note the similarity in location of the disulfydryl bonds and the general correspondence of the helical structure in the author's somewhat fictional drawings.

growth factors. These will be described later. Similarly the glycoproteins, thyroid-stimulating hormone (TSH), luteinizing hormone (LH), and follicle-stimulating hormone (FSH), along with human chorionic gonadotropin (hCG), are all very similar molecules. Indeed, one of their two subunits, the alpha subunit, is identical for all four hormones. The other subunit is solely responsible for hormone specificity. Even then, LH and hCG have identical biologic activities, but the latter hormone is normally present only during pregnancy.

4.3 • Mechanisms of Hormone Action

The Hormone Receptor

Some general characteristics of hormone action were introduced earlier, along with some broad categories of types of responses in the target tissues. Most hormone action can now be explained on the basis of what is known of the hormone receptors, so this section provides a fairly comprehensive overview of the receptor.

The receptor may be viewed as a *chemical transducer* that must be present in a tissue if that tissue is to be a target for the hormone of interest. Next, the receptor provides *selectivity* in the response system because it may be capable of interacting with a single hormone molecule or, at most, a very limited array of hormones with similar actions. For example, receptors for growth hormone can be occupied by growth hormones and some placental lactogens, but not by any other type of protein hormone. Third, the receptor may confer *specificity*; that is, the nature of the response to a given hormone's stimulation. The catecholamines introduced earlier bring about quite distinct responses in different tissues, depending on the precise nature of the adrenoreceptor in each of those tissues. For example, catecholamines stimulate heart muscle but may either contract or relax vascular smooth muscle. Different adrenoreceptors dictate that the target tissues react to the same stimulus in quite different ways.

Another aspect of specificity is to assure that the response is predictable, irrespective of how it is provoked. When steroid hormones were described, there were several examples of classes of steroid containing very weak and very potent members. The estrogen receptor, for example, can be occupied by estrone or estradiol-17β, and both steroids can bring about characteristic es-

trogen actions, because the receptor dictates specificity of response.

Many receptors are functionally coupled to enzyme systems that can provide great *amplification* within the response pathway. For example, some actions of catecholamines depend on the occupied adrenoreceptor being able to stimulate adenylate cyclase, the enzyme responsible for producing 3'5'-cAMP. The cyclase is located in the plasmalemma, close to the adrenoreceptor. A single catecholamine molecule occupies a single receptor at a given moment, yet hundreds or perhaps thousands of molecules of cAMP may be generated by this single molecule, thereby achieving amplification in the response pathway.

Location of Receptors

Receptors appear to be located within the plasmalemma or within the cytoplasm of the target cell. Those in the membrane are presumably proteins on the external face that are freely accessible to hormones present in the extracellular fluid. This is appropriate for large proteins that would not be able to gain access to the cytoplasm by diffusion through the membrane. Similarly, small but very polar molecules are unlikely to be able to pass through the hydrophobic interior of the membrane. The hormone molecules that are quite apolar, such as the steroids, can and do diffuse through membranes, and their receptors are located inside the target cells.

The location of receptors is consistent with the various mechanisms that couple the receptor to the response system. In the previously noted adenylate cyclase amplification system, the hormones and receptors that regulate adenylate cyclase have their primary interactions in the membrane, where this enzyme is located (Figure 4–16). Some hormones act by altering mem-

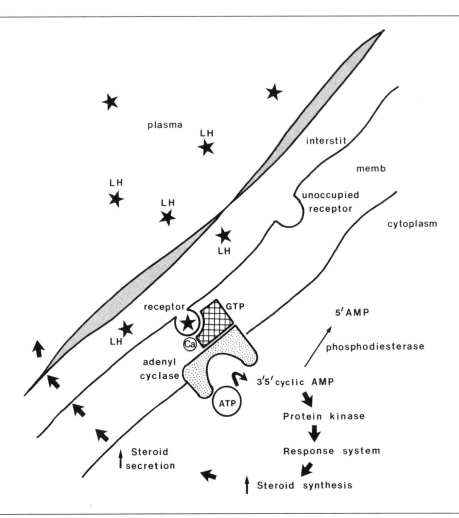

Figure 4–16. *3'5'-cyclic AMP mediation of hormone action.* Some hormones bind to receptors in the plasma membrane that are functionally coupled to adenylate cyclase. The coupling involves Ca^{2+} ions and GTP, a high-energy-containing compound related to ATP. The cAMP produced from ATP by the cyclase serves as an intracellular messenger to the response system. In many instances, cAMP activates another enzyme, protein kinase, which then phosphorylates proteins, including additional enzymes, to modify their function. The cAMP is also subject to rapid inactivation by enzymes that, in turn, are sensitive to common stimulant drugs such as caffeine. For example, luteinizing hormone (LH) acts by this mechanism in gonadal cells to influence the synthesis and secretion of steroid hormones.

brane permeability to particular ions such as Ca^{2+}, another second messenger. Again, if membrane channels mediate this response, it is logical that the hormone receptor is also located in the membrane.

Another aspect relates to the processes that terminate the action of the hormone. When the neuromuscular junction was described in Chapter 3, it was noted that acetylcholinesterase was an integral constituent of the motor end-plate and served to degrade the neurotransmitter after activating Na$^+$ channels in the muscle cell. Similar situations occur in endocrine systems, especially when the hormone is one of the primary or messenger hormones that have acute effects. The action has to be terminated quickly so that precise control can be achieved, and the most certain way to terminate the action is to degrade the hormone near the site of action. This certainly seems to be the case for catecholamines, but it is less certain for other messengers, partly because the methods of degradation are poorly understood. Steroid hormones that have been noted to react with cytoplasmic receptors are also degraded within the cell, usually by enzymes in the endoplasmic reticulum.

Nature of Receptors

Receptors are *macromolecules* that are conformationally mobile: they can move and change their overall shape and form. At least one form of the molecule is capable of enclosing the hormone to which it is receptive, and it can be demonstrated that this form is its most stable configuration. The receptor is most stable when bound to its hormone. Some details of receptor-hormone association are provided in Box 4–3.

By use of the methods outlined in Box 4–3, the *receptor populations* in different tissue and cell types can be determined, and it is quite evident that receptor numbers are themselves subject to regulation. The most striking consequences of

---

Box 4–3   The Behavior of Receptors

The binding of a hormone by its receptor occurs more readily than unbinding, or dissociation of the receptor-hormone complex. As for other simple binding systems, the receptor can be called the *binder* and the hormone can be called the *ligand*. The interaction of receptor and hormone is not energy dependent, so it is called *passive*. It is, however, concentration dependent and reversible, with the various forms of the reactants satisfying an equilibrium:

$$\text{Receptor} + \text{Hormone} \rightleftharpoons$$
$$\text{Receptor-Hormone Complex}$$

The equilibrium more correctly applies to concentrations, symbolized by [ ], though concentration of a constituent within a lipoprotein membrane is a rather abstract notion.

$$[R] + [H] \rightleftharpoons [RH]$$

This has two component parts:

$$[R] + [H] \rightarrow [RH] \quad \text{or association,}$$

and

$$[RH] \rightarrow [R] + [H] \text{ or dissociation.}$$

Equilibrium is the balance established between the two and, in addition to concentrations, time is a factor, because the association part-reaction has faster kinetics and proceeds more rapidly than does the dissociation part-reaction. If sufficient time is allowed for the differences in kinetics to be accommodated and it is assumed that the reactants, H, R, and HR, are perfectly stable and not degraded by the mechanisms described earlier, the equilibrium can be examined and the receptor population can be quantified. Such *receptor analyses* have been possible during the past decade.

the dynamic nature of receptors show up in a number of previously unexplained pathologies (Box 4–4).

In nonpathologic situations, marked variation in receptor numbers may occur, and factors underlying the dynamic nature of the receptors are starting to become known. One basis for change in receptor number is simply that of *ontogeny:* receptors may be absent until a specific *stage in development* is reached. For example, despite the high concentrations of growth hormone in fetal sheep blood, there seem to be no receptors present in liver, the key target tissue for this hormone during postnatal life, until some days after birth. The reverse is also true: receptors may disappear when the animal reaches a particular developmental stage. One form of receptor regulation occurring dynamically in target tissues can be called *autoregulation.* In this case the hormone itself is the cause of altered numbers of its own receptor. When the presence of the hormone acts to increase numbers of receptors, the term *up-regulation* is used. *Down-regulation* describes the situation when the presence of the hormone causes a decrease in receptor number. Examples of receptor regulation are provided in Box 4–5.

A wide variety of interactions occur between hormones. The classic examples are *synergism* and *antagonism.* For example, consider a response, say the weight of a tissue, that is af-

fected by two hormones, either together or separately. Synergism describes the situation in which the response to the two hormones is greater than the sum of the responses to each of the hormones when they act alone.

> For example, hormone A alone elicits a response of 10 units, and hormone B alone elicits the same kind of response, but of 6 units. Synergism exists when hormones A and B together bring about a response of greater than 16 (10 + 6) units (Figure 4–17).

When the hormones A and B elicit responses that oppose each other, they are said to be antagonistic. Hormone A might elevate plasma concentrations of glucose while hormone B might depress them: their actions are antagonistic.

Another interaction occurs when hormone A, while not bringing about a particular response, is nevertheless absolutely necessary for hormone B to elicit its response. For example, oxytocin stimulates uterine excitability and causes more frequent contractions, each of higher magnitude. It can only do so if the uterus has been exposed to estrogen. This was once called *priming:* the estrogen-primed uterus is responsive to oxytocin. It is now known that estrogen is responsible for the appearance of oxytocin receptors in the uterus. Estrogen itself cannot directly

---

Box 4–4 Pathologic Receptor Conditions

There is a form of *dwarfism* in humans, called Laron dwarfism, in which quite normal concentrations of growth hormone are present in the circulation. Dwarfism is usually due to abnormally low secretion rates and therefore circulating concentrations of pituitary growth hormone. Therapeutic administration of growth hormone to children of markedly short stature can usually promote growth and correct the problem. Laron dwarfs have no growth hormone receptors so their normal endogenous levels of growth hormone are ineffective.

Some forms of *diabetes mellitus* cannot be treated by injecting insulin. Patients in this situation are described as being insulin-resistant diabetics and many of them lack functional receptors.

Box 4–5 Dynamic Receptor Regulation

As an example of up-regulation, the number of estrogen receptors in estrogen target tissues is increased in response to estrogen exposure. Estrogens therefore promote the appearance of more estrogen receptors. Down-regulation is exemplified by many hormones, but is best known for gonadotropins such as LH. When LH targets are exposed to steady concentrations of LH, the number of receptors is quickly reduced. The explanation will be provided in detail later; for now it is sufficient to note that when LH binds to its receptor, the whole complex moves into the cell by a process called internalization. Fewer receptors are therefore left at the surface. The tissue is now less responsive than before to another exposure to the hormone. This provides yet another way of regulating the overall response of the control system.

Another method of receptor regulation entails *co-regulation*, whereby one hormone controls the number of receptors to another hormone, and the second hormone controls the receptors to the first. This is well exemplified by the major female gonadal steroids, estrogens and progestins. As noted earlier, estrogen promotes appearance of more estrogen receptors. It also stimulates the appearance of progesterone receptors. On the other hand, progesterone acts to reduce the numbers of both estrogen and progesterone receptors.

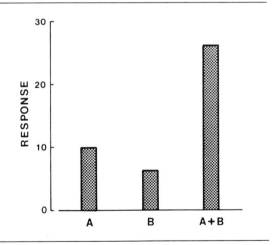

Figure 4–17. Synergism in hormone action. When given singly, hormones A and B evoke responses of 10 and 6 response units, respectively. The response to A plus B given together is 26, far in excess of the sum of the individual responses (10 + 6 = 16).

stimulate uterine contractions, but it does provide the receptors that enable oxytocin to stimulate the muscle. Actions such as the one described for estrogen may also be called permissive.

Receptor Activation

After the initial binding of hormone to receptor, a second process called *activation* is needed before a hormone response is obtained. Activation may involve triggering by the hormone-receptor complex of a second messenger system provided by adenylate cyclase and formation of 3'5'-cAMP. The receptor-hormone complex may serve to open chemically gated Ca^{2+} channels so that Ca^{2+} ions can flood into the cell to trigger Ca^{2+}-dependent processes such as vesicle fusion to the surface membrane, or Ca^{2+}-dependent acto-myosin interactions, as in muscle.

In steroid hormone action, the receptor-hormone complex, which forms in the cytoplasm, promptly *translocates* into the nucleus of the cell. This translocation cannot occur in the cold, despite the hormone and steroid being able to bind quite adequately, under laboratory conditions, at, say, 4 C. Immediately on warming to 37 C, the complex disappears from the cytoplasm and appears in the nucleus. This translocation step is therefore *energy dependent*. Recently, several membrane receptors to large, nondiffusible protein hormones have been found to move from the plasmalemma into the interior of the cell after occupancy by their appropriate hormones. This process, called *internalization*, is now partly understood and is described in some detail in Box 4–6.

Receptor Coupling

The final event needed for hormone action is the *coupling* of the activated receptor-hormone com-plex with the response system. This requirement is quite analogous to excitation-contraction coupling described for muscle. It has already been implied that elevated intracellular concentrations of 3'5'-cAMP or Ca^{2+} may mediate this coupling phenomenon. In one case, a group of enzymes called *protein kinases* serve to phosphorylate particular proteins to alter the properties of those proteins. The phosphate group is transferred from ATP to hydroxyl groups on serine or tyrosine, both of which are amino acids with hydroxyl groups, in substrate proteins. The protein kinases may be Ca^{2+} stimulated via the participation of calmodulin, the regulatory Ca^{2+} binder described in Box 3–8. Other protein kinases are cAMP dependent. In the presence of cAMP, the enzyme is activated and selected substrate proteins become phosphorylated. A number of hormone-regulated metabolic processes appear to be regulated in this fashion. Some enzymes are active only in the phosphorylated form; others may be active except when they are phosphorylated.

In the case of steroid hormones, the receptor-steroid complex translocates to the nucleus and interacts with the nuclear chromatin. The result is the selective *transcription* of portions of the DNA into specific messenger RNA (mRNA)

Box 4–6   Internalization of Receptors

When membranes were first described in Chapter 2, it was noted that some proteins are able to move laterally within the plane of the membrane. Some receptors, when occupied by their hormones, are activated and move to form *clusters* of receptor-hormone complexes at particular loci on the cell surface. Subsequently the membrane invaginates at these loci and *microvesicles* bud off and pass into the cytoplasm of the cell. These then fuse with lysosomes within the cell, and the hormones or receptors that have been internalized are processed by lysosomal enzymes. This mechanism provides an explanation for down-regulation. It also explains how some hormones are able to trigger a response inside the cell, even though their primary interaction with the receptor occurs at the plasmalemma, with no obvious participation of a second messenger. To do so requires that the processed hormone or receptor, now deep within the cell, initiate further regulatory events, perhaps at or near the nucleus. The details of such a proposed mechanism are not yet understood.

sequences. The mRNA leaves the nucleus to serve as a *template* at the ribosomes for protein synthesis. The hormone response then occurs as new proteins are synthesized, either to serve as enzymes in the target cell, to be anabolic constituents in steroid-controlled growth, or to be secreted as export proteins.

Many hormones are known to be *mitogens* for their target tissues, but very little is known about their precise mode of action. Presumably, using mechanisms similar to those already de-scribed, activation events must occur in the nucleus, but the result is *DNA replication* rather than transcription to mRNA. The cell cycle will be described in Chapter 8 and the phase when mitogens exert their actions will be identified. More complete clarification of this process during the next few years will become the most exciting part of endocrinology, with obvious consequences for growth biology, cancer biology, and animal science.

4.4 • Descriptive Endocrinology

This section provides a more conventional de-scription of the hormones of major interest in animal physiology. An attempt is made to sum-marize the nature, source, and principal actions of each of the hormones. The listing is certainly not complete and, given the rapidly changing nature of this field, it may not remain entirely accurate. The wide array of growth factors—molecules with demonstrable actions in various cell culture systems—includes some now well-accepted hormones, and these will be noted. Others still await adequate characterization before their role in vivo becomes established, and these will usually be omitted.

The Hypothalamic Hypophysiotropic Factors

These molecules are commonly called the hy-pothalamic releasing and inhibiting factors, or hormones, and most are peptides that are syn-thesized and secreted by hypothalamic cells into the *hypothalamo-hypophyseal portal system*. This is a local and highly specialized blood vascular bed that provides direct transport from part of the hypothalamus to the nearby anterior pituitary without passing back through the entire venous collection system (Figure 4–18). The molecules are presented to the pituitary in high concen-trations because of this portal system and it is unlikely that they have any direct systemic ef-fects, after passing through the general circu-lation. These hypothalamic factors provide the major form of regulation of the synthesis and/ or release of hormones from the anterior pitu-itary.

The first of the hypothalamic factors to be isolated and characterized was thyrotropin-releasing hormone (TRF), noted earlier as being the smallest of the peptide hormones. Though its likely presence was postulated 30 years ago, corticotropin-releasing factor (CRF), a controller of the secretion of adrenocorticotropic hormone (ACTH) and hence a key part of the control sys-

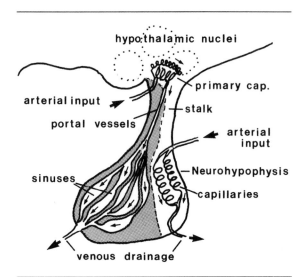

Figure 4–18. *The hypothalamo-hypophyseal portal system.* The pituitary gland is attached to the hypothalamus by the pituitary stalk. Axons of hypothalamic neurons, cytons of which are grouped as nuclei, pass through the stalk and terminate in the neurohypophysis, or posterior pituitary. Also, hypothalamic neurons secrete releasing factors into a primary capillary bed at the base of the stalk. These capillaries are drained through portal vessels that pass on to form blood sinuses in the anterior pituitary (shaded). The releasing factors act on cells of the anterior pituitary to influence hormone synthesis and secretion. Effluent blood from both portions of the pituitary collect into the venous system to reach the general circulation.

tem for the adrenal cortex (see Section 4.5, below), has been isolated only recently and appears to be a couple of small peptides.

Gonadotropin-releasing hormone (GnRH), a decapeptide that was characterized in the early 1970s, is especially interesting because this one factor exerts control over production of two pituitary hormones, LH and FSH. Various other hormones of nonhypothalamic origin contribute to the subtle regulation of secretion of these gonadotropic hormones and they will be described in detail in Chapter 10.

Prolactin-inhibiting factor (PIF) is especially noteworthy because, as the name implies, the control it exerts over prolactin (PRL) secretion is tonically of an inhibitory nature. Additionally, PIF is the best-known example of a nonpeptide hypothalamic hormone and almost certainly is dopamine, one of the biogenic amines shown in Figure 4–3. As an inhibitory factor, control over the pituitary is achieved by reducing its influence, thereby relieving the inhibition. This form of control was discovered quite early when the portal system was disrupted experimentally and resulted in increased secretion of PRL. Similar results occur in animals treated with tranquilizer drugs that interfere with the action of dopamine.

Another inhibitory factor found in the hypothalamus, along with several other tissues, influences the secretion of growth hormone (GH). GH is also called somatotropin, so this factor was called somatostatin. There is also a growth hormone–releasing hormone (GHRH), so control over GH secretion results from the interplay between somatostatin and GHRH. In recent years, molecules that are either exactly the same or very similar to the hypothalamic factors have been identified in nonhypothalamic locations, including the placenta, pancreas, and thyroid. Their function at these locations is not well understood.

Hormones of the Hypothalamus and Posterior Pituitary

The posterior pituitary, or neurohypophysis, is an extension of the hypothalamic neural tissue down into the vicinity of the anterior pituitary. It can be regarded as a specialized neurosecretory structure because it provides for intimate contact between the blood vessels that drain the pituitary and the axonal processes of neurons, the cytons of which are located high in the hypothalamus. The two major hormones of interest are oxytocin and ADH. It was noted in Section 4.2 that these peptides are structurally similar, and it is now appropriate to note that small differences exist in the amino acid sequence of the ADH molecules in certain domestic animal species.

Oxytocin is synthesized in the hypothalamus, travels down axons in combination with a carrier protein called *neurophysin,* and is stored in the posterior pituitary. The secretion of oxytocin provides a hormonal efferent limb to what is known as a neurohumoral reflex. Upon suitable neural input to the hypothalamus, oxytocin is released, along with the neurophysin, from the pituitary. It is not known if the neurophysin has any role once it has been secreted.

Oxytocin functions to promote contraction of myoepithelial cells surrounding the mammary alveoli and stimulates contractions in myometrium, or uterine muscle, provided the latter is suitably primed by steroid hormones. Specific details of the secretion and actions of oxytocin will be provided in Section 4.5 and then made use of in Chapters 10 and 11.

ADH, or vasopressin, is another peptide of the hypothalamus–posterior pituitary axis. It is synthesized in different hypothalamic nuclei from those producing oxytocin, and is transported axonally on another neurophysin. ADH, like oxytocin, is released as a humoral component of neurohumoral reflexes. ADH has major actions in controlling water resorption by adjusting permeability of the wall of the collecting duct in the kidney and somewhat related actions in water transport in epithelial systems in lower animals.

The hormone exerts potent pressor actions (blood pressure–increasing actions) in some species, notably birds, and this effect is the basis for the alternative name, vasopressin. Although this action is of significance in regulating arterial blood pressure in birds, it is of only minor consequence in mammals.

The Anterior Pituitary Hormones

Most of the protein hormones of the anterior pituitary serve as tropic hormones for other endocrine glands. They regulate the growth of these glands and then their hormone-synthesizing ca-

pacity. Tropic hormones, including TSH, ACTH, LH, and FSH, were traditionally bioassayed by their effects on appropriate target tissues in animals that had been surgically hypophysectomized, thereby creating deficiency states for this group of hormones.

PRL was assayed by its ability to initiate synthesis of milk by mammary tissues that were prepared experimentally with various other hormones. Alternatively, a bioassay based on the sensitivity to PRL of the crop in pigeons was widely used. This structure, part of the digestive tract, undergoes growth and massive secretory function to produce "crop milk," used to feed the squabs, or young pigeons.

GH is bioassayed by its effect, in young hypophysectomized animals, of stimulating whole body growth or, with more precision, of causing widening of the epiphyseal growth plate cartilages. It will be noted below that the response to GH is quite indirect.

Quite specific and ultrasensitive assay methods are now available for all of the pituitary hormones for most species of interest. These methods use radioactively labeled hormones and either specific antibodies prepared against the hormone of interest or receptor preparations made from known target tissues obtained from animals. For example, PRL concentrations in plasma can be measured by radioimmunoassay, if an antibody capable of binding the PRL of interest is available. Alternatively, a crude preparation of plasmalemma derived from mammary tissue will, under certain conditions, contain PRL receptors and can be used to quantify prolactin.

Growth Hormone

GH, or somatotropin, is secreted by the anterior pituitary, but there is still uncertainty about the hypothalamic mediators of secretion. The precise physiologic roles of GHRH and somatostatin are unclear. GHRH has been perhaps the most elusive hypophysiotropic molecule, in part because its concentration in the hypothalamus is only in femtomoles (10^{-15} moles) per hypothalamus. About 200 million hypothalami would be needed to extract 1 mg of the peptide!

The pituitary hormone GH is a polypeptide of some 21,000 daltons with generalized targets. Its action in promoting growth is likely to be mediated by secondary peptides termed somatomedins, or sulfation factors. These secondary factors are about 6,000 to 8,000 daltons and similar in structure to insulin, so they are now called *insulin-like growth factors*. They are produced in the liver, and probably some other tissues, in response to GH. In addition, they are produced in small amounts, probably independently of GH, in virtually all tissues of the body. They stimulate growth in young animals by stimulating the *growth plate chondrocytes* (see Chapter 8). They may act in an insulin-like fashion in protein synthesis and hence increase hypertrophy of muscle cells. This is particularly evident in *acromegaly*, when excess GH secretion, after longitudinal bone growth is completed at adolescence, leads to a gross increase in muscle size. GH has several ill-understood general metabolic actions, and causes altered renal handling of mineral ions (e.g., Ca^{2+} and PO_4^{3-}).

GH insufficiency before adolescence leads to *dwarfism*, and replacement therapy using human GH from the pituitaries of cadavers is a major therapeutic program in many countries. For years, attempts have been made to chemically synthesize human GH, but the task is enormous because nearly 200 amino acids must be linked together in a precise sequence. During recent years, recombinant DNA techniques have enabled insertion of the DNA sequence for human GH, bovine GH, and porcine GH into the genome of *Escherichia coli,* and the hormones have been produced by these modified bacteria. Such technology will enable production of adequate GH to treat all children in need of the hormone, an objective that has been impossible to achieve using hormone extracted from human pituitaries. Synthetic bovine GH was first administered to cattle at Cornell University in 1981 and has been followed by major studies investigating long-term administration to lactating cattle as a stimulant for milk production. Recent use of GH in growing pigs has shown that the hormone significantly changes the efficiency of nutrient use, leading to possibilities for markedly changing the composition of carcasses. Thus, deposition of fat is reduced while accretion of lean is stimulated.

Prolactin

PRL, another polypeptide of the anterior pituitary, is usually thought of in relation to lactation and mammary function, but the hormone is present in very primitive submammalian vertebrates, so other roles can be expected. There is some evidence that PRL regulates salt and water metabolism, that it can influence lipid metabolism, and that it may promote somatomedin production. Several tissues have PRL receptors, and while this makes it likely that they are PRL targets, little is known about the role of the hormone in these tissues. In the rat and dog, PRL is *luteotropic,* or stimulatory for the corpus luteum on the ovary, and necessary for progesterone secretion. A comparable role in other species seems to be unlikely. Less is known of the role of this hormone in males, yet PRL receptors occur in many of the accessory reproductive tissues of the male. As noted earlier, this finding suggests that these tissues are indeed targets for the hormone.

The unique feature of PRL is that hypothalamic control of its secretion is achieved by an *inhibitory* rather than stimulatory factor, called prolactin-inhibiting factor (PIF). Increased PRL secretion results from removing the influence of the hypothalamus from the pituitary. This can be achieved surgically by cutting the stalk that connects the hypothalamus and pituitary. It can also be achieved pharmacologically.

Some of these actions of GH and PRL may be displayed by *placental lactogen* from ruminant animals. The similarity in actions is due to the placental hormone having portions of its molecule containing GH active sites, or GH *determinants*, in addition to PRL active sites, or PRL determinants. GH, PRL, and placental lactogen also share much *homology*, or identity, of their amino acid sequence. It is likely that these hormones are all mutation products from some ancient common gene. Accordingly, it is convenient to consider these three hormones as making up a family of related molecules.

Adrenocorticotropic Hormone

Adrenocorticotropin (ACTH) regulates the growth and part of the secretory activity of the adrenal cortex. It is primarily concerned with the glucocorticoids such as cortisol and less concerned with mineralocorticoids such as aldosterone. The glucocorticoids promote *gluconeogenesis*, or production of glucose from amino acids (see Chapter 7), and they are *anti-inflammatory* and participate in chronic adaptation to stress (see Chapter 9). These hormones appear to regulate many perinatal adaptations such as the maturation of type II pneumocytes, the cells producing lung surfactant, in the fetus just before birth. They also induce new hepatic enzyme systems and alter placental steroidogenesis, thereby serving to control the onset of labor.

Cortisol is the main agent for negative feedback control on the hypothalamus to regulate ACTH secretion, presumably via corticotropin-releasing factor (CRF).

The synthesis of pituitary ACTH is a fascinating story by itself. A number of hormones similar to ACTH have been discovered over the years, and a great deal of sequence homology is evident between ACTH, melanocyte-stimulating hormone (MSH), lipotropic hormone (LPH), corticotropin-like intermediary peptide (CLIP), and the recently discovered endorphins. The endorphins are the so-called brain opiates. At present, it seems that all of these hormones are synthesized in one common precursor molecule called proopiomelanocortin. Depending on the sites of processing by specific proteolytic enzymes in the pituitary, different hormone components can be produced and released from this precursor. Little is known about the control over these enzymes, but it is already apparent that different products are released at different stages of development, and certain stimuli are capable of causing secretion of selected peptide products of the common precursor molecule. For example, in cattle, β-endorphin is secreted in response to painful stimuli, but not during labor and calving, conditions that human observers would consider to be stressful.

Thyroid-Stimulating Hormone

Thyrotropin (TSH) is under control by hypothalamic TRF and serves to regulate the size and secretory activity of the thyroid gland. Feedback control involves the thyroid hormones thyroxine (T_4) and triiodothyronine (T_3), which act on the hypothalamus to control TRF. When the synthesis of T_3 and T_4 is interfered with by various plant components acting as *goitrogens*, this feedback is relieved and TSH is secreted to try to increase thyroid function. This results in thyroid enlargement or *goiter*. The synthesis of thyroid hormones is a good example of biologic halogenation. The thyroid glands actively accumulate iodine and incorporate it into tyrosine, an aromatic amino acid, as part of the total synthesis to thyroxine. Thyroid cells are arranged as follicular layers and they secrete colloid into the cavity. The colloid can later be taken up and released into the circulation when the gland is stimulated by TSH. Most of the thyroid hormone is tightly associated with thyroxine-binding globulin (TBG) in the circulation. This transport mechanism results in thyroxine exhibiting one of the slowest half-times of any of the hormones. This means that acute increases and decreases in concentration in plasma are unlikely.

Thyroid hormones have generalized metabolic actions in many tissues and may be necessary for other hormones to show their actions. Some specific biochemical actions involve uncoupling of oxidative phosphorylation, resulting in metabolic energy being liberated as heat, rather than being conserved in the form of ATP.

TSH, LH, and FSH are glycoproteins; the peptide chains are heavily decorated with carbohydrate moieties. These glycoproteins are made from two protein subunits, one of which, the alpha subunit, is identical between the hormones. Distinctions therefore are due solely to the characteristics of the beta subunits. This is an important consideration for the development of ultraspecific immunologic assays for these hormones.

Luteinizing Hormone

LH is one of the pituitary *gonadotropins* involved in steroidogenesis, especially by the corpus luteum, and it is the *ovulatory hormone*. In primates especially, availability of LH seems to dictate the life span of the corpus luteum. In early pregnancy in primates, chorionic gonadotropin (hCG in humans), a molecule that closely resembles LH, serves as a luteotropin to "rescue" the corpus luteum and sustain its function into early pregnancy. hCG is viewed as a primitive hormone of the trophoblast, part of the system of fetal membranes (see Chapter 10). It is produced in the trophoblast even before implantation, and very careful analytical methods can detect hCG in women before implantation has started. With the possible exception of equine chorionic gonadotropin, there is no equivalent hormone in domestic animals.

Although LH is required for progesterone synthesis in the domestic animals, the life span of the corpus luteum may be terminated in some species by *luteolytic* agents, such as prostaglandins, that can override the stimulatory effect of LH. This is particularly important in relation to control of the estrous cycle in domestic ruminants, as will be discussed in Chapter 10.

LH and FSH are both secreted under the control of GnRH from the hypothalamus, but additional feedbacks by steroids and a protein hormone, inhibin, derived from the gonad, can act directly at the pituitary. Thus, while LH and FSH may be co-regulated, there is the opportunity for differential control as well. In part the differential control is due to the transduction by the pituitary of pulsatile signals of GnRH arriving from the hypothalamus. Both the frequency of "spikes" of GnRH and the average concentration of GnRH are important information carriers to the pituitary.

LH acts in target cells via specific membrane receptors that are functionally coupled to adenyl cyclase (see Figure 4–16). Thus, cAMP serves as the key intracellular or second messenger in the action of LH. The subsequent loci of action of cAMP are partly defined and include availability of cholesterol esters, side chain cleavage to generate 21-carbon steroids, and possibly later enzymatic steps in the synthesis of progesterone.

Follicle-Stimulating Hormone

FSH triggers then promotes development of follicles, maturation of the ovum prior to ovulation, and the synthesis of follicular steroids. The secretion of FSH, like that of LH, is under control by GnRH from the hypothalamus, and negative feedbacks by steroids and inhibin. Some actions of FSH and LH are cooperative and some are independent. Granulosa cells in the follicle are FSH targets and have specific FSH receptors. Testicular cells also have FSH receptors, and both gonadotropins are involved in androgen synthesis in the male. The only nonpituitary source of an FSH-like hormone is the endometrial cup in the pregnant mare and donkey. Enormous amounts of *equine chorionic gonadotropin*, or pregnant mare's serum gonadotropin (PMSG), are produced by equids, and it is one of the few hormones that can be purified in appreciable quantities from serum.

Thyroid and Parathyroid Hormones

Thyronines

The simple thyroid hormones, thyroxine and triiodothyronine, were described in Section 4.3 and mentioned above in relation to TSH.

Calcitonin

Calcitonin, a small 3,000-dalton peptide derived from C cells, or clear cells, in the thyroid gland, provides the opposing influence to parathyroid hormone (PTH) in calcium homeostasis. Confusion about its origin in different species resulted in its being given a variety of names, such as thyrocalcitonin and calcitonin. The hormone is secreted in response to high circulating concentrations of Ca^{2+}, and not TSH, as is the case for the other thyroid hormones. Another stimulus for its secretion is gastrin, a peptide hormone from the stomach. Calcitonin promotes uptake of blood calcium by bone-forming cells and hence provides for increased bone deposition. Additionally, this hormone seems to oppose the resorption of bone Ca^{2+} by interfering with PTH-mediated processes. The physiologic regulation of calcium homeostasis is described in the next section, and details of bone formation and breakdown are provided in Chapter 8.

Parathyroid Hormone

PTH is a large polypeptide of 84 amino acids that is secreted by the parathyroid glands, located near the thyroid. It serves primarily in calcium homeostasis by promoting calcium mobilization from bone depots. Action on the *osteocytes* is mediated by cAMP, which again serves as a second messenger.

A second action of PTH is in controlling the renal handling of phosphate by inhibiting tubular resorption of phosphate. PTH therefore increases phosphate excretion (*phosphaturia*) and hence lowers blood phosphate concentrations. This enables greater calcium concentrations to be achieved without precipitation of calcium phosphate. The product of calcium concentration and phosphate concentration is kept relatively constant. Another renal function of PTH is to promote synthesis of *1,25-dihydroxyvitamin D*, the active form of the vitamin for regulation of calcium metabolism.

PTH secretion is controlled directly by calcium sensors in the parathyroids. Secretion of the hormone increases in response to low blood calcium levels. Its action increases the concentration of Ca^{2+} ions which, in turn, feeds back to regulate secretion of PTH.

Hormones of the Gastrointestinal Tract

The humoral regulators of gut function include histamine, gastrin, secretin, pancreozymin-cholecystokinin (PZ-CCK), villikinin, and enterocrinin. There is now evidence for a family of peptide hormones, again with considerable sequence homology, that includes some of the foregoing along with some other hormones, the actions of which may not be confined to gut function. Thus, secretin, gut glucagon, and vasoactive intestinal peptide (VIP) are all closely related, and likely to have evolved from a common gene sequence. Some are more tentative hormonal species than others; their existence has been hypothesized to account for physiologic observations. Villikinin is considered to be responsible for contracting the sparse smooth muscle cells in the intestinal villi, a role related to the movement of lymph out of the lacteals toward larger lymphatics in the mesentery. Enterocrinin has been proposed to stimulate production of intestinal secretions. These hormones await isolation and purification. PZ-CCK is an interesting example of the confusion that may exist in the early stages of endocrine research when a crude extract displays a range of biologic activities. For some 15 to 20 years, two separate hormones, pancreozymin and cholecystokinin, were postulated to exist. The roles of these GI hormones will be discussed in Chapter 6. Many of the hormones have recently been found in the brain, a very puzzling discovery.

Adrenal Hormones

The adrenal gland (see Figure 4–8) produces different types of hormones in each of its two major portions. The cortex is a major steroidogenic tissue, producing an array of glucocorticoid and mineralocorticoid steroids. The medulla, a specialized portion of the sympathetic nervous system, produces catecholamines and the opiate hormone, β-endorphin.

Catecholamines

The *adrenal medulla* is a key neuroendocrine integration site. The medulla is controlled primarily by thoracolumbar outflow of the sympathetic nervous system. The ability to synthesize epinephrine from norepinephrine requires a cortisol-sensitive enzyme, phenylethanolamine-N-methyl transferase (see Figure 4–4). The enzyme transfers methyl groups from S-adenosyl methionine, a key 1-carbon donor, to norepinephrine, resulting in formation of epinephrine. Cortisol is provided to the medulla in high concentrations by a type of portal vascular system between the adrenal cortex and the medulla.

Catecholamines are stored in secretory granules in the medullary cells in enormous amounts. Upon appropriate sympathetic discharge, the hormones are delivered via the circulation to reinforce and prolong the action of the same transmitters released acutely from nerve endings. As a generalization, epinephrine is the major catecholamine released from the adrenal medulla, while norepinephrine is the major agent released from sympathetic nerve varicosities.

Catecholamines act at the level of membrane-bound receptors, some of which are linked to adenyl cyclase. A detailed analysis of the specificity of action of a range of synthetic catecholamines led to the first really useful statement of the receptor concept of hormone action about 40 years ago.

Adrenal Steroids

The steroids of the cortex were introduced in Section 4.2 and mentioned again in relation to ACTH earlier in this section.

The fetal adrenal cortex in primates has a dominant region, called the *fetal zone*, that is responsible for synthesis of a weak androgen, or male sex steroid, called dehydroepiandrosterone sulfate (DHEAS). This androgen, produced by the fetal adrenal gland, is 16-hydroxylated in the liver to 16-OH-DHEAS and then reaches the placenta, where it serves as the key precursor for the major estrogen of human pregnancy, estriol. This is the basis for the so-called *fetoplacental endocrine unit* (Figure 4–19).

Animals can survive with basal secretion of glucocorticoids, for example after removal of the pituitary, and therefore ACTH, providing they are unstressed. Removal of the adrenals, however, is usually lethal, mainly because of the loss of mineralocorticoid activity, although the loss of basal, or non-ACTH–stimulated glucocorti-

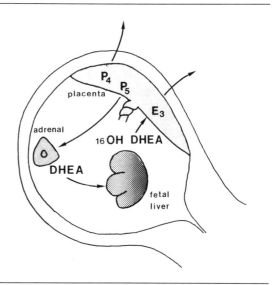

Figure 4–19. Feto-placental endocrine unit in primates. The placenta and fetus often cooperate in steroidogenesis by exchanging precursors. This diagram outlines the best characterized system—that which produces estrogens of pregnancy in women. The placenta produces progestins, including pregnenolone (P_5) and progesterone (P_4), which enter the fetal circulation and reach the fetal adrenal gland. The fetal zone of the adrenal cortex in primates converts pregnenolone into the weak androgen called dehydroepiandrosterone (DHEA). The reactions were depicted in Figure 4–11. DHEA is then converted by the fetal liver into 16α-OH-DHEA. This compound circulates back to the placenta and serves as a substrate for placental synthesis of the pregnancy estrogen called estriol (E_3). Estriol is finally secreted into the maternal compartment.

coid secretion, does contribute. Adrenalectomized animals can be maintained if they are given sodium chloride and are unstressed.

Aldosterone is the major mineralocorticoid and is involved in sodium and potassium homeostasis, mainly at the renal level. Control of aldosterone secretion is very complex and may involve circulating prostaglandins, angiotensin, and the enzyme renin, derived from the kidney in response to hypotension. This control system will be described in detail in connection with cardiovascular homeostasis in Chapter 5.

Pancreatic Hormones

The pancreas has a significant endocrine role in producing two major hormones of prime importance in metabolic regulation, insulin and glucagon. The venous drainage from the pancreas is into the portal vein, so secreted hormones are delivered directly to the liver. The liver is the most important target tissue for each of these hormones, although they do have important actions in nonhepatic tissues.

Insulin

Insulin is produced by beta cells of the pancreatic islets in response to a variety of stimuli, the most important of which is elevated blood levels of glucose. Several hormones can interact with glucose in influencing the insulin response, for example impaired insulin response in the presence of high levels of catecholamines. Insulin receptors are very widely distributed throughout many tissues that are known to be insulin sensitive, although those in liver are probably of greatest importance. Insulin promotes glucose and amino acid uptake by cells and subsequent incorporation into macromolecules such as glycogen and protein. In adipocytes, insulin is both *lipogenic*, meaning that it promotes triglyceride synthesis, and *antilipolytic*. The latter term is used to describe the inhibition of fat mobilization. (The

dynamics of the fat depots are addressed in Chapter 7.)

Insulin's best-known action is in reducing blood glucose concentrations. This is referred to as its *antidiabetic* role. Very high glucose concentrations, as for example in uncontrolled diabetes, result in *glucosuria*, or urinary loss of glucose. Glucose in the kidney filtrate closely follows the concentration in plasma; it is efficiently reabsorbed provided concentrations do not exceed about 170 mg/100 mL. When blood glucose concentrations exceed this glucose threshold—as they do in uncontrolled diabetes—reabsorption is incomplete and glucose is lost to the urine.

Insulin is synthesized as a precursor molecule called *proinsulin* (Figure 4–20) that is subsequently processed by removal of a connecting peptide to yield the final, two-subunit form of active insulin. Insulin has many close relatives that are structurally similar and often share homologous sequences of amino acids. Proinsulin, the somatomedins, and nerve growth factor (NGF) have similar form, while insulin and relaxin are very similar. The somatomedins were mentioned under growth hormone, and NGF is a *hypertrophic agent*, meaning that it is a stimulant of cell expansion but not division, for neural tissue.

The peptidase responsible for activating proinsulin to insulin is under the control of cAMP, and the secretion of insulin from granules in the beta cells seems to be triggered by Ca^{2+} ions. The structure of insulin differs very little from species to species, so hormone therapy for diabetics has been possible for decades using insulin extracted from the pancreas of cattle, sheep, and hogs. The discovery of insulin, its role in diabetes, and the development of insulin therapy was a milestone in endocrinology. Insulin is presently being produced by bacteria with the aid of recombinant DNA techniques, but sufficient amounts to replace animal-derived insulin will not be available for some time.

Although insulin plays a pivotal role in metabolic regulation and so influences the anabolic processes that underlie productive activities in farm animals, it is rarely used in animal science,

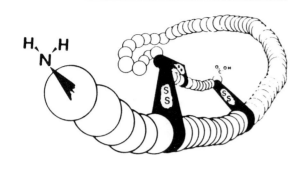

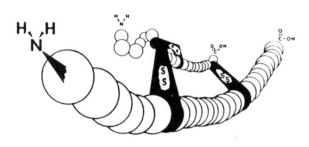

Figure 4–20. Proinsulin and insulin. Proinsulin is a single-chain peptide that is constructed in a helical or spiral fashion, shown above, and held together with three S–S bonds. Before secretion from the pancreas, the peptide is processed with the loss of part of the original chain, resulting in the formation of insulin, shown below. Insulin has two chains, connected with two of the original S–S bonds.

either therapeutically or to manipulate animal performance.

Glucagon

Produced by pancreatic alpha cells in response to low blood concentrations of glucose, glucagon, another small peptide hormone, is secreted primarily to balance the antidiabetic effects of insulin. Its prime target is the liver, where it has several actions such as *glycogenolysis*, or glycogen breakdown to glucose, in common with catecholamines. In addition, glucagon along with glucocorticoids facilitates the conversion of amino acids to glucose in a process called gluconeogenesis. Glycogenolysis is cAMP dependent and the glucagon receptor, although quite distinct from the catecholamine receptor, is also coupled to adenyl cyclase. It is less clear if cAMP mediates the gluconeogenesis response to glucagon.

Glucagon and insulin form an *antagonistic pair* of regulators. They are both controlled and act in a reciprocal fashion. The key aspects of this reciprocal control will be described in detail in Section 4.5. It is important to emphasize that the location of the pancreas and its venous drainage through the visceral portal system are crucial for the close regulation of the liver, serving in glucose homeostasis during both the absorptive and postabsorptive phases of digestion.

Another form of glucagon called *gut glucagon*, discussed earlier as one of the gastrointestinal hormones, is derived from the small intestine. It shares many properties with alpha-cell glucagon and until its presence was established with certainty, great confusion prevailed in the work using radioimmunoassays for glucagon, because both hormones were measured in these assays. It has been speculated that early release of gut glucagon, in relation to ingestion of a meal, could help provide a small amount of energy necessary for the remaining digestive activities.

Hormones of the Kidney

Erythropoietin is released from the kidney in response to renal tissue hypoxia, as may prevail in *anemia* and particularly severe parasite-related *hemolytic anemias*. In fetal life, erythropoiesis, or the manufacture of erythrocytes, is a function of the liver and spleen. while in adult life erythrocytes are produced by bone marrow. The actions of erythropoietin are still poorly understood but they involve control of cell divisions generating primordial cells capable of changing to white blood cells or to erythrocytes. The incorporation of elemental iron into hemoglobin iron can be used to monitor erythropoiesis. The concentrations of erythropoietin are increased in high altitudes as an adaptation to reduced P_{O_2}, or partial hypoxia, following hemolytic anemia as in several infectious conditions, after hemorrhage, and in several pathophysiologic states in which kidney oxygenation is impaired.

1,25-Dihydroxycholecalciferol

This molecule is the most active form of vitamin D_3 and is now best regarded as a hormone. Its formation is atypical of the hormones already described because the precursor molecule is obtained from the diet. After exposure to ultraviolet light impinging on the skin, vitamin D_3 is formed. This resembles the molecular form of a steroid or cholesterol derivative (Figure 4–21), but with a highly modified B ring. Vitamin D_3 is metabolized in liver to form 25-hydroxyvitamin D_3, and then converted in the kidney to the 1,25-dihydroxy form, which is the most potent.

The renal formation of the final active form is regulated by PTH, so conditions causing increased secretion of PTH, such as low blood concentrations of calcium, also lead to increased production of 1,25-dihydroxyvitamin D_3. The molecule serves to increase the absorption of calcium from the gut by specifically inducing synthesis of calcium-binding protein in the gut mucosa, and it favors calcium resorption from bone.

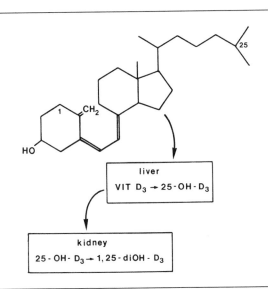

Figure 4–21. Metabolism of vitamin D. Vitamin D_3 is produced in cutaneous tissues of animals by ultraviolet-radiation-induced modification of a dietary precursor molecule. Note the similarity of the molecule to cholesterol (Figure 2–30) with some modifications in the B–ring. The liver hydroxylates vitamin D_3 to the 25-hydroxy metabolite, which is about 1.5 times as active as D_3. Under the influence of parathyroid hormone, renal tissue further hydroxylates 25-hydroxycholecalciferol to 1,25-dihydroxycholecalciferol, the most potent form of the vitamin (about 150 times that of D_3). Carbons 1 and 25 are identified on the parent structure.

Gonadal Steroids

Gonadal steroids are classified according to their biologic actions as androgens, estrogens, and progestins. Pregnenolone, a 21-carbon steroid, is the common precursor to all of these classes. Its synthesis from cholesterol occurs in tissues that are targets for tropic hormones, but also in the placenta of several species where there is no known tropic influence. As emphasized before, steroid interconversions proceed from progestins to androgens to estrogens (Figure 4–22). Some shuttling of precursors takes place be-

tween cells that have distinct tropic specificities. For example, androgens may be synthesized in response to one gonadotropin in one cell type, diffuse to neighboring cells, and, under the influence of a second gonadotropin, be converted to estrogens.

Similar shuttling occurs in the fetoplacental unit in primates, as noted earlier with reference to the adrenal hormones. The fetal adrenal cortex converts pregnenolone into androgens, and the androgens are secreted and are delivered to the placenta. Androgens are then converted to estrogens, many of which appear in the maternal circulation. A somewhat similar fetoplacental endocrine unit is present in equids where androgens, produced by the fetal gonad, are converted by the placenta into estrogens.

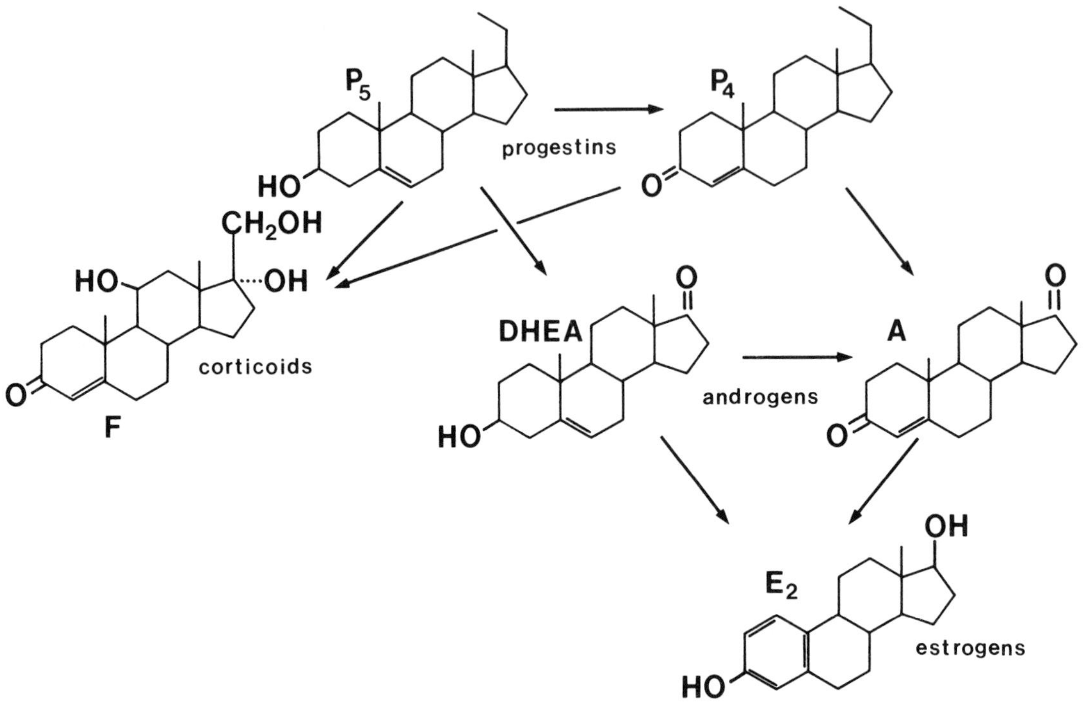

Figure 4–22. *Interconversions of steroids.* As emphasized in the text, steroid syntheses proceed from progestins to androgens to estrogens, except for the adrenal conversion of progestins into adrenal corticosteroids. The conversion of pregnenolone (P_5) to dehydroepiandrosterone (DHEA) represents the Δ^5 pathway; conversion of progesterone (P_4) to androstenedione (A) is the Δ^4 pathway. Cortisol (F) is shown as the corticoid and estradiol (E_2), as the estrogen.

The broad types of actions characteristic of the sex hormones will be described in Chapter 10.

Miscellaneous Hormones

Prostaglandins

Prostaglandins and closely related compounds fall into a class of paracrine agents that have some hormone-like actions but do not always act at distant tissues after secretion into blood. *Prostanoids*, a generic name for the whole family, are synthesized mainly from arachidonic acid, as described briefly in Section 4.2. A number of anti-inflammatory drugs are now known to be prostaglandin synthetase inhibitors. Aspirin, indomethacin, and meclofenamic acid are drugs in widespread use that act in large part by interfering with prostaglandin synthesis.

Some prostanoids have such short chemical and biologic half-lives that it is extremely difficult to study them. Their known range of activities is already broad, and knowledge about them is increasing. Some prostanoids influence smooth muscle, inflammatory responses, thermoregulation, platelet aggregation and clotting, and ion transport across membranes, and in many instances they play a role in hormone secretion and action.

Elsewhere in this text, mention will be made of prostaglandins affecting the function of the corpus luteum, control of aldosterone secretion, constriction of the ductus arteriosus in the new-born animal, stimulation of uterine contractions, and changing hypothalamic thermoregulatory setpoints, as in fever.

The Growth Factors

A whole array of peptides, of a size about that of insulin, have been identified as specific growth factors, and usually mitogens, for various cell types. Most of these factors have been discovered using cell culture techniques and then studied both in isolated cell systems and, to a lesser extent, in vivo. There is still very little known about the role of these agents in domestic animals.

Some of the factors, including the somatomedins mentioned in relation to GH, NGF, and relaxin, probably deserve to be designated as hormones. Others, including epidermal growth factor, platelet-derived growth factor, chondrocyte growth factor, fibrocyte growth factor, endothelial growth factor, and transformation growth factor still await adequate description or characterization before being added to the list of hormones.

These factors all appear to serve as chemical mediators, they often have a restricted range of tissues of origin and targets, and they act via receptors in those target cells. There will be some additional information provided about these factors in Chapter 8. It is this area of humoral regulation, especially with respect to the economically important domestic animals, that will be the focus of endocrine research of the future for animal scientists.

4.5 • Integrative Endocrine Control Systems

This section highlights major differences between endocrine and neural regulation by describing three major categories of endocrine control systems. Examples of each type will be provided, and in some cases endocrinopathies that expose disturbances to these control systems will be described. The full impact of this material may not be evident until much later in the text, when the various physiologic systems will have been examined in detail and integrated with each other.

Endocrine versus Neural Controls

The time course of the two control systems, relating input to output, is usually strikingly different, with endocrine regulation providing for a more prolonged response to a single input event. In endocrine regulation, the selectivity of targets obviously depends on the tissue distribution of receptors rather than on the neuroanatomic determinants that underlie neural selectivity. In most cases hormones enter the blood and are distributed throughout the circulation, yet only those tissues with receptors can respond to the signal carried by the hormone. An important specialization occurs in portal vascular systems, where hormone action is indeed largely restricted. The well-known portal systems provide for venous drainage from a *primary capillary bed* to pass to a second tissue with a set of blood sinuses before blood is returned to the general venous pool. Examples include the vascular link between the hypothalamus and anterior pituitary (see Figure 4–18), between the viscera and the liver, and between the adrenal cortex and its medulla. Hormones that are secreted into these portal systems are present in exceedingly high concentrations when delivered to their immediate targets, but they are drastically diluted when blood reaches the general circulation.

The major actions of the hypothalamic releasing factors are obtained in the anterior pituitary. However, it has recently become apparent that some nonhypothalamic tissues, for example the placenta, are able to synthesize the same peptides, but the importance of this flexibility is not known.

The visceral-hepatic portal system is an important means of selectively delivering materials to the liver, as will be made clear in the chapters concerned with digestion and metabolism. This portal system collects venous blood that has come from the digestive tract and the accessory digestive organs and passes it totally to the liver for initial processing. The gastrointestinal hormones and, most importantly, the pancreatic hormones insulin and glucagon, are all secreted into this portal bed. The liver is the most important target tissue for insulin and glucagon, although both hormones can and do exert significant actions in peripheral tissues after they have gained access to the general circulation.

The intraadrenal portal system provides for venous drainage from the outer cortex region of the adrenal to drain radially inward into the medullary portion before leaving the adrenal gland and entering the abdominal vena cava. Steroids released by the cortical cells are presented to the medulla in exceedingly high concentrations, and at present one major function for this arrangement is known. The enzyme phenylethanolamine-N-methyl transferase (PNMT), responsible for synthesis of epinephrine from norepinephrine, is induced by cortisol, the principal glucocorticoid of the cortex. In the rest of the sympathetic nervous system, norepinephrine predominates as the neurotransmitter, possibly because insufficient cortisol is available in nonmedullary locations to make PNMT available, as would be required for synthesis of epinephrine. As noted earlier, the adrenal medulla is really a highly specialized portion of the sympathetic nervous system; the arrangement described here serves as a superb example of cooperation between the nervous and the endocrine regulatory systems.

A characteristic of both neural and endocrine regulation is the frequent provision for co-regulation of a process by multiple, often antagonistic effectors. In the following examples, insulin and glucagon, and PTH and calcitonin, will be shown to provide cooperative controls. Recent studies are exposing great complexity in these actions, where part of the co-regulation may be synergistic, or permissive, with part being antagonistic.

Categories of Endocrine Control Systems

Neurohumoral Reflexes

The classic neurohumoral reflex consists of a neural afferent pathway, a central site of integration, and an efferent limb provided by the secretion and action of a hormone. The genital reflex and the milk ejection reflex, both described below, are the best-known examples of neurohumoral reflexes. A closely related control system is used to monitor and respond to the osmotic strength of the extracellular fluids and, to a somewhat lesser extent, the volume of blood in the circulatory system. In this case, ADH is the hormone mediating the effector responses.

The major receptive mechanism for osmoregulation is provided by *osmoreceptors* in the midbrain. Additional input is obtained from volume-sensing receptors in the low-pressure portions of the vascular system. The low-pressure vessels, the great veins, are also referred to as *capacitance vessels*. They are capable of accommodating a large proportion of the total volume of circulating blood. Stretch receptors in the walls of these vessels monitor distension and therefore indirectly monitor the volume of blood. With appropriate central integration, these inputs serve to regulate the hypothalamic neurons responsible for synthesis, transport, storage, and secretion of ADH from the posterior pituitary.

When *hyperosmotic* fluids perfuse the brain, or when *hypovolemia* (low blood volume) is detected in the circulatory beds, ADH is secreted to increase water retention by the kidneys. The hormone has specific receptors in the plasmalemma of cells of the renal collecting ducts. This will be described in detail in Chapter 5. The receptors are functionally coupled to adenylate cyclase, and 3'5'-cAMP, produced in response to ADH, serves to activate protein kinases that phosphorylate plasmalemmal proteins. The membrane is rendered more hydrophilic by this phosphorylation and hence becomes permeable to water.

Water is recovered out of the collecting ducts by osmotic forces from the hyperosmotic extracellular fluid in the kidney and is then made available back to the circulating body fluids. Water retention results in hemodilution, which expands the circulating blood volume and dilutes hyperosmotic solutions toward isosmotic concentrations. These two final results serve as negative feedbacks on the original input stimuli and so osmotic homeostasis is achieved. Failure of these mechanisms is seen in the major pathology, *diabetes insipidus,* described in Box 4–7.

In addition to this major mechanism, ADH can exert a minor *pressor* action. This means that it can elevate blood pressure directly, by actions on arterial smooth muscle. The increase in blood pressure tends to offset hypovolemia, although far more important methods of regulating arterial blood pressure will be noted in Chapter 5. The hormone ADH is also called vasopressin because of the action just described.

These reflexes are based on neural afferents bringing in information from *peripheral receptive fields.* Some additional input may be central, within the brain, as noted for osmoreception. The site of integration is within the endocrine secretory cell. The hormone constitutes the efferent or output limb of the reflex. The best-known examples are provided by reflexes involving oxytocin secretion. Two such reflexes that have elements in common are the *milk ejection reflex* and the *genital reflex of Ferguson.*

Stretch receptors, or similar receptors sensitive to vigorous tactile stimuli, activate afferent nerves entering the spinal cord via the sensory dorsal roots. After synapsing in the cord, ascending tracts relay information to the thalamic region of the midbrain (Figure 4–23). (The reader should refer to Chapter 3 if at all uncertain about the location of the thalamus.) At this level, additional inputs from higher centers in the brain are added. These depend on experience, training, and conditioning of the animal. Control is then exerted onto the cell bodies of hypothalamic neurons, causing the secretion of oxytocin from axonal processes of these neurons that extend deep down into the posterior pituitary. Oxytocin is released into the interstitium and hence into the circulation and is delivered to target cells in the uterine muscle or to specialized muscle-like cells surrounding the mammary alveoli. Under appropriate conditions, the target cells respond by contracting and the net effect is to increase intrauterine or intramammary pressure. Additional factors determine how well the target cells respond to the excitatory signal provided by oxytocin. These complications merely influence the effectiveness of the reflex, not the basic reflex mechanism.

Box 4–7   Diabetes Insipidus

The important pathology stemming from impaired secretion of ADH is called *diabetes insipidus* and is characterized by excessive urination, or polyuria, accompanied by excessive thirst and water intake, called polydipsia.

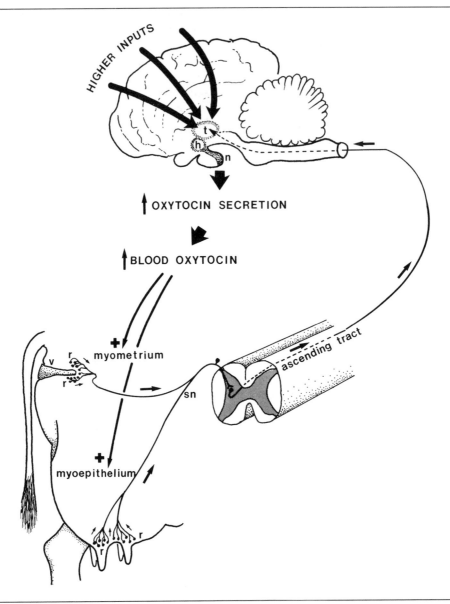

Figure 4–23. *Neurohumoral reflexes involving oxytocin.* The sensory portions of the milk ejection reflex and the genital reflex are shown in the lower part. Receptive fields (r) are located at the base of the teat and in the wall of the anterior vagina (v) and cervix. Afferent information, transmitted via sensory neurons (sn), ascends the spinal cord to the midbrain where it is integrated with higher inputs, such as sight, sound, and smell. These multiple inputs come together in the thalamus (t). Control is then exerted on the hypothalamic (h) neurons that regulate oxytocin secretion from the neurohypophysis (n). The hormone makes up the efferent arm of the reflexes; target tissues are myometrium or mammary myoepithelium. Note the proximity of these targets to the source of the original sensory inputs.

Note that in both cases, the receptors activating the afferent limbs are located very close by the final target or effector tissue of the efferent limb. For the genital reflex, stretch of the anterior vagina is the most potent stimulus. For the milk ejection reflex, the receptors are located near the base of the teat or nipple.

Although the hormonal component could possibly affect a wide range of tissues or organs, the effect of oxytocin is quite limited, because few tissues possess receptors capable of recognizing and responding to the hormone. Current research is focused on the nature of stimuli causing oxytocin release, properties of the sensory receptors, control over oxytocin sensitivity of target tissues, and factors that are capable of inhibiting the reflex. For example, it is known that the milk ejection reflex can be highly *conditioned*. The cow that squirts milk when its calf bellows is exhibiting a conditioned reflex. It is activating the efferent limb of the reflex by higher inputs. The higher inputs are projected from the cerebrum down to the thalamus, where they are integrated with the normal ascending afferent signals that have come in from the peripheral tissues. Conversely, milk ejection is impaired when animals are frightened or stressed. In this case a generalized sympathetic discharge causes vasoconstriction in the vicinity of the pituitary and secretion of oxytocin may thus be impaired. Peripheral vasoconstriction, or constriction of blood vessels in the mammary gland in this case, may impair delivery of the hormone to the myoepithelium. Mammary tissue is a derivative of ectodermal origins, and this vasoconstriction is a typical response of cutaneous tissues to sympathetic discharge. Some current aspects of this field are noted in Box 4–8.

Hierarchical Control of Endocrine Axes

A large number of endocrine controls are *nested*, with the first part involving the hypothalamus, the second involving the anterior pituitary, and the third involving a peripheral endocrine gland. Such systems allow for both neuroendocrine interactions and substantial amplification by stages. Most importantly, multiple loci are available for feedback controls. The final endocrine mediator may feed back at the pituitary, the hypothalamus, or possibly both. Endocrine axes of this general form typify the regulatory systems that involve tropic hormones of the pituitary. These include gonadotropins, TSH, and ACTH. The latter two will be detailed as examples. Further discussion of the gonadotropins will be deferred until Chapter 10, which deals specifically with reproductive biology.

Box 4–8   Oxytocin

There appears to be a basal or resting level of oxytocin secretion that was previously unknown. This may be quite independent of the basic reflex system. Oxytocin has recently been detected in the corpus luteum on the ovary in many nonpregnant animals, a surprising finding because the gland has little else in common with the hypothalamus. The function of oxytocin in the corpus luteum is poorly understood.

A continuing puzzle is exactly how oxytocin causes contraction of its target muscle or myoepithelial cells. The hormone initially acts on the cell surface membrane and causes depolarizations, possibly related to changes in Ca^{2+} influx, where Ca^{2+} acts as the inward current carrier to couple excitatory events with contraction.

The TRF-TSH-Thyroid Axis

Hypothalamic control in this example is exerted via TRF, noted earlier to be a simple peptide of three amino acids. The pituitary secretes TSH, a glycoprotein hormone, that controls the growth and secretory function of the thyroid gland. This target gland releases thyroxine (T_4), which may be converted to triiodothyronine (T_3) in order to bring about the overall actions of the axis. The thyroid hormones feed back at both the hypothalamus and the pituitary, and disturbances in this control system bring about striking pathologies (Boxes 4–9 and 4–10).

The CRF-ACTH-Adrenal Axis

Hypothalamic control of ACTH secretion in the pituitary was the original example of hypothalamopituitary regulation to be described. The nature of corticotropin-releasing factor (CRF) has evaded description until recently, but there are now two peptides of hypothalamic origin that appear to be capable of controlling ACTH secretion. ACTH is but one of the proteolytic products of the complex precursor molecule called proopiomelanocortin, and the ACTH portion is a 39-amino acid polypeptide.

ACTH stimulates growth and part of the secretory function of the adrenal cortex. Control is exerted on production of glucocorticoids and cortisol is the major steroid product involved in negative feedback to the hypothalamus.

The hypothalamo-pituitary-adrenal axis is further specialized because its activity varies in a predictable pattern every 24 hours. The *circadian rhythm* results in enhanced activity through the early to mid-morning each day. The integrity of the axis can be easily examined by a couple of drugs that provoke changes in the feedback processes. Metyrapone (Figure 4–24) is a drug that specifically inhibits hydroxylation at C_{11}, and so blocks cortisol synthesis. As plasma concentrations of cortisol decrease, so does the extent of feedback inhibition caused by cortisol. The hypothalamus is now unconstrained by feedback and permits increased secretion of ACTH. The adrenal responds by increased flux of steroid precursors through the pathways described earlier, but only as far as the 11-deoxy compounds. The 11-deoxysteroids are then secreted and can be measured in plasma. Metyrapone therefore provides a means of testing the secretory reserve capacity of the hypothalamo-pituitary portion of the whole axis.

Box 4–9   Thyroid Disorders

If T_4 synthesis is impaired as a result of chronic iodine deficiency, a real problem in parts of the world, or because of exposure to some plant toxins called goitrogens, the activity of the axis is unconstrained by feedbacks. Continued excessive secretion of TSH causes thyroid enlargement, or the development of *goiter*. Neonates exhibit goiter because of iodine deficiency in utero and the inability, in some species, of maternal T_4 and T_3 to cross the placenta. Abnormal neonates such as these signal the need to closely examine the iodine content of the diet. The introduction of iodized salt has been particularly effective in dealing with this type of thyroid deficiency, or *hypothyroidism*, in many parts of the world.

The most severe manifestation of hypothyroidism is seen as *cretinism* in newborns of mothers with untreated hypothyroidism, or in young children who were protected from it by maternal T_4 and T_3 until after weaning and subsequently become hypothyroid from iodine deficiency in childhood diets.

Box 4–10 Thyrotoxicosis: An Example of an Endocrinopathy due to Abnormal Function of the Immune System

Excessive thyroid activity, or *hyperthyroidism,* may result from tumors of the pituitary or thyroid gland. In these situations, normal homeostatic controls become disrupted. More frequently, extreme hyperthyroidism, or *thyrotoxicosis,* results from a peculiar consequence of the body's immune system starting to raise antibodies against its own tissues. These pathologies are classed as *autoimmune diseases* and the one involving the thyroid is well known. Antibodies are raised against the body's tissues and include some that specifically interact with the receptors for TSH in the thyroid. The antibody molecule binds to TSH receptors and activates them in a way that is indistinguishable from activation by TSH. The stimulated thyroid secretes T_4 and conversion of T_4 to T_3 proceeds. The thyroid hormones are, however, incapable of feeding back to suppress this form of stimulation. This is an example of an open control system that actually is out of control. All actions of T_3 and T_4 become exaggerated: basal metabolic rate is increased, there is excessive calorigenesis or heat production, blood flow is redistributed to the periphery to aid in heat loss, vasodilation of skin vessels occurs to aid skin blood flow, central arterial pressure falls, then heart rate increases to try and correct the hypotension. (The step-by-step deterioration will become more apparent after the description of cardiovascular adjustments is provided, in Chapter 5.) Eventually the heart fails because all attempts via increased cardiac output to restore normal blood pressure are counteracted by the peripheral vasodilation. Control or management of this disease is achieved by careful administration of goitrogens to disrupt T_4 synthesis and to bring plasma T_4 and T_3 levels back into a normal or euthyroid range.

A synthetic glucocorticoid, dexamethasone (Figure 4–24), can be administered to test the integrity of the feedback mechanism. This fluorinated steroid analogue is perhaps 100-fold more potent than cortisol and is an effective suppressor of the CRF-ACTH part of the axis. A dexamethasone suppression test consists of measuring basal (pretest) concentrations of cortisol in blood, then the postadministration concentration of cortisol. The dexamethasone inhibits CRF, then ACTH, then adrenal steroidogenesis, resulting in depressed concentrations of cortisol. If the levels of cortisol are not reduced, the feedback mechanism must be faulty.

Two major pathologies of this control axis, *Cushing's syndrome* and *Addison's disease,* are described in Box 4–11.

Autoregulated and Reciprocal Control of Regulator Pairs

This control mechanism depends on a single physiologic variable serving as the key input stimulus for the secretion of two hormonal regulators, each having opposing actions on that variable. There may be multiple inputs and there may be more than two humoral effectors. An appropriate balance between the actions of the output hormones provides homeostatic regulation.

This category describes the endocrine control systems that operate without direct neural or neuroendocrine input. These control systems are very dependent on feedback mechanisms for stability. As an example, the role of PTH and

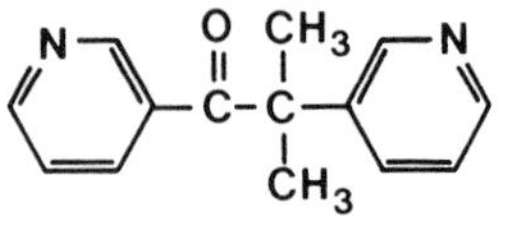

Metyrapone

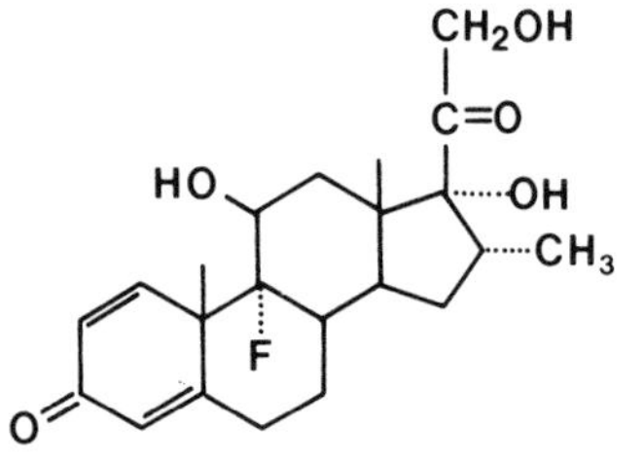

Dexamethasone

Figure 4–24. Metyrapone and dexamethasone. Metyrapone, a drug that inhibits the conversion of 11-deoxycortisol to cortisol, is used diagnostically to test the adequacy of the CRF–ACTH axis. It can also be used therapeutically to reduce cortisol synthesis in Cushingoid patients. Dexamethasone is a fluorinated synthetic steroid which acts as a very potent glucocorticoid. It is widely used in human and veterinary therapeutics.

calcitonin in exerting control over calcium homeostasis will be developed. Resident within the parathyroid cells themselves are calcium-sensing receptors. These could reasonably be called *calciumstats*. When hypocalcemia is detected, PTH secretion occurs in order that calcium stores can be mobilized to correct the deficiency. As normal or comfort-range concentrations are achieved, the original stimulus for PTH secretion is removed. The response of this system, increased extracellular concentrations of Ca^{2+}, serves as a negative feedback on the control of PTH secretion.

The hormone exerts multiple effects to mediate calcium entry into the circulating pool. A direct action is control by PTH over bone resorption, gut absorption, and renal conservation of Ca^{2+}. A particularly important indirect action is the control by PTH of renal conversion of 25-hydroxycholecalciferol to the active form of vitamin D_3.

The active form, 1,25-dihydroxyvitamin D_3, seems to act in the same general way as steroid hormones, although it is not a steroid. It induces a calcium-binding protein in the intestine that is important for Ca^{2+} absorption from the gut, in addition to actions favoring Ca^{2+} resorption from bone. The dynamics of bone growth and remodeling, including Ca^{2+} mobilization and deposition, are described in Chapter 8.

The physiologic regulation of *eucalcemia*, or normal concentrations of Ca^{2+} in extracellular fluids, is not due solely to the PTH-VIT D_3 control. A second regulatory arm is provided by calcitonin. This polypeptide is secreted by C cells in the thyroid rather than parathyroid gland, and it very promptly lowers circulating Ca^{2+} concentrations. It probably facilitates deposition in bone and interferes with Ca^{2+} mobilization by PTH. Its secretion is regulated by a calcium sensor capable of detecting higher than normal concentrations of the ion in extracellular fluids. Another form of control is achieved by the stomach-derived hormone, gastrin. Although gastrin is mainly concerned with control of secretory and motility functions of the stomach, it seems able to respond to the amount of Ca^{2+} in the digesta and then to exert an action on the thyroid C cells to increase secretion of calcitonin.

Negative feedback on calcitonin secretion is achieved by plasma concentrations of Ca^{2+} falling back into the normal range, thus removing the original stimulus for calcitonin secretion.

The regulation of blood glucose by largely reciprocal actions of insulin and glucagon will be detailed because this important regulatory system will be the focus of much of the material to be presented later in Chapter 7.

Insulin is secreted from beta cells within the islets of Langerhans, the endocrine portion of the pancreas. A major *secretagogue*, or stimulus for secretion, is elevated plasma glucose concentrations, and it is clear that some glucose-sensing mechanism, a *glucostat*, is present in the cells. Insulin is initially synthesized as proinsulin and must be proteolytically cleaved to the

---

Box 4–11 Adrenal Pathologies

Cushing's syndrome is the most severe form of hypercortisolism and can be brought about by excessive secretion of ACTH, and therefore of cortisol. It may be the result solely of adrenal hyperactivity, sometimes the result of an adrenocortical tumor.

Cushingoid patients present clinically with marked protein depletion and redistribution of body fat; they may appear to be pot-bellied, with very thin limbs. There is usually hair loss, a characteristic moon-face, and disturbed mineral metabolism; often these physical symptoms are accompanied by neurologic disorders. Some cases of adrenal hyperactivity may include disturbances in sex steroid production; the syndrome is called the *adrenogenital* condition. The consequences are bizarre and include androgenization, or masculinization, of female children, feminization of

boys, and often markedly precocious puberty. Comparable conditions have been described in domestic animals, but they are quite rare.

Adrenal insufficiency, or *Addison's disease,* is quite rare and was fatal prior to the availability of synthetic steroids, which now provide effective treatment. Lack of corticosteroids leads to generalized physiologic incompetence, with virtually no ability to tolerate even the mildest of stresses. One cause of the disease is atrophic degeneration of adrenal cortical tissue due to tuberculosis. One consequence is the failure to regulate sodium balance, because of loss of mineralocorticoids, but the gross symptoms are due also to loss of glucocorticoids. A bronze-like pigmentation of the skin develops and a progressive anemia and low blood pressure eventually cause death.

---

active hormone. Insulin is stored in granules in the beta cell, and the secretory mechanism involves granule migration to the apical region of the cell, fusion of the granule membrane with the plasmalemma, and release of the hormone. Both $3'5'$-cAMP and Ca^{2+} are involved in the control of insulin secretion.

Hypoglycemia results in secretion of glucagon from pancreatic alpha cells, again presumably in response to some type of glucostat capable of sensing glucose concentrations that fall below some setpoint. Both hormones are released into the visceral-hepatic portal system and pass directly to the liver. The actions of these hormones are probably better understood than those of any others but it is sufficient at this stage to note that glucagon acts to elevate plasma concentrations of glucose, while insulin does the

reverse. In part these actions stem from control of glycogen formation and degradation within the liver itself. The indirect and less obvious actions of these hormones are enormous in range and will not be analyzed in detail until later. The secretion of the hormones is closely linked with the digestive-absorptive process when nutrients are moving through the same portal vascular bed.

Early during digestion, a form of glucagon called gut glucagon is released from the small intestine to provoke a transient increase in blood glucose concentrations. It can be imagined that increased glucose availability, from previously accumulated stores, aids as an energy source for the digestive process. Glucose can be used in most tissues only if insulin is also present. Gastrointestinal hormones, including secretin and

Figure 4–25. Insulin secretion. The major secretagogues for pancreatic release of insulin are elevated blood concentrations of glucose, secretin, and glucagon. Insulin is released from the pancreas into the hepatic portal vein (P), and so it is delivered first to the liver, its primary target organ. Insulin also passes through the liver to influence most tissues of the body.

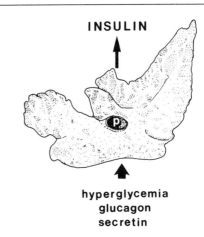

INSULIN

hyperglycemia
glucagon
secretin

Box 4–12   Insulin-Related Pathologies

The major pathology of the insulin-glucagon system is *diabetes mellitus,* a devastating disorder that takes many forms. In general, diabetes is caused by lack of or ineffectiveness of insulin. One form simply reflects impaired insulin secretion, or its complete absence. A glucose tolerance test exposes this problem because a standard oral or intravenous dose of glucose normally establishes a very consistent elevation, then clearance of glucose from the plasma. The rate of decrease to predose concentrations of glucose reflects the secretion and action of insulin to promote glucose utilization. If clearance is prolonged, assay of the samples drawn during the test for insulin concentrations will expose subnormal secretion of the hormone. If the insulin secretory response is normal but glucose clearance is still slow, this indicates a problem in the effectiveness of the insulin. When this is suspected, an insulin challenge test can be performed: a standard dose of insulin is administered to determine how rapidly and completely plasma

glucose concentrations are depressed. When this second test indicates a problem in insulin effectiveness, a diagnosis of *insulin-resistant diabetes* is usually made. One cause for this disease is another example of an endocrinopathy due to autoimmune disease. This example is similar to thyrotoxicosis, where antibodies are raised against receptors. In this case the antibody is against the insulin receptor but, unlike in thyrotoxicosis, this antibody blocks rather than stimulates the receptor. With the receptor effectively neutralized, endogenous insulin cannot act and neither can injected insulin. Such individuals require exacting dietary management rather than hormone therapy in order to survive.

Striking changes in insulin receptor populations have been described in some forms of *obesity* and in *anorexia nervosa.* It is likely that similar disorders occur in domestic animals, but they are not well known, and natural selection has probably served as an effective means of reducing their incidence.

Figure 4–26. *Reciprocal control of glucose by insulin and glucagon.* This simple control scheme shows the great flexibility possible when two regulators have opposing effects, and the stimulus for secretion of one serves to inhibit secretion of the other. Specifically, when plasma concentrations of glucose (shaded) exceed the comfort range (euglycemia is the term describing normal blood glucose levels), the hyperglycemic stimulus provokes insulin secretion and suppresses glucagon secretion. The secreted insulin serves to lower plasma glucose and thus serves as a negative feedback influence on the original disturbance. When hypoglycemia prevails, insulin secretion is suppressed and glucagon secretion is enhanced. Glucagon serves to increase plasma glucose toward the euglycemic range.

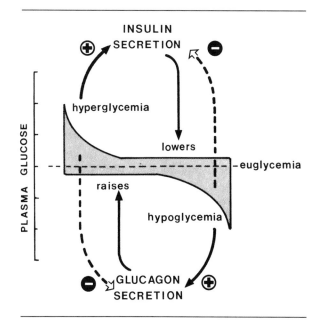

gut glucagon, along with a minor autonomic neural input to the pancreas, cause insulin secretion (Figure 4–25). This initial release of insulin during the early absorptive process probably primes the liver to facilitate efficient extraction of the flood of nutrients due to arrive when absorption gets under way. During absorption, there is net hepatic uptake of a variety of nutrients, under the dominant influence of insulin. Later, in what is called the postabsorptive phase, there is net hepatic release of nutrients, so between these two processes, the concentrations of key nutrients, or substrates, in blood are kept within acceptable limits (Figure 4–26). Disorders of insulin function are outlined in Box 4–12.

4.6 • Exercises

1. For the two hormones listed, identify the major physiologic variable they control and note the name of a hormone with opposing actions:

	Action	Other
Glucagon		
Calcitonin		

2. In the following sets of substances, one item in each set doesn't belong with the others. Identify the inappropriate entry and note why it is the odd one.

a. epinephrine, cortisol, histamine, norepinephrine

b. insulin, gastrin, PZ-CCK, secretin

c. LH, hCG, TSH, placental lactogen, FSH

d. GnRH, CRF, PIF, GHRH, TRH

e. progesterone, estradiol, relaxin, testosterone

3. One of the following general schemes for steroid transformations is correct. Identify it, then examine the schemes with the arrows reversed, when one other sequence becomes correct.

androgens → estrogens → progestins

progestins → androgens → corticosteroids

progestins → estrogens → androgens

corticosteroids → progestins → cholesterol

progestins → androgens → estrogens

4. There is widespread iodine deficiency in Nepal that affects animals and humans. Which endocrine system is most likely to be abnormal in the Himalayan yak in its home environment?

a. Identify the gland that is central to this system.

b. What gross changes are likely to occur in this gland?

c. What hormones produced by this gland are likely to be affected?

d. Will concentrations of these hormones be higher or lower than those in unaffected animals?

Vital Life Support Systems

5

5.1 • Integrated Systems and Homeostasis

The concept of homeostasis was introduced in Chapter 2, in relation to control systems that operate to preserve the internal environment. The following seven sections describe the major vital systems that cooperate with each other in supporting life. Their function can be described as being integrative, in that they are continually adjusted according to need and because changes in one system are usually accompanied by changes in the others.

Three key physiologic systems—*cardiovascular, respiratory,* and *renal* systems—play a dominant role in the preservation of the internal environment in face of external influences. They function cooperatively to try to maintain critical physiologic variables within acceptable comfort ranges. All three systems are primarily controlled by the autonomic nervous system,

with additional significant input from endocrine mechanisms. The vital physiologic systems yield endless examples of the application of the control systems, introduced in Chapters 3 and 4. Furthermore, the operation of these vital systems is intimately related to the structure of the component tissues and organs.

The adequacy of the function of the vital support systems is best assessed by a few key variables, the magnitude of which can readily be determined in the blood. Physiologists, clinicians, and animal scientists measure blood parameters and related variables such as heart rate, respiration rate, ease of respiration, and the like as *vital signs* in the animals (or humans) with which they work.

The circulation of blood provides linkage between the three vital systems, as is obvious in the example of gas exchange between the environment at large and the deep tissues. Indeed, Section 5.2 is devoted to a description of the integrative nature of blood and Section 5.4 will describe the important features of gas transport mechanisms.

In several earlier places in this text, the importance of water to the normal functioning of living systems was emphasized. Water is the most abundant molecule in the body, and it is the major solvent with a wide array of important properties, previously noted in Chapter 2. Cells are bathed in aqueous solutions making up the interstitial fluid, and most substances passing to and from the cells must traverse this compartment. Cells have rather stringent requirements for the concentration of solutes in the fluid in their immediate environment. In Chapter 2, the phenomena of osmosis and osmotic pressure were briefly introduced.

Osmotic pressure is a consequence of the total number of particles, dissolved in a solution. A 1 molar (1M) solution of glucose has the same number of particles as does a 0.5M solution of sodium chloride, or, more correctly, of sodium and chloride ions. Every molecule of sodium chloride dissociates into one Na^+ ion and one Cl^- ion, whereas the glucose does not dissociate. This logic can be extended further. Magnesium chloride, $MgCl_2$, dissociates to one Mg^{2+} ion and two Cl^- ions, for a total of three. Thus a 0.33M solution of $MgCl_2$, a 0.5M solution of NaCl, and a 1M solution of glucose are all said to be *isosmotic*. The three solutions each contain the same number of particles. The osmolarity of the extracellular fluids is closely monitored and is subject to fine adjustment by controlling water excretion and water intake. These mechanisms are crucial to the well-being of animals because of the behavior of cells in solutions of inappropriate osmotic strength.

Tonicity

When the osmotic pressure of blood is artificially lowered, as for example by diluting blood with distilled water, cells swell and lyse. The water dilutes the osmotic strength of the solution of proteins and ions. Water will be drawn into the cells from this now more dilute extracellular solution. The erythrocyte is a convenient cell to monitor osmotic rupture since the escape of hemoglobin is easily detected, and is called hemolysis. The cell membrane separates the intracellular "solution" from plasma; water moves by osmosis in an attempt to equalize concentrations of the solutes on either side. If no water movement occurs when erythrocytes are transferred to a salt solution, the latter may be considered to be *isotonic*. This term pertains to the effect of a solution on the integrity of the cell. Isotonic actually means "same tension" and, of course, tension refers to the degree of "stretch" of the plasmalemma, a consequence of change in intracellular volume.

Less concentrated solutions will lead to water movement into the cells, swelling and possibly lysis; such a solution is called *hypotonic*. Concentrated solutions draw water out of the cells, causing shrinkage, or crenation. Such solutions are *hypertonic*.

While this description reiterates material presented earlier on the need for osmotic regulation, it should be remembered that erythrocytes, because of their shape, are atypically tolerant of osmotic variation. Thus, if erythrocytes are damaged by a particular solution, it is likely that most other cells will be destroyed as well.

5.2 • Blood as a Tissue of Integration

This section reviews some of the material presented in various places in earlier chapters, then introduces a number of new aspects important to the operation of the major vital systems.

Blood volume is approximately 6% to 10% by weight (1 liter = 1 kg) of the adult animal. The adult pig is exceptional in having 3.5% to 4.5% of body weight as blood volume. The normal range of pH lies between 7.2 to 7.7, with a typical mean of about 7.4. Arterial blood may be slightly more basic and venous blood slightly more acid. This will be explained later in this section, when buffers are introduced.

slightly leaky circulatory system. Factors influencing the movement of fluids into and out of the blood vessels are described in the next section. When plasma protein concentrations are subnormal because of malnutrition or chronic blood loss, tissue edema will result from this movement of fluid out of the blood and into the interstitium. The plasma proteins also contribute to the *viscosity* of blood, an important hemodynamic factor, by influencing blood flow rate and the maintenance of intravascular pressure. Most importantly, plasma provides the *vehicle* for suspending, mixing, and transporting of blood cells.

Plasma

The noncellular component of noncoagulated blood is plasma, which accounts for 55% to 70% of blood volume. The plasma volume is determined by measuring the proportion made up by packed cells, the *packed cell volume*. The various constituents of plasma include gases, proteins, energy substrates, nonprotein nitrogenous molecules, inorganic salts, vitamins, lipids, and so forth.

Some important functions of plasma are obvious: the transport of glucose or of small hydrophobic molecules associated with the proteins. Lipids are generally hydrophobic and insoluble, but they can be transported efficiently when they are associated with plasma proteins.

A major function of the plasma proteins is to provide *colloid osmotic pressure* in the blood and thereby to reduce water movement out of the capillary beds and into tissue. The driving force for the efflux is simply the hydrostatic pressure present in the vascular bed, a result of the combined effects of the pumping action of the heart and peripheral resistance in the very

The Formed Elements

A brief review of material introduced in Chapter 1 is provided in Box 5–1. In cattle of about 500 kg live weight, blood volume is 40 L. There are approximately 7 million erythrocytes per cubic milliliter of blood. Thus the cell population is of the order of 2.8×10^{14}; the total surface area is about 30,800 m^2, or some 60 m^2 per kg body weight. Some comparative data are provided in Table 5–1.

As a result of their shape, the cells tolerate considerable osmotic swelling before they burst and release their contents. This rupture of erythrocytes is called hemolysis. The volume tolerance is important because blood is the primary tissue involved in water fluxes, especially within the visceral circulation, and it is continually subjected to fairly substantial inputs and outputs of water. Without the protection conferred by the unique shape of erythrocytes, the water fluxes and osmotic changes might disturb the integrity of the erythrocytes.

The shape also determines that the maximal

Box 5–1   Erythrocytes

Red blood cells in mammals are nonnucleated, flat to biconcave disks. The cells are small (4 to 9 μ in diameter) and readily deformed as they pass through capillary beds. The shape serves a number of additional purposes:

- Increased surface area relative to volume,

- Safety measure for erythrocyte swelling during osmotic changes, and

- Minimized diffusion distance into center from the surface.

The leukocytes, or white blood cells, were described briefly in Chapter 1. They will be described in more detail in relation to defense mechanisms in Chapter 9.

---

diffusion distance from the membrane into the interior of the cell is less than 1 μ. This is especially relevant for the gas transport function of the cells, described below.

Erythrocytes are produced in bone marrow by a process called erythropoiesis, under control by erythropoietin, a hormone released from the kidney in response to renal hypoxia, or inadequate tissue levels of oxygen. The formation of erythrocytes is also influenced by several vitamins and minerals. The cells are formed from *reticular cells*, a common primitive cell that gives rise to some leukocytes as well as immature erythrocytes called *reticulocytes*. The number of these cells in blood is diagnostically useful because the reticulocyte count is elevated in chronic anemia or other conditions when erythropoiesis is very active.

Under normal conditions a 500-kg bovid may be producing and destroying some 35 to 40 million erythrocytes per second!

The most obvious function of erythrocytes is in oxygen transport. This results from the loose affinity of the iron in hemoglobin for oxygen. The iron is normally present as the *ferrous* ion (Fe^{2+}) and can bind oxygen. Solids comprise about 35% of the erythrocyte, and hemoglobin makes up about 80% of that. Normal blood levels of hemoglobin range between 10 and 15 gm/100 mL. Subnormal hemoglobin concentration is referred to as *anemia*. Some other disturbances in oxygen-carrying capacity are noted in Box 5–2.

Box 5–2   Hemoglobin Disturbances

If the iron in hemoglobin is oxidized it becomes the ferric ion (Fe^{3+}). The resulting *methemoglobin* no longer carries oxygen. Hemoglobin binds carbon monoxide with great avidity, forming the compound known as carboxyhemoglobin, which cannot carry oxygen.

The oxidized (Fe^{3+}) methemoglobin form is encountered in animals as a result of nitrate poisoning and this can be of importance for domestic animals. It can also occur following administration of some drugs.

Table 5–1. Characteristics of Erythrocytes in Various Species

	Cattle	Horses	Pigs	Sheep	Goats	Dogs	Cats	Chickens	Humans
Body weight (kg)	500	500	100	40	30	20	3	2	70
Blood volume (L)	40	40	8	3.2	2.4	1.6	.24	0.16	5.6
Erythrocytes ($\times 10^6$/mm^3)	7	10	7	11	14	7	7	3	5
Diameter (microns)	6	5.5	6	4.8	4	7	6	11.2 × 6.8[a]	7.5
Surface area (microns^2)	110	84	113	66	50	121	113	183	162
Total erythrocyte area (m^2)	30,800[b]	33,600	6,328	2,323	1,680	1,355	190	80	4,536
Area normalized to body weight (m^2/kg)	62	67	63	58	56	68	63	44	65

[a]Chicken erythrocytes are oval.
[b]For comparison, the playing area of a football field is 4,180 m^2.

Blood Clotting

Blood coagulation results from conversion of *fibrinogen* to *fibrin*, under the influence of an enzyme called *thrombin*. Fibrinogen is a soluble protein that has a very high *axial ratio*. This means that, rather than being globular in shape, the protein is threadlike and has enormous length, relative to its diameter.

When converted to fibrin, the proteins intermesh and tangle upon each other, creating a meshlike or weblike matrix. Thrombin is normally present in plasma in an inactive form called *prothombin*. The activation of thrombin involves a cascade of controls that are the best example in biology of a *positive feedback system*. The very process of clotting acts to promote more clotting. Numerous factors are involved, but the ultimate event is the conversion of prothombin to thrombin, its active form, which is promoted by *factor X*, a proteolytic enzyme. The two major clotting mechanisms are briefly described in Box 5–3. Examples of bleeding disorders are given in Box 5–4.

The circulatory system has, in its small vessels, *mast cells*, which produce the endogenous anticoagulant *heparin*. This substance helps limit clot formation, and purified heparin is administered therapeutically to prevent or reduce clotting. Heparin is a complex mucoid substance commonly used in medicine. It is prepared by extracting byproduct tissues from animals, such as liver, collected in packing plants. The pharmaceutical preparation of heparin from this source is one of the many ways in which animals contribute to the welfare of human beings.

After clot formation in a ruptured blood vessel, the healing process begins. The clot is gradually dissolved, or fragmented, by the enzyme *plasmin*, and small portions are phagocytosed by leukocytes present in the blood.

An Introduction to Physiologic Buffering

Many molecules of physiologic interest exist in partially ionized states in water and in tissue fluids. Dissociation yields anions (negative) and cations (positive), the most important of which by far are hydrogen ions.

$$\text{Lactic acid} \rightleftharpoons \text{Lactate}^- + \text{H}^+$$

$$\text{Acetic acid} \rightleftharpoons \text{Acetate}^- + \text{H}^+$$

$$\text{Carbonic acid} \rightleftharpoons \text{Bicarbonate}^- + \text{H}^+$$

Box 5–3   Blood Clotting

Intrinsic coagulation mechanisms are initiated by blood contacting anything other than endothelial cells. These line the blood vessels, as noted in Chapter 1. A series of calcium-dependent processes results in fibrin formation, the gelling or crosslattice formation, and the trapping of blood cellular constituents.

The *extrinsic* mechanism involves release of thromboplastin from damaged tissue. This tissue-derived enzyme causes direct activation of factor X, which is much faster than all of the events involved in the intrinsic mechanism. Clot formation therefore occurs very rapidly. Clearly, this more rapid mechanism would be an asset to control massive hemorrhage in traumatized tissue.

Box 5–4   Bleeding Disorders

Some bleeding disorders are hereditary, such as *hemophilia,* and some result from deficiencies of vitamins or food components. Vitamin K deficiency interferes with hepatic production of clotting factors. Vitamin K action can be antagonized by war-

farin, a very effective rat poison, or by dicumarol, which is a natural constituent in some clover pastures and can be present in hay. This obviously can be of significance to domestic animals.

The differences between strong and weak acids and strong and weak bases, or H^+ acceptors, are described in Appendix A. Review this material if necessary. The dissociation equations indicate that mass action can drive these equilibria either way. The relative constancy in extracellular pH reflects what is called *physiologic buffering,* in which a range of dissociating molecular species acts to offset any potential change in H^+ concentration. Hydrogen ions are continuously generated by the various processes of metabolism. Sulfur and phosphorus, contained in many biologic/organic molecules, are metabolized to sulfuric and phosphoric acids. These strong acids are completely dissociated.

Many organic acids—nonesterified fatty acids from fat mobilization, lactic acid from muscular exertion, volatile fatty acids absorbed from fermentation digestion—although weak acids, still contribute substantial quantities of H^+ ions. However, by far the major source, normally balanced at the lung, is H^+ ions generated within blood, as follows:

$$CO_2 + H_2O \rightleftharpoons H_2CO_3 \rightleftharpoons HCO_3^- + H^+$$

If CO_2 retention in the body occurs, either transiently or chronically (as in cases of impaired pulmonary function), blood CO_2 concentrations rise above normal. By mass action (follow the reaction through to the right), this would elevate H^+ concentration, or decrease pH. In such cases acid excess can be removed only by renal mechanisms, as described in Section 5.6.

The key participants in buffering are HCO_3^-, protein$^-$, hemoglobin$^-$, and phosphates$^-$. These anions combine with H^+ and bring about neutralization:

$$Buffer^- + H^+ \rightleftharpoons H\text{-}Buffer$$

The bicarbonate concentration in extracellular fluids is high and is closely regulated by the kidneys. As HCO_3^- combines with H^+ and the carbonic acid breaks down to CO_2 and water, any sustained loss of CO_2, as in expired air, acts to remove H^+ (follow the reaction through to the left). This is facilitated because a fall in pH, excessive H^+ concentration, is a major stimulant for increased rate of respiration, and therefore CO_2 loss to the exterior is increased. These respiratory compensations will be described later in Sections 5.4 and 5.5.

Plasma proteins serve as buffers because of the population of negative charges they usually carry at physiologic pH. Thus, acting as anions, they can combine with H^+.

Hemoglobin that is not carrying oxygen, the *reduced hemoglobin* of venous blood, has a high affinity for H^+. Venous blood also has a high concentration of CO_2 as a result of active tissue metabolism. However, because:

$$CO_2 + H_2O \rightleftharpoons H_2CO_3 \rightleftharpoons HCO_3^- + H^+$$

the H^+ so generated is largely but incompletely taken up by the reduced hemoglobin. This is yet another buffering action. Thus the pH of venous blood is only slightly less than that of arterial blood. This all reverses at the lungs when CO_2 is blown off and hemoglobin becomes oxyhemoglobin.

Phosphate acts as a buffer by shifting between two forms:

$$HPO_4^{2-} + H^+ \rightleftharpoons H_2PO_4^-$$
$$\text{(base)} \qquad \text{(weak acid)}$$

In similar fashion, ammonia produced by deamination of amino acids can take up H^+ ions to form the ammonium ion (NH^+_4):

$$NH_3 + H^+ \rightleftharpoons NH_4^+$$

This is exactly what happens when ammonia gas is dissolved in water to form ammonium hydroxide solutions and it is an important method by which the kidneys eliminate H^+ from the body.

Acid-Base Balance

The normal distribution of acids, or H^+, and bases, or OH^-, or HCO_3^-, is strictly regulated. There is little allowable range in pH in the extracellular compartment. Considerable disturbance can, however, occur for reasons related to metabolism and respiration.

Metabolic acidosis can cause serious production losses in animals and can arise from:

- excessive ketoacid production,
- failure of renal HCO_3^- reabsorption, and

- diarrhea, with fecal loss of HCO_3^- derived from pancreatic and intestinal secretions.

In all cases, HCO_3^- concentration is subnormal and H^+ concentration is excessive. The acidosis may stimulate respiration to increase CO_2 loss. The normal concentrations are usually recovered only after compensatory renal acid secretion.

Metabolic alkalosis usually results from excessive acid loss such as from vomiting (loss of HCl), or from excessive renal H^+ excretion. The homeostatic adjustments are similar to but reversed from those in metabolic acidosis.

Respiratory acidosis occurs when pulmonary excretion of CO_2 is less than the rate of production. Blood concentrations of CO_2 increase and this is called *hypercapnia*. This may be due to depression of the respiratory center in the medulla oblongata. Alternatively, there may be some mechanical problem in ventilation that prevents normal removal of CO_2.

Respiratory alkalosis usually results from hyperventilation as a result of disturbed function of the respiratory center, or that evoked consciously such as excessive forced deep breathing. This is called *voluntary hyperventilation*. The resulting pH change is sufficient to disturb the state of ionization of several ions, and potentially hazardous side effects can occur, for example respiratory arrest and tetanic contraction of muscles.

This material is merely introduced at this point and will be developed further, later in this text. Much of the control of acid-base status involves the three major physiologic systems to be described in the following few sections. The reader is not expected to become proficient in this area until all of the relevant systems have been described.

5.3 • The Cardiovascular System

Cardiac Structure and Function

The following material summarizes the key aspects of the myocardium that were presented in Chapters 1 and 3, in the context of heart muscle as an excitable tissue. The emphasis is now placed on the function of this highly specialized tissue. Some of the details provided earlier are reviewed before they are developed in relation to the regulation of cardiac function.

Structure of the Muscle

Cardiac muscle grossly appears syncytial; however, the cells are mononucleate but provided with very tight electrocoupling at the cell junctions, or the intercalated disks. Distinct striations are evident. It can be assumed at this level of treatment that the intracellular mechanisms described for skeletal muscle are broadly applicable to cardiac muscle. That is, Ca^{2+} is needed to couple excitation and contraction, and the role of regulatory proteins, the function of cross-bridges, ratchet mechanism for filament sliding, and adenosine triphosphate (ATP) hydrolysis are all essentially as described for skeletal muscle in Chapter 3.

Electrophysiology

A major distinction between muscle types is evident in the form of excitation at the sarcolemmal level. In most cardiac muscle cells, there is *no steady resting potential*, but rather a slow drift to a threshold then the rapid generation of an action potential. The cell stays depolarized for a long time, some 150 to 500 msec, compared to the 1 to 2 msec in skeletal muscle. It remains refractory to generating further action potentials throughout this prolonged phase of depolari-

zation. The contraction develops, is maintained longer than in twitch muscles, then decays to rest before repolarization occurs to the *recovery potential*. Initially, Na^+ channels open and Na^+ pours in until sodium inactivation limits the extent of depolarization. K^+ efflux starts, but, in contrast to the situation in skeletal muscle and in nerves, it is then arrested, and so a sustained depolarization occurs. During this phase, Ca^{2+} enters the sarcoplasm and couples excitation to contraction. It seems likely that Ca^{2+} ions from outside the cell, together with those from sarcoplasmic reticulum, provide for excitation-contraction coupling. When the contraction is complete, K^+ efflux continues and repolarization is achieved. This long refractory period prevents temporal summation and provides for an obligatory relaxation phase, which permits heart filling. Without this protection, a steady cycle of relaxation and contraction could not occur and the heart would be unable to act as a pump.

Because the cells are so tightly electrocoupled, the activity of the cell population as a whole tends to be dictated by the cells with the fastest rate of firing. The specialized cardiac cells forming the sinoatrial (SA) node, or *heart pacemaker*, are *autorhythmic*, simply because of the instability of the resting potential and the slow drift of potential up to threshold. This drift is due to changes in K^+ permeability of the membrane, but finer details remain unknown. The autorhythmicity persists in completely isolated cells that continue to ''beat'' in cell culture. The rate of firing is determined by the rate of drift in potential from the recovery value. Note, this cannot be called a resting potential.

The intrinsic activity of the SA node is subject to influences from the autonomic nervous system. Most importantly, parasympathetic, cholinergic innervation from the vagus provides a means of slowing down the firing rate of the SA node.

This is a most important example of inhibitory motor innervation. It will be recalled that this type of control does not exist for skeletal muscle.

Although the SA node normally provides the pacemaker role, if for some reason any other myocardial area develops excessive excitability and begins firing more frequently than the SA node, this new area can take over the pacemaker function. This is a well-known aspect of caffeine intoxication. Some other aspects of abnormal pacemaker function are noted in Box 5–5.

The atrioventricular (AV) node is another coordinating group of cells located on the right atrium near the junction with the ventricle (Figure 5–1). The AV node is not normally autorhythmic because it picks up action potentials, originating in the SA node, that travel across the atrium by cell-cell contact. From the AV node these impulses are propagated to the bulk of the ventricular cells via the specialized cardiac muscle cells of the bundle of His and terminal Purkinje fibers. The AV node imposes a short delay on the action potentials, then the bundles provide for rapid and near-synchronous distribution of excitation to the myocardiocytes of the ventricles. Because of this arrangement, atrial contraction precedes ventricular contraction, and so the heart is designed and functions as a pumping organ. Damage to the AV node or the His bundle system causes partial or even complete dissociation of events in the atria and ventricles. These "heart conditions" are diagnosed with a great deal of precision by *electrocardiograms*.

Electrocardiography

The earlier discussion of excitable tissues (see Chapter 3) introduced the fundamentals of ions carrying charges, ion flows therefore being current flows, and differences in charge concentrations being the basis of potentials or voltages. The flow of current through a conductor generates an *electric field* that can be detected some distance away from the conductor. The propagation of action potentials through the myocardium likewise generates fields that can be detected at the body surface, in the form of the electrocardiogram (ECG).

The clinically useful ECG in reality represents the summation of action potential events from all parts of the heart, from the first depolarization at the SA node through to the last stage in the ventricular muscle. The compound signal in the ECG varies according to the placement of the electrodes over the heart and according to the relative spatial orientation of the heart to the rest of the body.

As shown in Figure 5–1, the *P wave* corresponds to depolarization of the SA node and cell-cell propagation over the atria. The major *QRS wave* reflects ventricular depolarization, then

---

Box 5–5   The Sinoatrial Node

If the SA node became dysfunctional, the atrial cells would take over the pacemaker role and the rate of contraction of the heart would decrease by 10 to 20 beats per minute. If the SA node and atrial tissue were both compromised, there would still be a safeguard, with the ventricular tissue able to take over pacing but at a much reduced rate (20 to 45 beats per minute).

Similarly, a device can be implanted to provide an electronically regulated stimulation to the heart, such as the nuclear pacemaker. Output may be at the SA node if this is defective or may be directly to the ventricles if there is a conduction block out of the AV node.

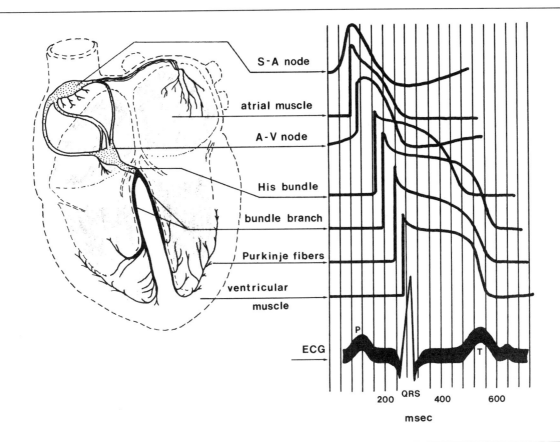

Figure 5–1. Composite electrocardiogram. The composite electrocardiogram (ECG), detected at the body surface, derives from electric fields associated with the passage of action potentials through the body of the heart. The pattern of depolarization—from the sinoatrial (S-A) node, across the atria to the atrioventricular (A-V) node, and through the His bundle and the Purkinje fibers to the ventricular muscle mass—is depicted by the tracings at right. Note the time axis, which indicates the delays within a single cycle and the relatively long period of depolarization at all locations distal to the A-V node. (Modified slightly and redrawn from the original by permission of the publisher. From Netter, F.H.: *The Ciba Collection of Medical Illustrations,* Vol 5, Summit, NJ: Ciba Pharmaceutical Products, 1969.)

the *T wave* corresponds to repolarization of the ventricles. This composite diagram illustrates many of the aspects already described:

- There is a time progression in the electrophysiologic events.

- The delay imposed by the AV node is evident.

- The prolonged depolarization of the ventricular components is quite obvious.

The Cardiac Cycle

The cardiac cycle denotes the sequence of events occurring during filling *(diastole),* and emptying *(systole).* Starting at diastole, when the heart is relaxed and filling, the cycle (see Figure 5–2) is as follows:

- The ventricles relax and intraventricular pressure falls;

- Backpressure in the arteries (aorta and pulmonary artery) snap the semilunar valves shut and generate the "dup" part of the "lub-dup" heart sound;

- Atrial contraction starts first and pumps blood into the relaxed ventricles;

- Ventricles are now filled and the contraction wave passes to the ventricles (the delay is explained above), and ventricular pressure starts to rise;

- During this phase of systole, valves between the atria and ventricles are closed (the "lub" sound) and pressure builds up to and then beyond residual arterial pressure;

- The valves to the arteries open and ventricular contents are forcibly ejected;

- The ventricles relax and the cycle starts with refilling of the relaxed atria.

Regulation of Cardiac Output

Cardiac output is defined as the volume of blood pumped through the heart each minute. It is expressed in units of mL/min or L/min, and is derived from the product of *heart rate* times *stroke volume:*

Figure 5–2. The cardiac cycle. This figure shows phases of the contractile cycle of the heart. The early stage of ejection (1) is followed by a major contractile effort (2); both phases constitute systole. During diastole, the atria fill (3), and the ventricles become distended (4). Because of Starling's Law, the volume at this stage—called *end diastolic volume*—largely determines the force of the subsequent systole.

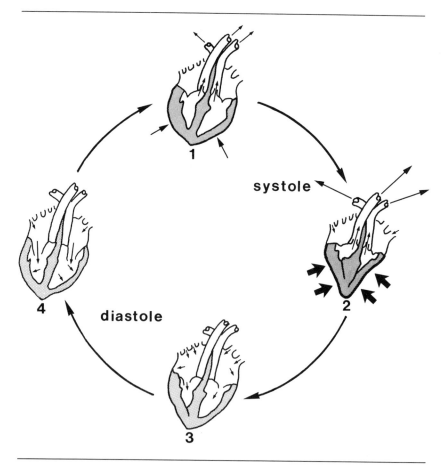

Cardiac
Output = Heart Rate × Stroke Volume
(mL/min) (beats/min) (mL/beat)

Heart rate is measured in beats per minute and stroke volume is expressed as volume of blood pumped per beat. Physiologically, adjustment of heart rate is achieved primarily by regulating the tonic vagal influence on the SA node. This vagal influence, or *vagal tone,* normally serves to hold the excitability of the pacemaker cells in check. The vagus nerve carries motor cholinergic fibers from the cardioinhibitory center of the medulla oblongata.

If the vagus nerve is sectioned, the typical response to the loss of motor traffic is an acceleration of heart rate, referred to technically as *tachycardia.* Atropine, as a cholinergic blocking agent, similarly causes tachycardia when administered to animals. On the other hand, acetylcholine or related agonists will slow down the rate of beating. This is called *bradycardia.* The vagal influence is said to be tonic because it is normally operative. Feedback influences that serve to increase heart rate are integrated at the cardioinhibitory center and result in less traffic of inhibitory action potentials being delivered via the vagus to the SA node.

There is a minor sympathetic influence on heart rate, mediated by epinephrine and norepinephrine. These catecholamines, obtained from either sympathetic nerve endings in the myocardium or by delivery via the circulation, after being released by the adrenal medulla, directly increase excitability of the cells. Any increase in excitability of SA node cells is manifested in more rapid drift of potential from the recovery value up to threshold. As a result, action potentials are released more frequently from the SA node, each one giving rise to a discrete heart beat.

In addition to regulation of the rate of heart beating, a great deal of flexibility in cardiac output is obtained from regulation of the volume of blood pumped at each stroke. By and large, this is varied by altering the *force* of each contraction, with more or less blood being drawn in from the great veins and delivered out at each systole.

Part of the regulation of stroke volume depends on *venous return,* which in turn depends on posture, regulation of the amount of blood pooled in the veins, or capacitance vessels, and the level of respiratory activity. With cyclic changes in the degree of vacuum prevailing in the thoracic cavity (see Section 5.5), changes also exist in the extent to which blood is drawn or "sucked" back to the heart.

One aspect of myocardial function, particularly important in regard to changing stroke volume is known as *Starling's law of the heart.* Starling's law recognizes that the contractility of the myocardium increases in relation to the degree of distension of the chambers at the end of diastole. Distension of the chambers is equivalent to greater stretching of the myocardiocytes that make up the walls of the chambers. If more blood is returned, filling and distension will be greater, and therefore the force of contraction is appropriately increased. This phenomenon is *intrinsic* to the muscle itself and, in comparison with other muscle types that have been described, is more a characteristic of smooth than of skeletal muscle.

Because the myofilaments in myocardium are organized in a way that shows up microscopically as striations, a characteristic of skeletal muscle, yet have the capacity to contract more forcefully when stretched, cardiac muscle is clearly intermediate in properties between the two major classes of muscle.

The strength of contraction is also subject to an *extrinsic* control mediated by catecholamines. The catecholamines act to reinforce the excitation-contraction coupling mechanism, possibly by their effect on excitability that was noted earlier, and a more powerful contraction results. Because this results in the potential for pumping greater than normal volumes of blood, venous return to the heart becomes even more important. It is not surprising, therefore, that the same sympathetic influences tend to cause partial constriction of the veins, so less blood is pooled and more is made available back to the heart.

The Heart as a Pump

The left and right sides of the heart function virtually simultaneously, and blood is ejected from both ventricles during systole. The right ventricle supplies the pulmonary artery and so delivers nonoxygenated blood to the lungs for gas exchange. The left ventricle supplies the aorta with oxygenated blood for delivery to remaining tissues. Return from the lungs via the pulmonary veins supplies the left atrium with freshly oxygenated blood; the right atrium collects nonoxygenated blood from the bulk of the body tissues via the venae cavae, or great veins.

The major pulmonary vessels provide an exception to the generalization that arteries carry oxygenated blood and veins carry nonoxygenated blood. There is, however, no exception to the statement that arteries carry blood, under substantial pressure, away from the heart, while veins bring it back, usually under minimal and sometimes slightly negative pressure.

The Peripheral Circulation

There are two major aspects of the properties and controls operating in the vascular system: arterial blood pressure and resistance to blood flow. Both are important in maintaining an adequate perfusion of the tissues. The controls of arterial pressure and flow at the vascular level are closely integrated with the central control of cardiac output.

Maintenance of Blood Pressure

Arterial pressure arises from the pumping action of the heart being opposed by resistance of the vessels through which the blood flows. Formal treatment of the flow of fluids in a tube is pure hydrodynamics and is described by *Poiseuille's equation:*

$$\text{Flow} = \frac{(\text{Pressure difference}) \times r^4 \times \pi}{8 \times \text{length} \times \text{viscosity}}$$

From this statement, several principles can be abstracted:

- Flow between two locations is proportional to the pressure differential existing between those locations;

- Flow increases in proportion to the fourth power of the caliber of the tube;

- Flow decreases if the tube is longer;

- Flow decreases if viscosity of the fluid increases.

Several physiologic mechanisms exist to regulate flow. The pressure differential can be increased either by more forceful contraction of the heart or by reducing the peripheral resistance of the small blood vessels. The diameter of the blood vessels changes in a systematic fashion from the aorta through the arterial tree down to the finest diameter vessels. The capillaries have approximately 1/3,000 the diameter of the trunk arteries in an animal of about 60 to 80 kg live weight. If the diameter of a vessel decreases by 50%, flow will decrease 16-fold, or by a factor of 2^4. All other factors being equal, and of course that is not strictly true, blood flow through a unit length of a capillary should be $3,000^4$-fold, or $1/81 \times 10^{12}$, less than through an equivalent length of aorta. Capillary flow rate can be directly visualized under a microscope and indeed it is miniscule and may periodically cease altogether.

Blood flows faster through shorter vessels, so as the diameter of the vessels is decreased for anatomic reasons within the branching of the arterial tree, the vessels are usually much shorter to offset this effect.

Blood viscosity is determined mainly by the density of the formed elements, expressed as the packed cell volume, though the plasma proteins do contribute to blood viscosity. An anatomic specialization, described in Section 5.6, results from the arrangement of branches in the renal arteries that effectively *skim* off cell-poor blood of lower viscosity to send into the glomeruli of the kidneys. The lower cell content means lower viscosity and therefore permits higher rates of flow.

> The principles underlying hydrodynamic flow are quite analogous to those expressed in Ohm's Law for electrical current flow: *Flow is directly proportional to the pressure difference and inversely proportional to the resistance of the conducting system.*

The driving force for the circulation of blood is clearly the muscular effort of the heart. However, the heart relaxes between each contraction, and something else is required to sustain pressure in the arteries between each systole. The architecture of the arterial vessels changes with distance from the heart, as shown in Figure 5–3.

The major arteries have heavy *fibroelastic* walls, while arteries of smaller caliber have proportionately more smooth muscle. The fibroelastic vessels are deformed outward by the peak arterial pressure during systole. This stretching generates tension in the vessel wall. The vessels recoil during diastole and, in so doing, they transmit the recoil potential back onto the blood contained within the lumen. This translates to a maintenance of pressure within the vessel. However, it doesn't totally even out pressure fluctuations because systolic pressure always exceeds diastolic pressure. Sufficient diastolic

Figure 5–3. Comparative structure of the blood vessels. These cross-sections provide an approximate indication of the diameters and wall thicknesses of major blood vessels (see numerical data for greater accuracy). The cellular nature of the wall varies with the mechanical stresses these vessels experience and certain functional specializations. The walls of the aorta and major arteries are fibroelastic (fe), providing strength and recoil potential upon deformation during each systole. This maintains arterial pressure during diastole, an important factor in the maintenance of blood flow despite the cyclical nature of cardiac contractions. The smallest arteries and arterioles have walls predominantly made up of smooth muscle (sm), subject to regulation by hormones and the sympathetic NS. The degree of smooth muscle contraction is the main determinant of peripheral resistance, and in part determines regional blood flow, as well. The capillary wall is essentially pure endothelium (endo), providing a leaky, semi-permeable barrier between the vascular system and the interstitial space. The smallest vessels on the venous side, venules and small veins, have some smooth muscle but are mainly fibrous (f) in nature. The walls are readily deformed (they lack the elasticity of major arteries) so these vessels can accommodate large volumes of blood under minimal pressure. The larger veins and venae cavae are still quite distensible but contain appreciable amounts of smooth muscle (sm). These capacitance vessels hold much of the total volume of blood in the circulation; the actual amount is regulated by veneconstrictor influences on the smooth muscle.

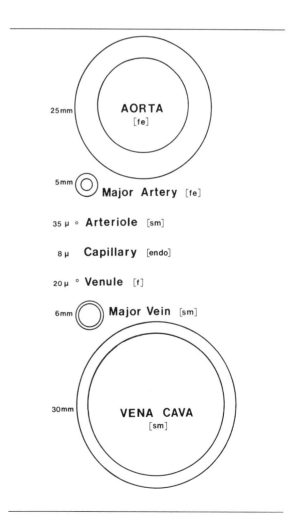

pressure remains, however, to sustain blood flow. The cycle of stretching then recoil serves to conduct pulse pressure along the vessels: this is what is palpated when one's pulse is counted.

The smooth muscle in the walls of the smaller arteries and arterioles are subject to control by neural and chemical influences. The state of contraction of the circular layer of muscle in the vessel wall determines the diameter of the vessel. Pressure within these vessels is drastically reduced compared to that in the trunk arteries, but extensive branching results in the total cross-sectional area for flow being markedly increased. Naturally, this is a requirement of a branching system that delivers blood to virtually all cells of the body. At the tissue level, further branching occurs prior to supplying the capil-

laries, the finest units of the circulatory tree. The consequences, in terms of velocity of flow and pressure, are depicted in Figure 5–4.

The capillaries are leaky tubes of a single layer of endothelial cells. These connect the arterial to the venous sides of the circulation. Structurally they are ideally suited for materials exchange between blood and interstitial fluid because of the minimal diffusion barrier of a single layer of cells, the leaky junctions between the cells, the capillaries' relatively long length, and their small diameter. The diameter requires many of the blood cells to deform in order to transit the capillary and hence flow along the length of the capillary is slow, another factor aiding the completeness of exchange of materials.

These structural properties of the capillary

Figure 5–4. Hemodynamics in the vascular system. This figure illustrates changes in pressure, relative total cross-sectional area, velocity of blood flow, and percentage distribution of blood volume in the major portions of the blood vascular system. Pressure is greatest in the arterial system (aorta, A; trunk arteries, TA; small arteries, SmA). It decreases abruptly in the arterioles (Ar), before the capillary system (Cap). The vast number of capillaries offsets their small diameter (see Figure 5–3) so that total cross-sectional area is greatest at this level. The bulk of blood volume (indicated by the percentages at bottom) is always found in the venous system (venules, Ven; small veins, SmV; large veins, LV; trunk veins, TV). These vessels have distensible walls and are known as capacitance vessels.

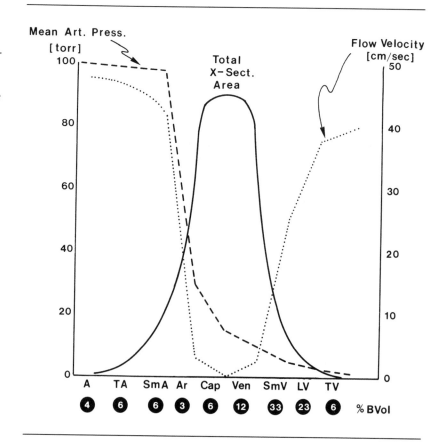

are disadvantageous, however, because of the possibility that hydrostatic pressure within the blood could rupture the delicate vessels.

The arterioles, over which most of the pressure drop occurs (see Figure 5–4), are assisted by *precapillary sphincters* in the task of protecting the capillaries from excessive pressure. The sphincters open and close to determine if flow actually occurs in a particular capillary; at no time would every capillary in the body be open.

Blood can bypass the capillary beds entirely by flowing through arteriovenous *anastomoses* (Figure 5–5). This has particular significance in thermoregulation, in addition to its protective function for the capillary beds. Shunting of blood through anastomoses in the peripheral tissues such as skin is used to dissipate heat (see Chapter 9).

After passing into the venous side of the vascular system, blood accumulates in vessels that are noticeably more distensible than the arteries. The bulk of blood volume can be found at any one instant in the venules and veins (see Figure 5–4). These relatively inelastic vessels distend without great recoil potential and so are called *capacitance vessels*. The veins do have a sparse investment of smooth muscle in their walls (see Figure 5–3), and their caliber can be controlled by sympathetic activity. As noted earlier, this neural control enables some degree of regulation of the venous return of blood to the heart.

Venous blood flow occurs, despite only a minimal pressure gradient that can be traced back to the arterial side, and thence to systole. Most of the arterial pressure is dissipated by the time blood reaches the small veins. Veins are structurally adapted by having *valves*, mere flaps of fibrous tissue, that allow blood to pass unidirectionally toward the heart. Skeletal muscle tone, particularly in the limbs, acts to squeeze blood along past the venous valves.

Thoracic and abdominal movements during breathing create periods during which negative pressure is transmitted into the vessels. These also serve to draw venous blood toward the heart, and are described as the *thoracic pump* and the *abdominal pump*. Venous pooling may be excessive during immobilization, especially when one

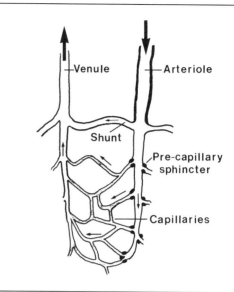

Figure 5–5. The capillary bed. Capillaries are the finest caliber blood vessels, merely the size of erythrocytes in diameter, with walls consisting only of a single layer of endothelial cells (illustrated in Figure 5–13). They are structurally weak and protected from excessive hydrostatic pressure from the arterial system by pre-capillary sphincters found in the smallest of the arterioles. The sphincters open and close under local controls in the vicinity of the capillaries; at any given time, most capillaries will be closed. Blood can bypass the capillary bed by passing through shunts (arteriovenous anastomoses), vessels of wider diameter that permit high flow rates, but do not provide the completeness of materials exchange that is typical of the capillary.

is standing quite still; the deficiency in venous return compromises cardiac output and so can be a cause of fainting.

Capillary Function and Tissue Fluid

The capillary beds are the low-pressure components of the blood vascular system that provide for materials exchange between elements of the blood and the interstitial fluid bathing cells in the tissues. Various capillary organizations may occur, with characteristic permeability differences in different tissues.

Capillaries are structurally well suited for providing a minimal diffusion barrier for gases and other dissolved materials. Some filtration also takes place, so the capillary must be regarded as a *leaky semipermeable membrane*, because large plasma proteins can and do exit in some capillary beds.

Some of the forces operating in diffusion have already been considered. Filtration pressure is essentially the net result of the outwardly directed forces minus the inwardly directed forces. These are related by *Starling's law of filtration:*

Factors favoring movement out of the vessel and into the interstitium are:

- Hydrostatic pressure within the vessel (P_{hv})

- Interstitial colloid osmotic pressure (P_{ci})

Factors favoring movement into the vessel from the interstitium are:

- Interstitial hydrostatic pressure (P_{hi})
- Plasma colloid osmotic pressure (P_{cv})

The net filtration force leading to fluid movement out of the capillary is obtained from:

$$(P_{hv} + P_{ci}) - (P_{hi} + P_{cv})$$

Of these four variables, only P_{hv}, or hydrostatic pressure within the vessel, changes appreciably along the length of the capillary. As shown in Figure 5–6, net fluid movement is from the capillary to the interstitium at the arterial end, but this is reversed toward the venous end and becomes an inward movement. A more complete derivation of the filtration forces and

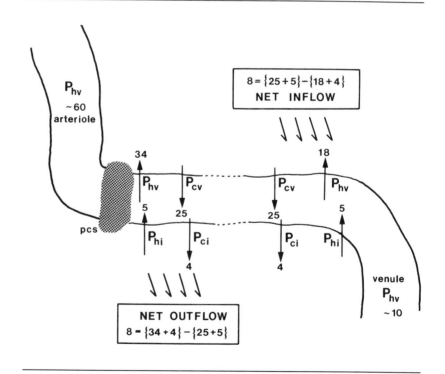

Figure 5–6. Starling's filtration forces. This figure provides some values, expressed in torr, of the major variables influencing liquid movement into and out of a capillary. Note the gradient in hydrostatic pressure within the vessels (P_{hv}) from the arteriole, past the precapillary sphincter (pcs), across the length of the capillary, and into the venule. The interstitial hydrostatic pressure (P_{hi}) for most capillaries is comparable at either end, as shown here, but varies with location in the body. Colloid osmotic pressure of the plasma (P_{cv}) and interstitium (P_{ci}) are given typical values. The computation of inward and outward forces, in this case leading to no net movement of fluid, is detailed in Box 5–6.

an explanation of the numbers used in Figure 5–6 are given in Box 5–6.

Normally, filtration into the tissues is somewhat in excess of the tendency for return from the tissues at the venous end, and there is an overall fluid transfer into the tissue from the circulation. Lymphatic drainage provides the means for returning this excess tissue fluid to the circulation. The amount of fluid leaving an individual capillary and reaching the interstitium is minute. However, there is such a large number of capillaries in the body that, totaled for all, the equivalent of total plasma volume leaves the circulation and enters the interstitium every minute. Obviously, much of this is re-

covered osmotically within the capillary by the mechanisms just described. The return of tissue fluid, or lymph, back into the plasma pool must account for the remainder. Any interference with lymphatic return will result in excessive extravascular accumulation of fluid, a phenomenon called *edema*.

A series of blind-ended, very permeable capillaries provides the uptake sites for lymphatic drainage. Lymphatics, like veins, have valves to help direct flow back toward the great veins, but all pumping arises from squeezing effects of muscle systems and the thoracic pump, arising from respiratory changes in thoracic pressure. Venous return and lymphatic drainage ob-

---

Box 5–6   Starling's Filtration Forces

The hydrostatic pressure in the immediate precapillary and postcapillary vessels has been measured by various techniques, and values of the order of 30 to 35 torr (1 torr = 1 mm Hg) are reasonable for the arterial side, while values less than 20 torr are obtained on the venous side. Colloid osmotic pressure inside the capillary (P_{cv}) remains at about 25 torr throughout. Only in the capillaries of the gut wall and in some renal capillaries is there any substantial change in osmotic pressure along the length of individual capillaries. This potential complexity can be ignored for the present. In the tissue, colloid osmotic pressure is about 4 torr, reflecting the relative paucity of proteins in the interstitial fluids, as noted in Chapter 2. Hydrostatic pressure in the interstitial fluid (P_{hi}) varies with location in a standing animal but is constant over the length of a single capillary.

Filtration force at the arterial end is therefore:

$$34 \text{ (hydrostatic, outward)}$$

$$- 25 \text{ (colloid osmotic pressure, inward)}$$

$$+ 4 \text{ (interstitial colloid osmotic pressure, outward)}$$

$$- 5 \text{ (interstitial hydrostatic, inward)}$$

or a net force outward of 8 torr.

At the venous end, forces inward are:

$$25 \text{ (colloid osmotic pressure)}$$

$$+ 5 \text{ (interstitial hydrostatic)}$$

$$- 18 \text{ (capillary hydrostatic)}$$

$$- 4 \text{ (interstitial colloid osmotic pressure)}$$

or a net inward force of 8 torr.

In this case, the tendency for fluid to leave the capillary and enter the interstitial space at the arterial end is exactly matched by the opposite tendency at the venule end. In most capillary beds, there is a net loss of fluid into the interstitial space.

viously have elements in common. Both depend on forces extrinsic to the cardiovascular system to ensure movement of fluid back toward the heart.

In the pulmonary vascular bed, the net filtration pressure is such that fluid does not normally accumulate in the perialveolar tissue. Pulmonary edema is a pathologic condition that impairs efficient gas exchange across the epithelial-endothelial wall of the alveolus.

Control of the Peripheral Circulation

Enormous opportunity exists for precise control of the peripheral vessels so that central arterial pressure can be maintained and the special *perfusion* needs of particular tissues can be satisfied. An array of neural and chemical means exists to achieve this control; and as might be expected, regulation of the vessels is closely integrated with control of cardiac function. Autonomic nervous control of the peripheral vessels is probably the most important mechanism, but its description will be deferred so that the overlaps with cardioregulation can be emphasized.

Chemical or humoral regulation is best separated into two classes: control of vessel relaxation and control of vessel constriction.

Vasodilators

Vasodilators are agents that act to relax peripheral arterial smooth muscle, thereby overriding the tonic (i.e., usually present) vasoconstrictor or sympathetic neural activity. Some vasodilators are "local" agents with restricted regional actions that serve to influence regional tissue blood flow. Examples of locally acting vasodilators include increased H^+ concentration, increased CO_2 concentrations, increased temperature, increased lactate or adenosine, and increased histamine, especially in damaged tissue. Some vasodilators are more typically "hor-

mone-like," although still mainly concerned in local, or intraorgan, controls. For example, active exocrine secretory tissues such as salivary and sweat glands release an enzyme called kallikrein, which generates, from a plasma protein precursor, a 9-amino acid peptide called *bradykinin*. Bradykinin is a potent vasodilator compound, best known because of its role in producing the redness and warmth associated with some inflammatory reactions. In salivary tissue the production of bradykinin and an active exocrine secretion are initiated by parasympathetic activity. With a high level of water flux into the secretory ducts, it is entirely reasonable to provide a method for increased blood flow to the gland.

Vasoconstrictors

Vasoconstrictors are agents able to contract vascular smooth muscle, irrespective of the state of tonic sympathetic activity. The catecholamines norepinephrine and epinephrine usually exert vasoconstrictor actions, but the delivery of these hormones via the circulation is normally less important for overall vasomotor control than is their release from sympathetic nerve endings in the tissues comprising the walls of the small arterioles. Although epinephrine is known to vasodilate blood vessels in skeletal muscles, it is a vasoconstrictor of most vascular beds. The difference in target tissue response is due to subtle adaptations and specializations in the catecholamine receptors in different tissues.

The biogenic amine serotonin is an example of a "local" vasoconstrictor. Serotonin is released from platelets when they aggregate on damaged vessel walls. Serotonin, by constricting flow through a damaged vessel, contributes to *hemostasis* in traumatized tissue.

The major circulating *pressor* agent is *angiotensin II*, an octapeptide derived from a precursor peptide angiotensin I, which in turn is split off plasma α_2-globulin by the kidney-derived enzyme *renin*. Renin is secreted into the circulation by the kidney as a compensatory mechanism in response to low arterial pressure (hypotension) sensed locally in the kidney (Box

5–7). Along with the kidneys' more obvious role of regulating water balance and therefore plasma volume, the renin-angiotensin system is a good example of the cooperative mechanisms displayed by the vital internal organ systems.

Neural Control

A general sympathetic innervation under control of the medulla oblongata is responsible for tonic control of the degree of constriction of the arterioles, and therefore of total peripheral resistance. This is the major determinant of arterial blood pressure. The medullary integrating area is the *vasomotor center.* It receives various inputs: a combination of descending, local, and ascending peripheral sensory information. Descending or cortex-derived inputs are responsible for characteristic pressor responses to certain emotions, such as the high blood pressure of anger, while depressor reactions may be associated with other selected emotions and are known to be a cause of fainting.

There is some input from the respiratory centers, as will be discussed later. The major input to the vasomotor center is from *baroreceptors* in the walls of the aortic arch, carotid sinus, the left and right atria, and the left ventricle (Figure 5–7). High intraluminal pressure serves to distend the elastic wall of these structures and the distension activates stretch receptors.

Stretch receptors in the wall of any distensible vessel or organ function as pressure receptors. Afferents from the baroreceptors travel in the glossopharyngeal and vagus nerves and serve as *inhibitory* influences on the vasomotor center.

A relatively minor sensory input to the vasomotor center is provided by *chemoreceptors* in the carotid and aortic bodies, the locations of which are also shown in Figure 5–7. These structures are highly vascularized tissues in the walls of the great arterial vessels. They are especially rich in receptors capable of detecting blood pH and/or concentration of CO_2. These chemoreceptors and their afferents exert major control on the inspiratory center for regulation of respiration.

Vasomotor tone, or the steady discharge of sympathetic motor signals to the arterioles, is reflexly adjusted to maintain blood pressure, as sensed by the baroreceptors. A *depressor response*, or a decrease in mean arterial blood pressure, results from the reduction in peripheral resistance. When stimulated by hypertension, the vasomotor center is inhibited and efferent sympathetic activity is reduced to cause *passive* vasodilation. This is achieved merely by reducing the vasoconstrictor tone. The response is facilitated by baroreceptor-mediated stimulation of the cardioinhibitory center. This leads to enhanced vagal efferent activity, a reduction in rate of firing of the SA node and therefore a consequent bradycardia. Carefully consider what is happening in this good example of a coordinated response between two mechanisms:

Reduced vasomotor tone allows the small arterioles to relax. The resistance of the blood vessels to the flow of blood is reduced. The slowing of the heart directly reduces cardiac output.

The combined effects of bradycardia

Box 5–7   The Kidneys and Blood Pressure

Any experimental constriction of the renal artery activates the renin-angiotensin mechanism and causes a pressor response. If a partially constricting clamp is placed on the renal arteries, *hypertension* develops. This has been useful as a model for research purposes in the study of cardiovascular diseases.

Figure 5–7. Receptive fields for cardiovascular regulation. Afferents from baroreceptors in the vessel walls lead to the vasomotor center (VMC) in the medulla oblongata of the brain. Their input is inhibitory on the VMC, which regulates vasoconstrictor tone of the arterioles. Baroreceptor input is excitatory on the cardioinhibitory center (CIC) that controls vagal influence on the heart. Activation of the baroreceptors leads to reduced vasoconstrictor tone (from the VMC) and increased cardioinhibitory traffic (from the CIC) to the heart. Afferents from the chemoreceptors in the carotid bodies and the aortic bodies have some influence on the VMC and CIC, but they are more important for regulation of respiration (Section 5–5). The major receptive fields are in the aortic arch where the impact of each systole on the arterial wall is greatest, and in the region where the common carotid artery divides to supply the internal and external carotids.

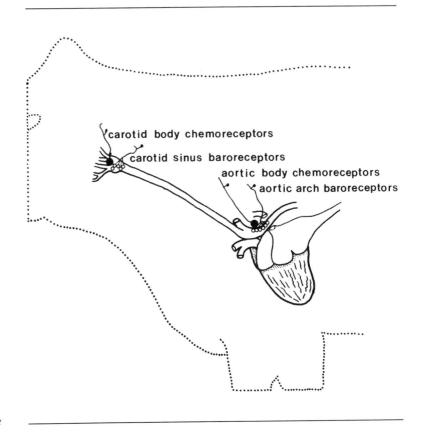

carotid body chemoreceptors
carotid sinus baroreceptors
aortic body chemoreceptors
aortic arch baroreceptors

and reduction of peripheral vasoconstrictor tone reduces blood pressure. The reduction in pressure serves then as a negative feedback to achieve homeostasis.

The interplay of factors determining mean arterial pressure is illustrated in Figure 5–8. As was emphasized earlier, pressure is the result of the pumping action of the heart working against total vascular resistance. The reader should be quite familiar with all of the variables and controls contributing to stroke volume, heart rate, arteriolar tone, and blood viscosity.

An example of a disorder involving regulation of mean blood pressure, indeed one that is likely to affect many readers at a later age, is noted in Box 5–8.

Box 5–8 Chronic Hypertension

In chronic hypertension, a common circulatory disorder, the processes described in the text all operate, but they do so at a higher *setpoint*. Blood pressure is maintained homeostatically in exactly the same way, and with the same degree of precision, but it is held at a consistently higher level than normal.

Figure 5–8. *Factors contributing to arterial pressure.* Mean arterial pressure is influenced by two major determinants: *cardiac output* and *total peripheral resistance.* Each is in turn the result of the interplay of variables that can be altered physiologically and pathologically. Use this figure for summary and review purposes. If components of this control chart are unclear, return to the description in the text for a more complete explanation.

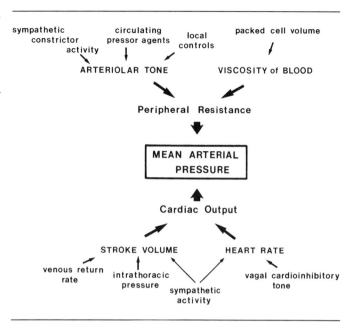

5.4 • Gas Transport

It was noted in Section 5.2 that hemoglobin participates in buffering H^+ ions and that its ability to do so varies with its oxygenation state. This results from a conformational change in the protein when it takes up O_2, with the release of one H^+ ion. Similarly, reduced hemoglobin (hemoglobin that has given up O_2) has a high affinity for H^+. A "solution" of oxyhemoglobin is thus more acid than reduced hemoglobin. This phenomenon is termed the *Haldane effect:*

$$Hb \cdot H^+ + O_2 \rightleftharpoons HbO_2 + H^+$$

As noted earlier, this buffering role of hemoglobin minimizes pH differences between arterial and venous blood.

There are two important consequences of these properties of hemoglobin. Increased acidity in peripheral tissue resulting from general metabolic processes, by mass action, assists in displacing O_2 from hemoglobin and making it available for diffusion into the tissues. This phenomenon is called the *Bohr effect:*

$$\overset{\text{available to tissue}}{Hb \cdot H^+ + O_2 \rightleftharpoons HbO_2 + H^+} \underset{\text{tissue acidity from metabolism}}{}$$

Increased partial pressure of oxygen (PO_2) in the pulmonary vascular bed aids in H^+ release and, through the buffering by HCO_3^-, facilitates CO_2 release from blood and makes it available for diffusion into the alveolus of the lung:

$$Hb \cdot H^+ + O_2 \rightleftharpoons HbO_2 + H^+$$
from alveolar air

$$CO_2 + H_2O \rightleftharpoons H_2CO_3 \rightleftharpoons HCO_3^- + H^+$$
yielded up to alveolar air

The amount of oxygen combined with hemoglobin is mainly controlled by P_{O_2}. The concentrations of gases are described in terms of P_{O_2} and P_{CO_2} in Box 5–9.

In addition to P_{O_2}, pH (via the Bohr effect) and temperature both influence what is called the *oxygen dissociation curve*. This is the relationship between the degree of association of O_2 with hemoglobin, expressed as the percentage saturation, for different P_{O_2} values. Because O_2 combines with Hb to form HbO_2, increased P_{O_2} should increase formation of HbO_2 merely by mass action.

The shape of the saturation curve (Figure 5–9) also means that as hemoglobin takes up O_2 in the lungs, blood P_{O_2} remains low, and so diffusion of alveolar O_2 down a concentration gradient and into the blood is facilitated.

In peripheral tissues, where tissue P_{O_2} is lower than arterial P_{O_2} (Figure 5–10), O_2 diffuses out of the capillaries, following its concentration gradient. The supply of O_2 for diffusion into the

---

Box 5–9   Properties of Gases

Physical principles dictate the behavior of gases in contact with the liquids, including body fluids, in which they can dissolve. At reasonable altitudes and in reasonable environments, the atmosphere is composed of about 21% O_2 and 0.03% CO_2 in a bulk volume that is mainly nitrogen. The following principles or laws are important in understanding the behavior of gases:

Boyle's law: At any given temperature, the product of the volume of a gas times the pressure it exerts is constant.

Partial pressure: Partial pressure is the pressure that would be exerted by one component of a mixture of gases if that component were present alone in the container.

Dalton's law: The pressure exerted by a gas mixture equals the sum of the partial pressures of the gases making up the mixture. The pressure exerted by gas *A* in a mixture of *A* + *B* + *C* + . . . + *X* is independent of the pressure of *B* or *C* or *X*.

Henry's law: The amount of gas dissolved in simple physical solution at any given temperature is proportional to the pressure of the gas in the atmosphere contacting the liquid.

The amount of gas in blood is expressed as a partial pressure. For example the P_{CO_2} in venous blood is about 46 torr, and this is sometimes called the *blood gas tension*. When the liquid is in contact with an atmosphere and the gas equilibrates between the two phases according to Henry's law, the partial pressure can then be determined. Blood, within a closed system of blood vessels, is obviously prevented from direct contact with the atmosphere. However, for the purposes of calculation, it is easiest to consider that the dissolved gas does exhibit a partial pressure even in a closed vascular system. There is additional complexity in any consideration of gases and blood because of the chemical reactions that occur between CO_2, O_2, and blood constituents. The gases are not simply dissolved in the blood.

Figure 5–9. *Oxygen association–dissociation curve.* The degree of saturation of hemoglobin with oxygen varies with the partial pressure of the oxygen (the oxygen tension, see Box 5–9). Note that the shape of the curve means that percent saturation of the hemoglobin remains relatively constant at above P_{O_2} of about 70 torr. This means that the total oxygen carrying capacity of the blood (almost entirely in the hemoglobin bound form) is only slightly affected by quite substantial reductions in P_{O_2}.

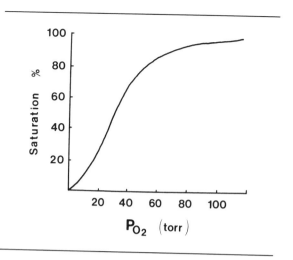

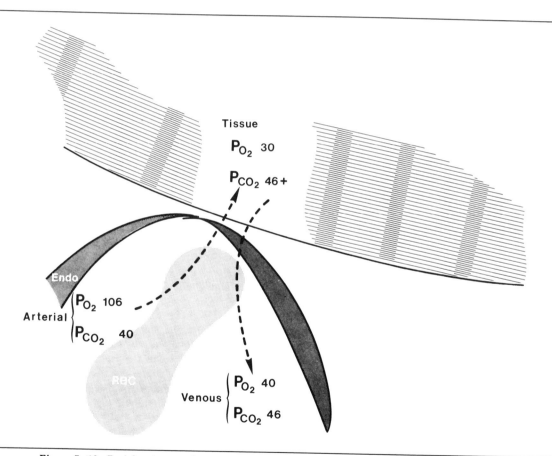

Figure 5–10. *Peripheral gas exchange.* The marked gradient existing between P_{O_2} in arterial blood and P_{O_2} in the tissue (106 to 30 torr) enables the latter to extract oxygen out of the blood and across the endothelium (Endo). P_{O_2} in blood is buffered by hemoglobin in the erythrocyte (RBC) giving up O_2. P_{CO_2} in the tissue is a little higher than arterial P_{CO_2} (46 compared with 40 torr), but carbon dioxide diffuses very readily and in blood is converted to carbonic acid (H_2CO_3), so venous P_{CO_2} is in equilibrium with that of the tissue.

solid tissues is continuously replenished by O_2 obtained from hemoglobin by dissociation. The Bohr effect assists this transfer of O_2. Additional factors facilitate the yielding up of O_2 from HbO_2 in metabolically active tissues. As shown in Figure 5–11, as temperature rises, O_2 dissociates more completely. That means that there is less O_2 bound in the form of HbO_2 at any given value of PO_2. Active tissues also produce more CO_2, and capillary blood is said to be hypercapnic, or has a higher PCO_2. Now, because:

$$CO_2 + H_2O \rightleftharpoons H_2CO_3 \rightleftharpoons HCO_3^- + H^+$$

from active tissue

made available to tissue

$$Hb \cdot H^+ + O_2 \rightleftharpoons HbO_2 + H^+$$

it is apparent that the Bohr effect operates to favor O_2 availability.

An important adaptation of the fetus stems from the different type of hemoglobin it possesses until after birth. *Fetal hemoglobin* has much higher affinity for O_2 than does adult hemoglobin. Because of this, fetal hemoglobin becomes saturated with O_2 at lower PO_2, and this aids in extracting O_2 from the maternal circulation, across the diffusion barrier of the placenta. Fetal tissue PO_2 is much lower than in maternal tissue, so the gradient maintains the supply of O_2 to the fetus:

Maternal Blood → Fetal Blood → Fetal Tissue

However, while PO_2 seems to be very low (i.e., *hypoxemic*), the total O_2 content of the blood is not so low. Fetal hemoglobin is just more completely saturated at the lower PO_2 than is maternal hemoglobin.

The same principles as those enumerated above are critical for efficient oxygenation of the fetus. These include relative *hypercapnia*, elevated fetal *temperature*, marginal *acidosis*, low PO_2 in blood, and *relative hypoxia* (reduced oxygenation) in the tissues. The biology of the fetus, including its special circulatory system and the changes that occur at birth, will be described in some detail in Chapter 10.

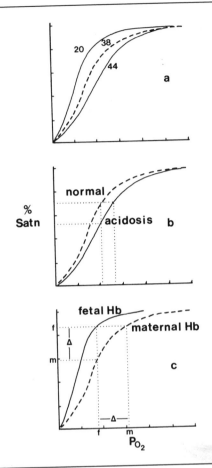

Figure 5–11. *Adjustments to the hemoglobin dissociation curve. a:* The dissociation curves show, under experimental in vitro conditions, that oxygen dissociates from hemoglobin to a greater degree at elevated temperatures, at any given value of PO_2. Thus, oxygen is made available for diffusion more readily at elevated temperatures. The converse is true at temperatures lower than physiological values. *b:* Acidity has the same effect as elevated temperature (Bohr Effect or Shift). The elevated temperature and acidity typically found in active tissues increases the availability of oxygen. *c:* Fetal hemoglobin has different oxygen saturation properties than adult hemoglobin; the fetal pigment is more completely saturated at substantially lower values of PO_2. The oxygen carrying capacity of fetal blood can therefore be met while fetal PO_2 is kept at lower levels than maternal PO_2. This gradient in PO_2 favors oxygen transfer from maternal to fetal blood across the placenta.

Box 5–10   Oxygen Dissociation Curve

The oxygen dissociation or saturation curve (Figure 5–9) shows that most combining of Hb and O_2 occurs at a Po_2 of about 60 torr. The plateau abve 65 to 70 torr is important because it ensures that nearly complete saturation of hemoglobin still occurs even though Po_2 may have fallen substantially from typical arterial O_2 tensions of about 100 torr. This is exactly what prevails at high altitudes when Po_2 in the air breathed by animals is reduced. If exposure to low Po_2 persisted chronically, other adaptations would occur, such as increased erythropoiesis to increase the circulating red cell population. This characteristic of the saturation curve is therefore mainly a short-term protective device. The increase in Pco_2, by producing H^+, contributes to increased dissociation of $Hb \cdot O_2$ via the Bohr effect.

5.5 • External Respiration

This section examines the reasons for and advantages of breathing, introduces some aspects of the mechanics of external respiration and gas exchange between the atmosphere and blood, and considers the key elements in the regulation of respiratory activity. The reader should attempt to integrate this material on respiratory activity into the functioning of the other vital life support processes.

Why Breathe?

Large multicellular animals cannot depend on simple diffusion mechanisms to exchange gases between tissues en masse and the environment; nor does their internal environment tolerate being subjected passively to variations in the external environment. The mutual participation of the circulatory and respiratory systems circumvents this potential hazard. Simultaneously, respiratory mechanisms provide for a number of more specialized functions:

- Respiration provides a continuous supply of oxygen for general metabolic needs, as in oxidative phosphorylation.

- In the processes of energy production, respiration recycles lactate as part of the Cori cycle.

- Respiration removes excess carbon dioxide produced by metabolism and aids in the maintenance of acid-base balance. In ruminants, other gases produced within the rumen may be absorbed into the blood and eliminated by respiratory activity.

- Respiration contributes to thermoregulation (see Chapter 9) by providing a means of dissipating body heat through two mechanisms: *conductive*, or direct heat flow, to warm incoming atmospheric air to body temperature; and *evaporative*, by vaporizing moisture in the airways to saturate the incoming air.

- Respiration provides a mechanism for vocalization, and provides an air stream for minimizing thermal trauma of the buccal cavity from ingestion of very hot food and drink.

- Through the generation of positive or negative pressure, respiration aids in the function of the digestive tract (see Chapter 6), and in the process of parturition at the end of pregnancy (see Chapter 10).

For the present, this introduction is mainly concerned with the passage of gases from inspired air across the moist membrane of the lung and into the blood, and vice versa. Diffusion mechanisms, introduced in Chapter 2, are applicable, with concentration differences for each gas providing the driving force. The nature of the diffusion barrier will be briefly considered; the structural components of the airways and then the mechanics and control of ventilation will then be described.

The Alveolar Membrane and Gas Exchange

The *alveoli*, or terminal air sacs of the airways (Figure 5–12), provide approximately 100 m^2 of surface area and an average separation between capillary blood and air of just a few microns

Figure 5–12. The lung and pulmonary alveoli. The upper diagram shows the right lung of a sheep viewed mediastinally, or from the left. The bronchial tree is shown in dotted outline as it is not visible in the intact lung. The lobes are apical (a); cardiac (c); diaphragmatic (d); and mediastinal (m). The fine terminal structures of the airways are shown in the exploded views. Note that along with the pneumocytes, or alveolar epithelial cells, capillaries are integral components of the alveolar wall.

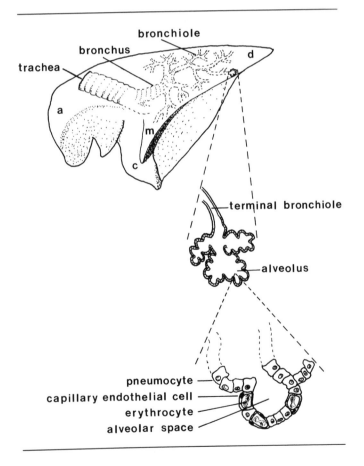

(Figure 5–13). This capillary bed is probably the richest of all tissues in the body and may contain up to 25% of blood volume during quiet rest. Gas exchange across the moist diffusion barrier of the alveolar membrane is described as follows:

$$\text{Velocity} = k \times \frac{(\text{Pressure diff.}) \times (\text{Gas solubility})}{\text{Square root of gas density}}$$

where k, the diffusion constant, varies directly with the exchange surface area and inversely with the thickness of the diffusion barrier.

Of these variables, the pressure differential and exchange area can and do alter physiologically. The thickness of the membrane is altered in some pathologies. Figure 5–14, illustrating P_{O_2} and P_{CO_2} gradients, indicates that the differential between deoxygenated blood and alveolar air is approximately 60 torr for oxygen and approximately 6 torr for carbon dioxide. This 10-fold greater gradient for oxygen is offset by the 20-fold greater solubility of carbon dioxide. Since the gas densities are similar, it can be concluded that carbon dioxide diffuses out of the blood a little more readily than oxygen diffuses in.

Because alveolar air is continuously but incompletely exchanging with the air moving in and out of the airways, and because blood is continually moving through the capillaries, calculation of the amount of gas exchanged is rather complicated. At rest, blood transits a pulmonary capillary in 0.7 to 0.9 second, a time that is quite adequate for gas exchange. During exercise or activity, this accelerates to as little as 0.3 to 0.4 second, and it may then be a limiting factor for complete exchange. Efficient exchange still occurs, however, because the air-to-blood gradients in partial pressure are larger during exercise. Additionally, cardiac output increases during exercise, so more capillaries become perfused and more of the lung's available exchange area is in use.

The Airways

The alveoli communicate, via *respiratory bronchioles* that are devoid of muscle, to small *bron-*

Figure 5–13. Fine structure of the alveolar–capillary membrane. A capillary with two erythrocytes is shown separated from the alveolar air space by a thin process of an adjacent pneumocyte, or alveolar epithelial cell. The free surface is covered by a thin liquid layer, called lung fluid. The diffusion barrier between air and plasma is detailed above; the thicknesses of the component layers are given in microns.

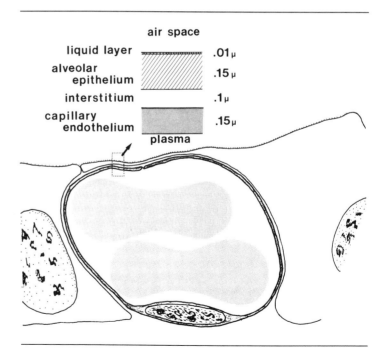

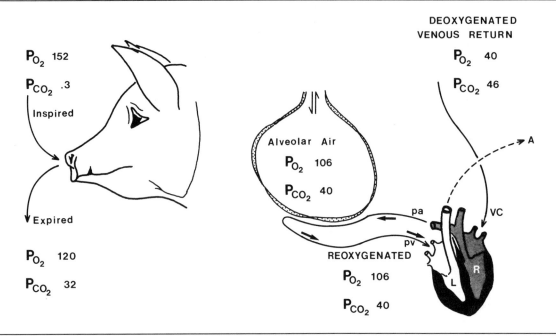

Figure 5–14. *Gradients in partial pressures.* Values for P_{O_2} and P_{CO_2} in the air passing into and out of the pulmonary system and in oxygenated and deoxygenated blood are given in torr. Blood returning from the body's tissues to the right (R) side of the heart in the venae cavae (VC) is deoxygenated. It passes through the pulmonary arteries (pa) to perfuse the capillary beds in the lung for gas exchange. The reoxygenated blood returns to the left (L) side of the heart through the pulmonary veins (pv). It is then distributed to the body via the aorta (A). Alveolar air has relatively constant composition, virtually the same as that of freshly oxygenated blood in the pulmonary vein. The most obvious difference in the blood before and after passing through the lungs is the increase in P_{O_2}. The largest gradient between inspired and expired air is the increase in P_{CO_2}. Of course, expired air contains mostly inspired air that never reached the exchange area in the alveoli.

chioles, as part of a complex branching tree, ultimately to the *main bronchi,* and then to the common *trachea.* The arrangement (Figure 5–15) provides for a progressive decrease in caliber of the airways and a marked increase in total surface area as air passes down the system from the exterior. These "tubes" are lined with a ciliated mucous membrane that warms and moistens the incoming air. The cilia filter out particulates and sweep them away from the terminal branches.

The trachea is semirigid because it possesses incomplete cartilaginous rings. On the dorsal side, the cartilage is replaced by a fibrous muscular wall so that the trachea is not occluded when the head moves. This arrangement also enables a large food bolus to move through the immediately adjacent esophagus without the resistance that could arise if rigid rings completely encircled the trachea. These rings are usually ossified in birds.

The intermediate-sized bronchioles have muscular walls that are under autonomic neural control. The *larynx,* or site of communication of the respiratory tract and buccal cavity, is under dual autonomic control. Parasympathetic nerves

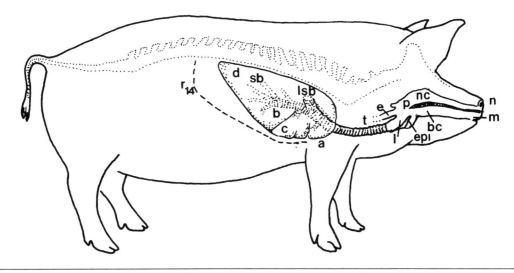

Figure 5–15. Gross anatomy of the airways and pulmonary system. The major components of the external respiratory apparatus of the hog include the nasal cavity (nc); buccal cavity (bc); mouth (m); nares (n); pharynx (p); epiglottis (epi); esophagus (e); larynx (l); trachea (t); right stem bronchus (b); left stem bronchus (sectioned, 1sb); secondary bronchi (sb); apical lobe of the lung (a); cardiac lobe (c); diaphragmatic lobe (d). The 14th rib is shown in dotted outline (r_{14}). The pharyngeal region (p) is common to both the digestive and respiratory systems. The larynx (l) is the entry to the trachea, which divides into left and right bronchi then into smaller secondary bronchi. Still finer airways within the tissue of the lungs were depicted in Figure 5–12.

bring about constriction while sympathetic nerves control relaxation of the laryngeal muscles.

The Thorax

Except for special maneuvers when control is exerted on the glottis, the mechanical driving force for pulmonary ventilation reflects alterations in the volume of the thorax, with the lungs passively following chest movements. Briefly review the description of the thoracic viscera that was provided in Chapter 1.

The thoracic cavity is lined with a mesothelial membrane called the pleura. On the lung surface this is the visceral pleura, on the inner wall of the thoracic cage it is the parietal pleura,

and on the diaphragm it is the diaphragmatic pleura. The pleural cavity, or the space between the visceral and other portions of the pleura, is small (Figure 5–16), but it is always moistened with *pleural secretions* to provide lubrication between the tissues. This fluid layer tends to cause adhesion between the visceral and parietal pleuras because of surface tension (see Chapter 2), and forces are required to break this attachment. A balance exists between the tendency of the lungs to fill the available space, and the resulting stretch that this confers on the tissue. The stretch represents the *recoil potential*. This is a force, or potential force, that tends to collapse the lung back to a resting state with little or no stretch. The force is called intrapleural pressure, and it is negative with respect to atmospheric pressure. Typical values are -3 torr during expiration, -10 torr during quiet breathing, and -30 torr in deep inspiration.

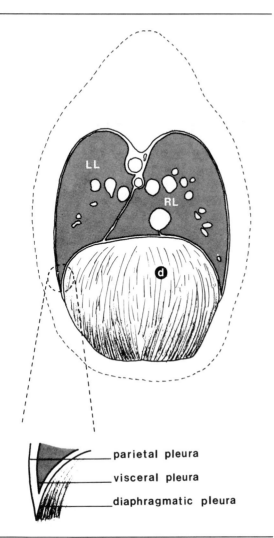

parietal pleura

visceral pleura

diaphragmatic pleura

Figure 5–16. The pleura and pleural cavity. This transverse section of the equine thorax shows the various portions of the pleura enclosing the small pleural cavity—an example of a serous or internal cavity first described in relation to mesothelium in Chapter 1. The body wall is shown in dotted outline; this section is through portions of the left and right lungs (LL and RL) and shows the ventral portion of the diaphragm (d). The ventrolateral extremity is exploded to indicate the parietal pleura lining the thoracic wall, the visceral pleura covering the lung, and the diaphragmatic pleura on the thoracic surface of the diaphragm.

The increase in negativity is normally achieved because diaphragmatic contractions flatten the normally forward, dome-shaped structure, thereby increasing thoracic volume by downward and outward displacement of the abdominal contents (Figure 5–17).

This is exactly what prevails during quiet abdominal breathing. More active breathing introduces a component of rib cage activity. Muscles attached to the superficial surface of the ribs, called the external intercostals, contract and slightly rotate the ribs outward, and so thoracic diameter is slightly increased. In very deep inspiration the sternum can move ventrally and the vertebral column can move. Both of these movements further increase thoracic diameter.

The inspiratory muscles do nothing directly to the lung tissues. The work simply overcomes the elastic recoil resistance of the lungs and the elastic resistance of the costal cartilages. Similarly, during normal expiration, there is no active muscular participation. The work component arises from recoil and the release of the elastic recoil potential.

Forced expiration may involve active contraction of the internal intercostal muscles and compression of the thoracic cavity by contracting the ventral abdominal muscles.

There is never total exchange between the air spaces and the atmosphere during a single breath. This could only be achieved if the alveolar components were in between a set of input airways and a distinct set of output airways. Certain parts of the respiratory system of birds have this arrangement. In mammals only about 10% of the alveolar contents is exchanged during normal quiet breathing. This is the reason why alveolar air stays relatively constant in composition and why "dead space" air is fairly constant. Dead space refers to all of the air in the pulmonary system that is not actually in the alveoli.

Expired air is a mixture of dead space air and alveolar air. Alveolar air is partially mixed

Figure 5–17. The diaphragm. Excursions of the diaphragm are shown in relation to the thoracic wall (tw) and the lateral margin (lm) of this respiratory muscle. During inspiration (ins) the diaphragm flattens (arrows) from its forward, domed position in expiration (ex) thereby increasing the volume of the thoracic cavity.

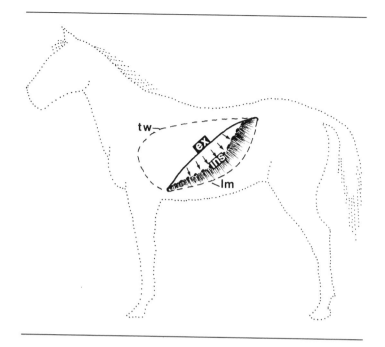

with incoming air from the dead space volume. Both physical mixing and rapid diffusion occur between these air volumes and so composition at any one location remains relatively constant. Some typical values for P_{O_2} and P_{CO_2} in inspired, alveolar, and expired air are given in Figure 5–14.

Respiratory Performance

Numerous indices of pulmonary function are used, and specific definitions may be helpful when reading other materials about respiration. The parameters are defined in Box 5–11 and illustrated in Figure 5–18 as fractions, or percentages, or the total lung capacity. It is not necessary to learn these terms for the present description of respiratory physiology.

The parameter of greatest interest is *respiration rate*, or the number of breaths per minute. Normal ranges of respiration rates for a selection of species are given in Table 5–2.

Table 5–2. Rates of Respiration

Species	Breaths per Minute
Humans	12–30
Cattle	12–28
Sheep	14–24
Goats	13–20
Pigs	15–25
Horses	8–16
Dogs	20–30
Cats	25–44
Rabbits	35–55
Chickens	ca. 13

Pulmonary Mechanics

As introduced in Chapter 2 in the description of important physicochemical properties of water, the cohesive intermolecular force displayed by liquids, called surface tension, is the basis for

Box 5–11   Respiratory Parameters

Tidal volume: The volume of air moving in and out during normal quiet breathing, or *eupnea*.

Minute respiratory volume: The product of tidal volume times respiration rate, or breaths per minute.

Inspiratory reserve volume: Maximal additional volume of air that can be voluntarily taken in, over and beyond the normal tidal volume.

Expiratory reserve volume: Maximal reserve volume that can be forcibly expired at the end of a normal expiration.

Residual volume: The air that remains in the airways after maximal forced expiration, and so cannot be removed.

Vital capacity: The maximal volume that can be inspired after a maximal expiration, or the maximum that can be expired after a maximal inspiration. Vital capacity is the arithmetic sum of tidal volume plus inspiratory reserve volume plus expiratory reserve volume.

Total lung capacity: The sum of vital capacity as above plus the residual volume.

Functional residual capacity: The volume of air left in the lungs after a normal expiration. This must equal expiratory reserve volume plus residual volume.

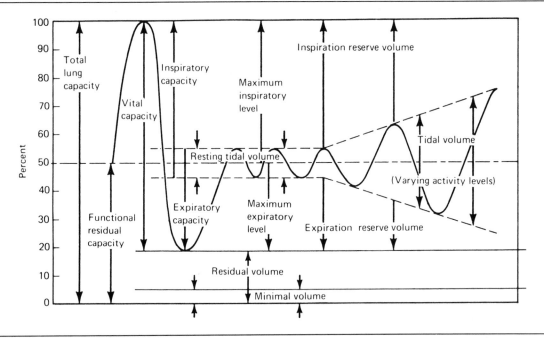

Figure 5–18. Respiratory volumes. This figure illustrates the parameters described in Box 5–11. The most important item to note is the variability or range of tidal volume, from the resting level to some 50% of total lung capacity, depending upon need from exercise or activity. (Reproduced by permission of the publisher. From Bone, J.E.: *Animal Anatomy and Physiology,* Reston, VA: Reston Publishing Company, 1979.)

drop formation. Such forces are unequal at air-liquid interfaces and the result of unequal forces is to favor collapse of the surface into the smallest possible area. Surface tension is a force acting inward and perpendicular to any plane, tangent at the surface. In a bubble, this inward force is the cause of, and is opposed by, an outwardly directed force that is called pressure. The Laplace equation, introduced in Box 2–1, describes the relationship between pressure (P), tension (T), and radius (r):

$$P = \frac{2\omega T}{r}$$

where ω is the property of the wall.

Review the information in Box 2–1, because without some understanding of surface tension, it is impossible to understand the mechanics of respiration.

Surface Tension and Pulmonary Surfactant

The principle of surface tension is clearly applicable to the lung. During inspiration, intrapleural pressure decreases to about 6 to 8 torr below atmospheric pressure (Figure 5–19). The lung alveoli expand into this partial vacuum and draw air into them. The alveoli are lined with a thin layer of liquid. If this liquid were water, the alveoli would collapse because of surface tension during expiration when alveolar volume was small. Inspiration would then require a much greater negative pressure to be developed in the intrapleural space in order that the alveoli could inflate; this would result in exhausting muscular effort.

Specialized alveolar cells, called type II pneumocytes, synthesize and secrete a phospholipoprotein complex with surface-active properties, known as *pulmonary surfactant*. Its surfactant power varies with its effective concentration at the air-liquid interface. For a given

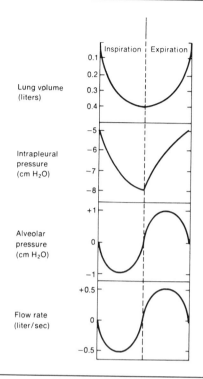

Figure 5–19. Pressure–volume relationships in the thorax. The relationship between rhythmic changes in negative intrapleural pressure and alveolar pressure, resulting from expansion of the thoracic cavity by the respiratory muscles, determines the flow of air and resultant lung volume. Data apply to human respiration. (Reproduced by permission of the publisher. From Wilson, J.A.: *Principles of Animal Physiology*, 2nd edition, New York: Macmillan Publishing Co., 1979.)

volume of alveolar fluid, inflation and deflation of the alveoli change the "area" of this lining of fluid, and the ability of a given amount of surfactant to change surface tension varies with the respiratory cycle. As alveoli become smaller during expiration, the surfactant molecules are packed with greater effective concentration across the liquid-air interface and so become more effective. By reducing surface tension at this time, the risk of alveolar collapse is minimized. Another advantage stems from there being less tendency for vascular fluid to be drawn across the alveolar membrane into the lung.

The major cause of neonatal loss of premature animals, humans included, stems from the *respiratory distress syndrome* (RDS). Immature fetuses do not have competent lungs because they lack surfactant. The alveoli tend to remain collapsed and even heroic inspiratory effort, gasping and grunting, still fails to cause inflation. Hypoxia, then eventually anoxia, with carbon dioxide accumulation from the futile respiratory exertion, cause death.

This phenomenon will be expanded as part of the treatment given to fetal and neonatal physiology in Chapter 10.

Neural Regulation of Respiration

Respiratory activity is normally quite involuntary but brief episodes of voluntary control can be imposed. It is not possible to establish terminal apnea by consciously not breathing. In such a life-threatening situation, the involuntary mechanisms will always break through to prevent hypoxic damage to the central nervous system. An anatomically ill-defined group of neurons in the medulla oblongata functions as a respiratory center to integrate the alternation of *active* phase of inspiration and *passive* phases of expiration. Regulation is exerted on both rate and depth of ventilation.

The nature of central control of respiration has been learned by the combined use of the classic techniques of physiologic investigation. These include transections within the neural system, electrical recording of action potential traffic, and electrical stimulation of parts of the nervous system to examine what can mimic the normal control process.

The earliest studies depended on transections of the brain stem and spinal cord. The findings can be summarized briefly:

- Spinal section caudad to the thoracic region is without effect on normal breathing.

- Spinal section within the thoracic region evokes responses that depend on the level of transection. The respiratory accessory muscles, for example the intercostals, receive motor input from spinal nerves along the length of the thorax.

- Section in the lower cervical area deactivates all respiratory accessory muscles but does not interfere with contractions of the diaphragm.

- Section above cervical segment 4 abolishes diaphragmatic contractions and respiratory arrest is absolute. The diaphragm is innervated by the phrenic nerve, which leaves the spinal cord at cervical segment 4.

- Brain stem section above the medulla oblongata does not affect normal respiration.

These observations can be interpreted to indicate that the respiratory center lies in the lower brain stem, actually within the *medulla oblongata*. Innervation of the diaphragm is from cervical segment 4, via the *phrenic nerve*. The intercostals are innervated by *thoracic spinal motor nerves*. The phrenic nerve passes down the neck and traverses the thoracic cavity in order to reach the diaphragm.

Recordings from compound motor nerves such as the phrenic and thoracic spinal nerves indicated that phasic action potential firing occurred only during inspiration. This reinforced the notion that inspiration is active and that expiration is usually passive.

Use of extrinsic electrical stimulation exposed the complexity of the afferent drives to respiration. Appropriate stimulation of ventral portions of the medulla oblongata causes *apneusis*, the technical term for inspiratory cramp, or arrest, in deep inspiration, with inhibition of expiration. Stimulation of the ventral medulla results in continuous action potential traffic passing down the phrenic nerve. Further stimulation progressively results in the respiratory accessory muscles becoming involved. These observations led to the ventral medullary area being named the *inspiratory center*.

When stimulation was applied more anteriorly and dorsally, respiration was also arrested, but in this instance the arrest occurred in full expiration. There was complete cessation of action potentials in the phrenic nerve. These more dorsal areas are called the *expiratory center*. The expiratory center is in communication with the inspiratory center. The former periodically inhibits the latter so that expiration can take place. During continued experimental stimulation of the expiratory center, the inhibition will last only about 3 minutes, because eventually the activity of the dominant inspiratory center breaks through.

The respiratory center thus has two components but they function in a coordinated manner to provide alternation of respiratory activity. There are additional influences from peripheral sensory endings and complex "higher" influences, derived from the pons, that modify the basic activity of the medullary centers.

The most important feedback type of control is achieved through the *Hering-Breuer reflex*. Sensory neurons in the vagus nerve, cranial nerve X, carry inhibitory signals back to the respiratory centers from stretch receptors in the lung tissue. These afferent signals arrest inspiratory efforts when the degree of stretch in the lung indicates a potential danger to the tissue if expansion were to proceed any further. When this afferent function is interrupted, for example by cutting the vagi, breathing deepens and slows. This is called *hyperpnea*. The vagi also carry afferents from chemoreceptors in the aorta (see Figure 5–7).

Additional respiratory inputs arise from the baroreceptors and various chemoreceptors, and from diffusely located pain and touch receptors. A major control is obtained from local chemoreception within the brain. The cytons of the respiratory center are extremely sensitive to the gaseous composition of the blood perfusing the brain.

crease in carbon dioxide content, or P_{CO_2}, in inspired air will increase arterial blood P_{CO_2} and then increase the depth of breathing. Maximum ventilation rate can increase 20-fold in intense exercise.

Although these changes result from increased P_{CO_2}, the actual mediator at the neuron may well be pH, because any elevation in P_{CO_2} will usually lower pH.

$$CO_2 + H_2O \rightleftharpoons H_2CO_3 \rightleftharpoons HCO_3^- + H^+$$

Increased pH, perhaps resulting from *voluntary hyperventilation*, or forced deep breathing, can result in *apnea*, or a cessation of breathing, until P_{CO_2} increases and pH falls. The apnea is followed for a while by a characteristic pattern of episodic breathing before normal breathing is resumed.

Oxygen lack can provoke acute changes in respiration but the oxygen content of inspired air must decrease substantially, from the normal 21% down to about 14% to 15%, before changes in respiration become evident. Certain chemoreceptors monitor and respond to any decrease in blood oxygen levels, or *hypoxemia*. The first response is increased depth of respiration. However, increased depth of respiration causes increased ventilatory loss of carbon dioxide, so blood P_{CO_2} falls and the P_{CO_2} stimulus to respiration is lessened. Overall, a sudden marked reduction in oxygen content of air sets up periodic breathing activity. This reflects a balance being established between the stimulatory effect of hypoxemia and the inhibitory influence of hypocapnia, or low blood P_{CO_2}. The respiratory center is, however, much more sensitive to changes in P_{CO_2} than in P_{O_2}.

Chemical Regulation

Respiratory activity is subject to regulation by various receptors that monitor the properties of arterial blood. Of the various possibilities, P_{CO_2} is by far the most important, and any slight in-

Summary of Neural Control of Respiration

- Inspiration is the active phase of breathing.

- The initiating influence is the inspiratory center, partly in response to P_{CO_2}, sensed locally in the brain, and partly from chemo-receptors in the arterial tree.

- Motor, or efferent, output is via the phrenic nerve to the diaphragm.

- Lung stretch receptors are activated as the lungs expand and sensory information returns to the expiratory center via afferent neurons in the vagus.

- The expiratory center inhibits the inspiratory center until the lungs deflate enough to terminate stretch receptor activity. If the expiratory center is grossly stimulated, there may be active recruitment of the expiratory muscles along with the inhibition of inspiration.

5.6 • The Renal System and Its Contribution to Homeostasis

All higher animals have developed specialized *excretory* systems that function to preserve the internal environment. In mammals, the renal system contributes to water balance, ion balance or "mineral metabolism," removal of nonvolatile metabolic wastes and complexed toxins, and pH homeostasis. Kidneys participate in support of other physiologic systems as well. The kidney produces erythropoietin in response to hypoxia, thereby stimulating production of red blood cells. Renal hypotension results in renin secretion and production of angiotensin, the potent vasoconstrictor agent, described earlier in Section 5.3. Additionally, angiotensin causes release of aldosterone, the major mineralocorticoid from the adrenal cortex. This steroid increases sodium retention and increases potassium excretion by effects back on the kidney.

The main functions of the kidneys to be considered here concern urine formation. Urine is stored in the bladder and is periodically eliminated from the body by urination, or *micturition*.

Anatomy and Structure

The urinary system is made up of a set of abdominal and pelvic viscera: the *kidneys*, the *ureters*, the *bladder*, and the *urethra* (Figure 5–20).

The kidneys receive 20% to 25% of cardiac output, yet they represent a mere 1% of live weight. This enormous blood flow comes in through a short system of renal arteries that branch off the aorta almost at right angles (see Figure 5–20). Because blood cells tend to concentrate in the center of a vessel, the blood plasma is "skimmed" off by these sharp branches and so has a relatively lower packed cell volume in the renal circulation than elsewhere. The viscosity of the blood is less because of the fewer cells, and vascular resistance is low because of the short blood vessels. Both of these factors contribute to the exceedingly high rate of renal blood flow.

The functional units of structure in the kidneys are the lobules, organized in concentric layers. The outer zone, or *cortex,* lies over the inner zone, or *medulla;* and the central area, or *pelvis,* is where the urinary ducts come together to form the ureters. The ureters, one from each kidney, transport urine to the bladder. The bladder is a highly distensible, smooth muscle–walled reservoir that in turn communicates to the exterior through the urethra.

The functional unit for urine formation is located across all of the kidney layers (Figure 5–21) and is called the *uriniferous tubule,* or *nephron* (Figure 5–22). The nephron originates at Bowman's capsule, a flasklike, blind-ended portion of the tubule surrounding the knot of capillaries known as the *glomerulus.* The capsule feeds directly to the proximal convoluted tubule, then to the descending limb of the loop of Henle, extending deep into the medulla. The nephron

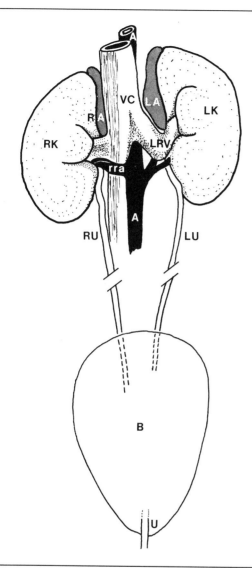

Figure 5–20. Organs of the urinary system. The mammalian urinary system consists of paired kidneys (RK and LK) and ureters (RU and LU) supplying the bladder (B), and a single urethra (U) draining the bladder. This ventral view shows the vascular arrangement at the major trunk vessels (aorta, A; vena cava, VC; left renal vein, LRV; right renal artery, RRA), the relative position of the adrenals (RA and LA), and the origin of the ureters.

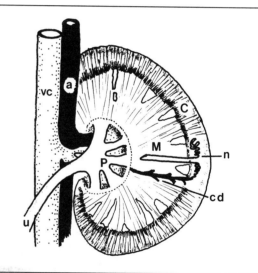

Figure 5–21. Structure of the kidney. This figure shows the relationship between the cortex (C), medulla (M), and pelvis (P), and the origin of the ureter (U). The renal artery and veins also meet the kidney in the pelvic area. The major trunk vessels are the aorta (a) and vena cava (vc). Thousands of nephrons (n) lie across the cortex and medulla, and drain centripetally via collecting ducts (cd) into the pelvis. This illustration is a dorsal view with the right kidney sectioned in the frontal plane.

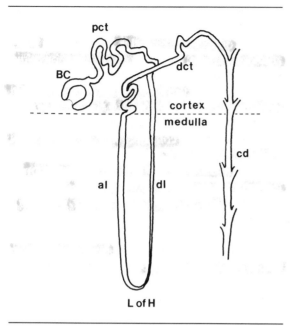

Figure 5–22. *The nephron.* The nephron originates in Bowman's capsule (BC; see Figure 5–24 for more detail) and leads directly into the proximal convoluted tubule (pct). The loop of Henle (L of H; includes descending limb, dl, and ascending limb, al) and the collecting duct (cd) are connected by the distal convoluted tubule (dct). Bowman's capsule and convoluted tubules lie in the renal cortex.

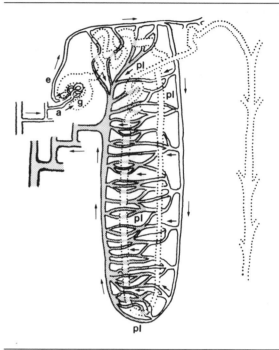

Figure 5–23. *Renal vasculature.* The arterial supply to the glomerulus (g) is a low resistance, high flow region. Branches from the renal artery are short and at acute angles, resulting in plasma skimming, as noted in the text. The glomerulus is supplied by afferent arterioles (a). Beyond the glomerulus, efferent arterioles (e) impose vascular resistance; this contributes significantly to filtration forces operating in the glomerulus. Efferent blood then perfuses a plexus of vessels (pl) intimately associated with the nephron (dotted outline) before being collected into the venous system (shaded).

continues around the "hairpin bend" and then the ascending limb of the loop brings it back to the cortex. In the cortex, the nephron continues as the distal convoluted tubule, then it turns back toward the medulla and joins with others, forming larger structures called collecting ducts. The collecting ducts become progressively larger in size and fewer in number because of fusion with others before the renal pelvis is reached. Finally, urine leaves the kidney via the ureter, which passes caudally to the bladder. The bladder does nothing toward urine formation but merely stores it, awaiting urination.

The arterial supply to the kidney (Figure 5–23) enters in the pelvic region and fans out to form a series of interlobular arteries. At about the level of the junction between the cortex and the medulla, another series of smaller arteries, called intralobular arteries, branch off to supply

the glomeruli. These last vessels are the *afferent arterioles* and they divide to form the glomerulus (Figure 5–24). This rich capillary bed is nestled within Bowman's capsule, the latter being the beginning of the structures making up the uriniferous tubule.

On the distal side of the glomerulus, the capillaries coalesce to form *efferent arterioles*. This is a quite unusual arrangement for blood vessels because, in most capillary beds, the exiting vessels are small venules, not secondary arterioles. The efferent arterioles are subjected to a degree

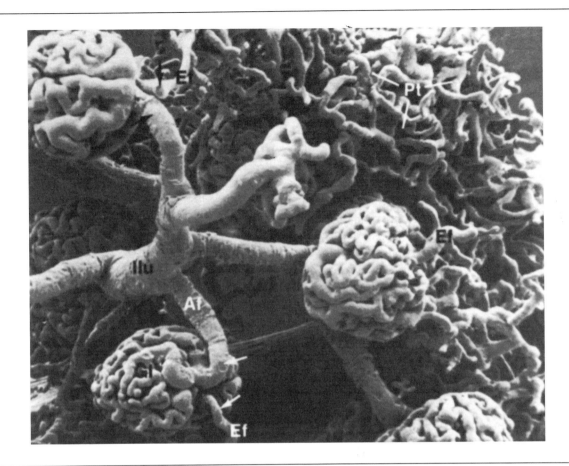

Figure 5–24. *Vascular organization of the glomerulus.* This scanning electron micrograph of a corrosion preparation of blood vessels was made by perfusing plastic into the major vessels, allowing polymerization, and then digesting all tissue prior to microscopy. The capillary knot forming the glomerulus (Gl) is supplied by an afferent arteriole (Af) and drained by an efferent arteriole (Ef). Note the difference in caliber of these vessels, the basis for the elevated hydrostatic pressure in the glomerulus and hence very high filtration rate into Bowman's capsule. The peritubular plexus (Pt), lying within the medullary zone of the kidney, is also evident to the right. (× 295. Reproduced by permission of the publisher. From Kessel, R.G. and Kardon, R.H.: *Tissues and Organs: A Text-Atlas of Scanning Electron Microscopy,* San Francisco: W.H. Freeman and Company, 1979.)

of vasoconstrictor tone. This serves to increase the hydrostatic pressure within the glomerulus and is a major factor aiding filtration at that location.

The efferent arterioles pass radially inward toward the medulla (see Figure 5–23), where a secondary series of branchings make up the *med-ullary plexus* of vessels. The plexus surrounds the nephrons and ramifies throughout the cortex and medulla of the kidney. The plexuses lead to efferent venules, to small veins, and to progressively larger veins. Venous blood finally leaves the kidney via the renal vein and is collected into the posterior vena cava.

Function of the Nephron

The initial step in urine formation is filtration at the glomerulus. The cell barrier separating capillary blood from the lumen of the capsule behaves just like any other leaky capillary. It is freely permeable to water and small molecular weight solutes. Proteins are usually not filtered, but the concentration of small solutes in the filtrate is essentially the same as in the blood plasma, from which it is obtained. Bulk flow of materials by filtration across the glomerulus is enormous and represents about 20% of the renal blood flow, or a staggering 180 L of fluid filtered per day in a 60 to 70-kg animal. Obviously, the vast bulk of this fluid is reabsorbed, or the animal would spend most of its time drinking and voiding.

The driving force for filtration is quite simple. As in other capillary beds, it is the sum of Starling forces, described earlier in Section 5.3:

Forces favoring filtration:

P_{glom} (glomerular capillary blood pressure)

COP_{Bowman} (colloidal osmotic pressure in Bowman's capsule)

Forces opposing filtration:

P_{Bowman} (capsular fluid pressure)

COP_{glom} (colloidal osmotic pressure in glomerular capillary)

The *net filtration pressure* is:

$$P_{glom} + COP_{Bowman} - P_{Bowman} - COP_{glom}$$

Because there are normally no proteins in the capsular fluid, COP_{Bowman} is usually zero. Therefore:

Net filtration pressure
$$= P_{glom} - P_{Bowman} - COP_{glom}$$

Typical values for these quantities are:

$$50 \text{ torr} - 10 \text{ torr} - 30 \text{ torr} = 10 \text{ torr}$$

Note that capillary hydrostatic pressure ($P_{glom)}$, given here as 50 torr, is substantially in excess of the value provided earlier for typical capillary pressures. This difference is a result of the atypical vascular anatomy of the kidney, described above. *The arterial divisions supplying the glomerulus facilitate high flow rates and maintenance of high pressures.*

In the equation and its solution provided above, colloidal osmotic pressure within the capsule is given the value zero. This is normally the case because proteins are effectively retained within the capillary. In pathologies where permeability of the filtration barrier is increased, protein may be lost to the capsule during filtration and then there may be a real capsular osmotic pressure due to the protein. This would add to the filtration drive and increase the net filtration pressure. When protein is present in urine *(proteinuria)*, dehydration, hypotension and hypovolemia, or reduced blood volume can all be expected.

Tubular Processes: Absorption and Secretion

Some transport processes are *active* and require the expenditure of metabolic energy to move the solutes against concentration gradients. Others are not energy-consuming at the transport site and can be considered *passive*. An example is simple diffusion across a permeable membrane in an attempt to maintain constant concentrations on either side of the barrier.

Active transport systems are carrier mediated, or employ pump devices similar to the Na^+-K^+–ATPase pump, described earlier. This particular pump transports two substances, so the handling of Na^+ requires that K^+ be transported in the opposite direction. Active transport mechanisms have a finite capacity that can be saturated. If *transport rate* or *flux* is linearly related to concentration, then flux will increase as concentration increases. However, once the carrier is saturated, further increases in concentration cannot be handled because flux is maximal. This is illustrated in Figure 5–25.

In diabetics, whose control over plasma glucose concentrations is poor, any marked increase in plasma concentration causes parallel increase in glucose concentration in the filtrate. Glucose is reabsorbed by a carrier-mediated system, up to a particular concentration. Concentrations in the filtrate that exceed the transport maximum cannot be reabsorbed and so glucose is lost from the body in the urine. This is called *glucosuria*. A simple urine glucose test can serve as an aid to the diagnosis of diabetes.

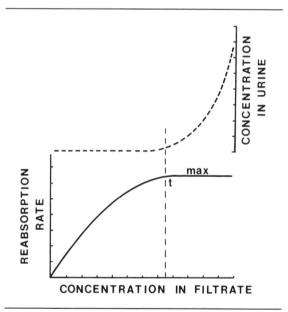

Figure 5–25. Carrier-mediated transport. The rate of transport (or flux), expressed as mass per unit time, increases with increased concentration up to the threshold concentration (t) that saturates the carrier mechanism; flux is then maximal. Any further increase in concentration in the tubular fluid cannot be transported and results in the increasing appearance of the solute in urine (see upper curve).

In addition to active transport, the nephron engages in passive transport, in which the driving force for solute movement is simply one of a concentration gradient across a permeable membrane. Other passive transport mechanisms include osmotic movement of water, when the solute cannot cross the membrane, and ion movements driven by electrochemical imbalance across a membrane. This means that if positively charged species move across a membrane, negatively charged ions will move along with the positively charged ions in the same direction, or different positive ions will move in the opposite direction. For example, in the nephron Na^+ ions are usually accompanied by Cl^- ions; if one of these is pumped across the nephron wall, the other will usually follow it passively.

Tubular function calls on all of these transport mechanisms. The following description separates out the events occurring as filtrate leaves the capsule of the glomerulus on its way to the renal pelvis and thence to the bladder.

The kidneys are specialized for the production of *hyperosmotic* urine. This means that the osmotic strength of the urine, a reflection of its concentration of osmotically active substances, is greatly in excess of that in plasma. This minimizes the obligatory water loss needed to sweep certain products out of the body. Some desert-adapted species have the ability to produce superconcentrated urine and the obligatory urine water loss is so low that these animals need never drink water. They obtain sufficient water from metabolism for water balance. Because high osmolarity prevails in the inner or medullary portion of the kidney, these cells are especially adapted to withstand osmotic pressures that would damage normal cells (see Section 5.2). The radial gradient in osmolarity from outer to inner regions of the kidney is illustrated by the shaded areas in Figure 5–29.

The flow of tubular contents through the loop of Henle, down into and then out of the region of high osmolarity, provides the basis for a very effective "multiplier device." This is the basis for the *countercurrent mechanism* for concentrating the filtrate. This mechanism will be considered in some detail.

First, the epithelia lining different portions of the tubule have different properties with regard to materials transport. Second, wherever possible, solutes, which are ions or small molecules, will attempt to equalize concentrations by moving down concentration gradients. Water will move because of osmotic drag (see Chapter 2), if the barrier is permeable to water. Third, charge balance will always prevail.

As filtrate flows from the capsule into the proximal convoluted tubule, the filtrate is isosmotic with plasma and with the interstitial fluid in the renal cortex. Sodium is actively pumped out of the tubule and water follows passively to maintain osmotic balance. About 75% of the filtrate volume is reabsorbed by the time fluid reaches the loop of Henle (Figure 5–26).

The loop provides the basis for the countercurrent mechanism because fluid moves in opposite directions in the two limbs. A profound osmotic gradient exists from the cortex down through the medulla. It is maintained because Cl^- is actively pumped from the tubule into the interstitial fluid on the ascending side; Na^+ follows passively for electrochemical reasons. There is no active transport either into or out of the descending limb, but water, Na^+, and Cl^- can move passively (Figure 5–27).

Water flows out from tubular fluid that was originally isomotic with plasma into the interstitial space that is progressively more hyperosmotic the closer it is to the "hairpin bend," deep in the medulla. The driving force is purely osmotic and results in the remaining fluid in the tubule becoming more concentrated.

In addition to water moving out, NaCl moves in, because its concentration gradient is from interstitial to intratubule, and the wall is freely permeable to both Na^+ and Cl^-. This solute transfer further increases the fluid osmolarity inside the descending limb so that it closely mirrors the concentration in the interstitium.

With all of this movement of material, it is important to understand how the osmotic gradient is maintained, because this gradient is absolutely critical to the concentrating function. Firstly, as noted above, Cl^- is actively pumped into the interstitium in the ascending limb and

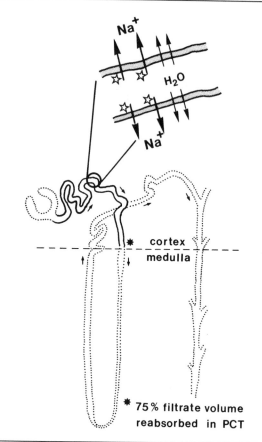

Figure 5–26. Processing of filtrate in the proximal tubule. Active transport in the proximal convoluted tubule (PCT) of the nephron recovers Na^+ and Cl^- ions from the filtrate. Energy-consuming ion pumps transfer solute from the lumen of the PCT into the interstitium of the renal cortex where osmolarity is comparable to that of the plasma. The tubule wall in this region is freely permeable to water and substantial volumes are transferred. The driving force is purely osmotic and results in about 75% of the filtered volume being removed from the lumen of the nephron before the fluid passes down the descending limb of the loop of Henle.

Na^+ follows electrochemically, but water cannot leave in this region. This would seem to set up a futile cycle of Cl^- and Na^+ leaving the ascending limb merely to enter the descending limb, and so on. This surmise is largely true, but it provides the real basis for the concentrating function of the countercurrent mechanism. Be-

Figure 5–27. The countercurrent mechanism. In the loop of Henle, the descending limb (right), which is freely permeable to Na$^+$ and Cl$^-$, permits salts to move passively down their concentration gradients into the lumen of the tubule from the hyperosmotic interstitial fluid of the renal medulla. Water moves in the opposite direction to try to balance the osmotic strength inside and outside. In the ascending limb (left), the ions are actively pumped out of the nephron and into the interstitium. In this region, the wall is impermeable to water. The fluid contents are therefore diluted (made hypoosmotic relative to the interstitial fluid) by the selective removal of ions.

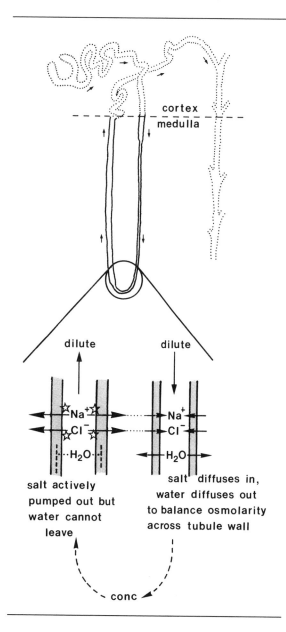

cause the medullary or peritubular plexus of blood vessels extends down into the medulla, and blood flows in a counter direction to the flow of fluid in the loop, some further concentrating is achieved by osmotic gradients from the interstitium into blood in the capillaries. Interstitial solute is picked up by the blood and water is taken along osmotically.

What is most important is the fact that selective removal of NaCl, but not water, effectively dilutes the fluid remaining in the ascending tubule without requiring any increase in its volume.

As illustrated in Figure 5–29, the fluid is hypoosmotic, or more dilute, relative to interstitial fluid by the time it enters the distal convoluted tubule. The lining of the nephron in this region is again permeable to water, so the osmotic gradient drags water out of the tubule until the remaining fluid in the nephron is isosmotic with the interstitial fluid. This is taking place in the cortex, where interstitial osmotic pressure is known to be equal to that of plasma.

As the tubule fluid reaches isosmolarity with the interstitial fluid, further Na$^+$ reabsorption takes place. This final component of Na$^+$ reabsorption is subject to close control by the adrenal mineralocorticoid hormone aldosterone (Figure 5–28). As before, Cl$^-$ follows passively, or to a certain extent H$^+$ or K$^+$ may be secreted into the tubular fluid to balance Na$^+$ removal. If these events cause a net loss of solute, tubular fluid osmolarity decreases once again and water will move passively to redress the situation.

Water can move out of the distal portion of the tubule and the collecting ducts only when antidiuretic hormone (ADH) is present. If there is no ADH present, water uptake is limited, despite the osmotic gradient, and copious volumes of dilute urine are produced. This is known as *diuresis*. However, if a water debt is sensed and ADH is secreted from the hypothalamohypo-

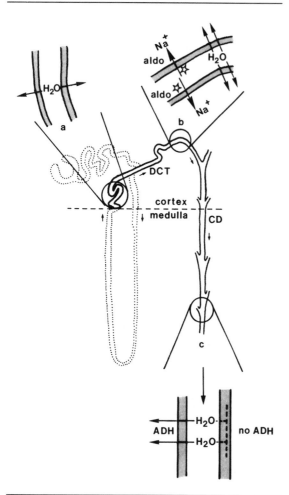

Figure 5–28. Distal tubular processes. Fluid reaching the distal convoluted tubule (DCT) is hypoosmotic relative to the interstitial fluid because of the diluting process that occurs in the ascending limb of the loop of Henle (see Figure 5–27). The tubule wall in the DCT is freely permeable to water (a); water leaves the lumen of the nephron for osmotic reasons. Final active recovery of Na$^+$ in the DCT (b) is subject to control by aldosterone (aldo); still more water follows passively. Concentrated fluid then moves into the medullary portion, called the collecting duct (CD), where final adjustment to osmolarity is made (c). Water is selectively recovered from the CD into the interstitium, again for osmotic reasons, but only when antidiuretic hormone (ADH) renders the wall of the CD permeable to water. The highest osmolarity possible in the urine so produced is that of the deep medullary interstitium.

physeal axis, the walls of the distal convoluted tubule and collecting ducts are made highly permeable to water (see Figure 5–28). A very concentrated urine of small volume is then produced. This final concentrating occurs because the collecting ducts pass back down through the renal medulla and the very high interstitial osmolarity again drags water out from the duct.

The driving force for the final concentration of the urine is again osmotic. Regulation is achieved by endocrine control of the permeability to water. The upper limit for urine concentration is determined by the osmolarity of the medullary region.

Summary of Transport in the Nephron

- Na$^+$ or Cl$^-$ is actively pumped out of the lumen at all places except the descending limb of the loop of Henle.

- Whenever possible, water also moves in an attempt to maintain osmolarity. It cannot leave the ascending limb where Cl$^-$ is being actively reabsorbed.

- Osmolarity in the ascending limb is less than that of the interstitial fluid at the same level (see Figure 5–29), and active removal of Cl$^-$(Na$^+$ passive) drives the countercurrent system.

- Na$^+$ removal in the distal tubule is regulated by aldosterone and K$^+$ or H$^+$ may be secreted into the tubule to achieve electrochemical balance.

- If ADH is present, water flows out of the tubule to match Na$^+$ movement and additional water is removed by the osmotic gradient prevailing around the collecting tubule, as it descends back into the renal pelvis.

Bladder Function and Micturition

The bladder communicates to the exterior by means of a single urethra. The voiding of urine

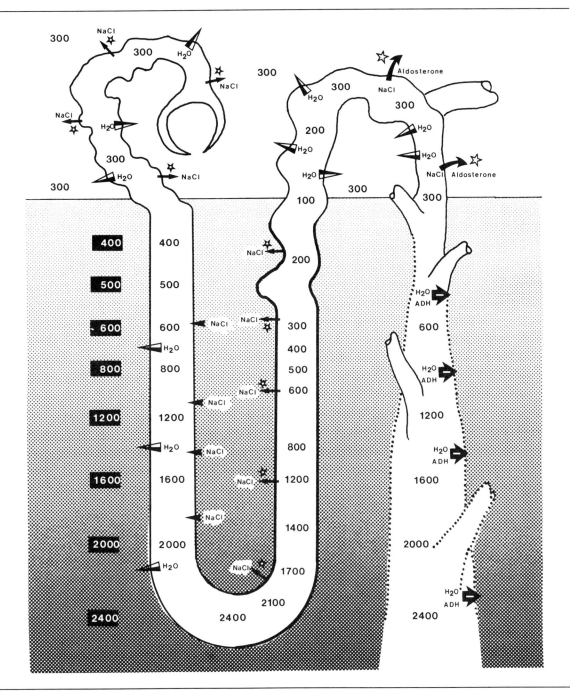

Figure 5–29. *Osmolarity changes within and outside the nephron.* This figure shows, by means of shading density, the radial gradient in osmotic strength of the interstitial fluid in the renal medulla. The osmolarity of the contents of the nephron is in equilibrium with the interstitium until the fluid reaches the ascending limb where it becomes progressively more dilute inside compared to outside. The passive movement of water and salts is shown with arrowheads, and active transport, with stars next to arrows. Aldosterone-dependent sodium recovery in the DCT and ADH-dependent water recovery in the CD are indicated. In the final stages of processing filtrate into urine, the fluid may reach, but not exceed, the osmolarity of the adjacent interstitium.

is achieved by contraction of the smooth muscle of the bladder wall and relaxation of a skeletal muscle sphincter in the urethra. The ureters, arising from each kidney, pass through the bladder wall in an oblique manner so that when the bladder contracts, the ureters are passively closed off. Thus urine is prevented from being refluxed back up the ureters. Bladder filling results in the wall being placed under tension, and this is monitored by stretch receptors as part of an afferent spinal reflex.

The bladder receives parasympathetic motor innervation from the sacral outflow of the autonomic nervous system. The external urethral sphincter, being skeletal muscle, is innervated by typical somatic nerves of spinal origin. When the bladder is distended, parasympathetic motor traffic increases and causes the bladder to contract. The sensory information is delivered via synapses in the spinal cord to enhance this parasympathetic outflow and to simultaneously inhibit the otherwise tonic motor outflow to the sphincter.

Obviously, there is considerable voluntary control over these events. Higher influences descend via ventral tracts in the spinal cord and impinge upon the neurons of the reflex just described. Micturition can be inhibited by these higher inputs by their inhibiting the motor innervation of the bladder wall and enhancing the constrictor tone delivered to the sphincter. Voluntary urination is achieved by relieving the inhibition on the parasympathetic neurones and by inhibiting tonic outflow to the sphincter. The bladder then contracts and the sphincter relaxes.

Renal Participation in Acid-Base Balance

Earlier descriptions of other systems that serve to regulate pH in the body focused on the ability of the HCO_3^- ion to combine with H^+, eventually liberating carbon dioxide to be expired. Reactions involving other anions such as lactate and

phosphate were noted, but all of these merely complex H^+. None of the foregoing mechanisms eliminates H^+ ions from the body.

The major contribution of the kidneys to pH regulation is by their being able to secrete H^+ as part of specialized tubular mechanisms. In essence the process involves:

$$HPO_4^{2-} + H^+ \rightleftharpoons H_2PO_4^-$$

where dibasic phosphate (HPO_4^{2-}) can be filtered from plasma in the glomerulus, but once reduced to monobasic phosphate ($H_2PO_4^-$) it cannot be reabsorbed further along the nephron.

The process also involves:

$$NH_3 + H^+ \rightleftharpoons NH_4^+$$

where ammonia, produced in tubular cells by deamination of amino acids, diffuses into the tubular fluid and, once reduced to the ammonium ion, cannot diffuse back out.

The kidney's role in acid-base balance is intimately related to reabsorption of Na^+, an essential function described earlier, and the presence of HCO_3^- as a normal solute in the glomerular filtrate. It is possible to regard the mechanisms as providing for trading of H^+ for Na^+ and possibly K^+. To some extent, HCO_3^- is recovered while Cl^- is excreted.

To follow the events shown in Figure 5–30 requires going round and about a little. Start with Na^+ uptake from the tubule fluid into the tubule cell (step 1) in exchange for H^+ moving the other way (step 2). This excreted H^+ combines with filtrate HCO_3^-, which is driven toward CO_2 + water (step 4). The CO_2 diffuses into the tubule cell (step 5), where it promptly combines with water to form H_2CO_3 (step 6), then dissociates (step 7) because H^+ ions are continually being secreted (step 2). The HCO_3^- generated in step 7 moves along with Na^+ (step 8) to provide electroneutrality as the Na^+ is reabsorbed into the blood capillary.

Although this scheme has oversimplified events somewhat, it illustrates the principles underlying renal excretion of H^+. The amount of H^+ ions lost to the urine is subject to adjustment,

Figure 5–30. *Tubular ion exchanges.* The role of the tubule cell in recovering Na^+ in exchange for H^+ by means of the bicarbonate–carbonate system is shown. The numbers identify steps that are described in detail in the text. This exchange is the major method used by the body to eliminate excess H^+.

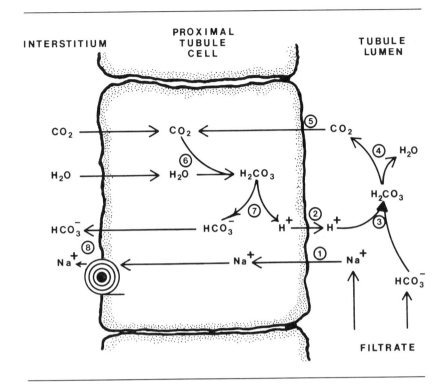

Box 5–12   Renal Acid-Base Mechanisms

In the earlier discussion of buffers, metabolic and respiratory alkalosis and acidosis were mentioned. The kidney can help deal with these conditions by the mechanisms just described.

Metabolic acidosis: Metabolic acidosis might be provoked by diarrhea, with excessive fecal loss of HCO_3^- of pancreatic origin. A respiratory compensation might be to increase ventilation rate and expel more carbon dioxide. This would consume H^+ via the bicarbonate-carbonate buffer system. A more effective compensation is achieved by increased H^+ excretion in urine, increased

Na^+ reabsorption, and so increased recovery of HCO_3^- to offset the loss.

Respiratory alkalosis: A comment was made earlier regarding voluntary hyperventilation leading to alkalosis with its potentially hazardous consequences. One immediate compensation results from the transport mechanism (step 8) being opposed by excessive plasma HCO_3^-. This serves, by mass action, to oppose tubular cell generation of H^+ (step 7). There is less H^+ available for step 2, and so the reactions described by steps 3 and 4 are held in check. HCO_3^- is therefore lost from the body in the urine.

depending on the amount of H$^+$ being produced by metabolic and respiratory mechanisms. At the end of Section 5.2, several situations that challenge acid-base balance were noted. The na- ture of compensatory renal adjustments to a couple of these imbalances is described in Box 5–12.

5.7 • Circulation, Respiration, and Excretion in Chickens

The life support systems of birds will be described briefly using the domestic chicken as the type species. In general, the requirements of these systems are similar to those for mammals, but considerable structural specialization has attended their evolution.

Cardiovascular

The blood of chickens contains relatively few erythrocytes (about half the concentration found in mammals), the cells are smaller, and they retain their nuclei. Circulating erythrocytes are capable of continued synthesis of hemoglobin. The lymphocyte is the dominant leukocyte and there are no platelets because thrombocytes occur as intact cells. Blood cell formation is confined to the sparce amount of marrow found in just a few of the bones, as noted in Section 1.7. Chickens lack definitive lymph nodes equivalent to those of mammals, but there are specialized lymphoid tissues associated with the digestive tract (which be described in Section 6.10).

Chickens have a high metabolic rate and, because of the low oxygen carrying capacity of the blood, the needs of tissues are met by the cardiovascular system operating at a higher rate of performance than is typical for mammals. High perfusion rates are sustained by increased arterial pressure resulting from elevated cardiac output and, in turn, elevated heart rate (see Figure 5–8). Accordingly, the mass of the left ventricle is large when compared to that of mammals and the right auricle, serving as a major capacitance structure, is larger than the left. A major specialization of the avian heart is the extension of the Purkinje fiber system to supply the atria as well as the ventricles.

Respiration

The most striking deviation from the mammalian form is observed in the external respiratory apparatus. It was noted earlier that birds lack a separate thoracic cavity because the diaphragm is essentially absent. The thoracic cage is relatively inflexible and intercostal muscles, which rotate the ribs in mammals to alter intrathoracic volume, are also missing. Thus there is no means by which a blind-ended lung structure could be inflated as in the manner described for mammals.

The airway in the chicken passes from the nasal space, which is incompletely separated from the beak cavity, across the pharynx and larynx and through a trachea, which possesses bony rather than cartilaginous rings. The two lungs are nonlobular, lack alveoli, are attached to the ribs with connective tissue, and do not inflate and deflate to any great extent. Air movement is through rather than reversibly into and out of the lungs. The lung mass contains a branching system of progressively finer caliber tubes that then fuse into larger spaces and supply air to the *air sacs* (Figure 5–31). The chicken has nine air sacs. Four pairs are located in the abdominal region, the posterior and anterior thoracic region, and in the lower neck, while a single sac lies medially near the clavicles. The air sacs form a continuous, interconnecting pathway from the lungs to the pneumatic bones.

Air movement is achieved by rhythmic relaxation of abdominal, thoracic, and pectoral muscles which expand the whole body cavity and draw air in. Contraction of these muscles permits expiration. If chickens huddle together, a behavioral adaptation to cold (see Chapter 9), their ability to breathe is impaired and suffocation may result.

The Urinary System

Chickens lack a bladder and urethra so the urinary tract consists solely of a pair of kidneys and two ureters. The kidneys are located ventrad to the fused transverse processes of lumbar and sacral vertebrae making up the synsacrum. In

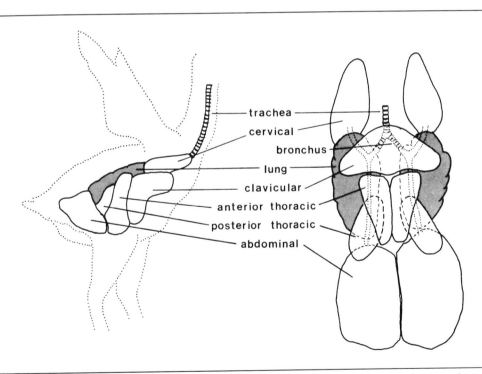

trachea

cervical

bronchus

lung

clavicular

anterior thoracic

posterior thoracic

abdominal

Figure 5–31. The respiratory apparatus in chickens. These two views illustrate the complex system of airways in the chicken. The trachea supplies bronchi which then communicate with lungs (shaded) and the air sacs. The pneumatic bones, described in the text, are not shown.

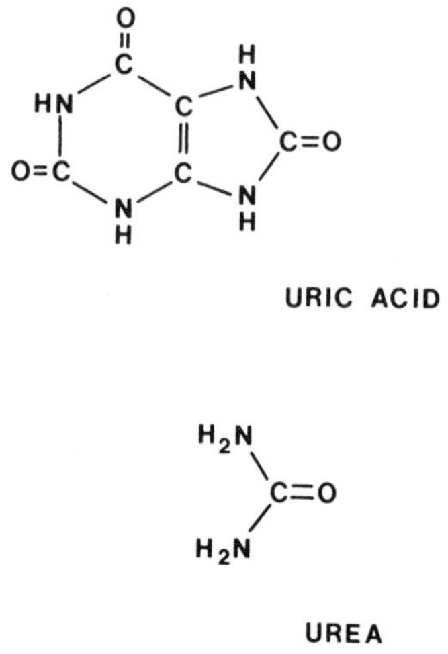

Figure 5–32. Uric acid and urea. Uric acid, the essentially insoluble nitrogenous excretory product of birds, is shown at top. Urea, the far more soluble equivalent product in mammals, is below. Although there is considerable similarity in these structures, their vastly different solubility properties confer adaptive advantages to the animals that employ one or the other as a means of detoxifying ammoniacal products of metabolism. Refer to Chapter 7 for further discussion of nitrogen metabolism.

URIC ACID

UREA

contrast to mammals, each kidney is supplied by three arteries and there are differences in the arterial organization within the organ. Avian kidneys possess two types of nephrons, one has deep medullary loops as in mammals while the other type does not extend beneath the cortex. The ureters pass to the middle segment of the cloaca (described in more detail in Section 6.10).

The principle excretory product is a semisolid paste of uric acid crystals (Figure 5–32). Uric acid is an essentially insoluble salt that, in contrast to highly soluble urea, can be eliminated with minimal water loss. The use of uric acid as a terminal excretory product for nitrogen

metabolism may have evolved as a mechanism for species that undergo embryonic development within an egg where water conservation is of critical importance.

Chicken "urine" accumulates in the cloaca and is periodically voided along with feces.

5.8 • Exercises

1. What component of blood largely determines its viscosity?

How is the amount of this component usually expressed?

What pathologic condition describes a substantial deficiency of this component?

Blood flow velocity is *increased* or *decreased* (strike out one) when viscosity is reduced from normal.

In one vascular bed in the body, the anatomic organization of the angles of the major arteries and a simple hydrodynamic principle enable viscosity to be lowered, with an important consequence on the rate of perfusion of that particular organ. Describe where this occurs and why it is important.

2. In what units is cardiac output (CO) expressed?

What two major variables contribute to CO? Give the names and units of measurement for each.

Think carefully about the general nature of the circulation, then decide what proportion of cardiac output passes through the lungs (circle one):

10%–15%   15%–35%   35%–50%
50%–75%   100%

3. Write out and interpret the equation for the carbonate-bicarbonate buffering system.

Distinguish between the Haldane effect and the Bohr effect. Which of these describes the phenomenon whereby H^+ ions aid in making oxygen available from HbO_2 for use by the tissues? Illustrate the example just given with a simple equation.

What happens to the pH of blood during forced rapid and deep breathing?

What compensatory renal mechanism is invoked to help restore normal blood pH?

4. Review the following examples of interactions and cooperation between the vital life support systems.

a. The thoracic pump aiding venous return to the heart.

b. The kidneys helping preserve the osmotic strength of body fluids.

c. The endocrine role of the kidney in blood pressure homeostasis and in controlling the oxygen-carrying capacity of blood.

d. The overlaps in function of the vasomotor center and the cardioinhibitory centers of the medulla.

e. The meaning of the hemoglobin dissociation curve, and how it is influenced by temperature and pH.

f. The relationship between the muscular work of respiration and the phenomenon of surface tension.

Digestive Mechanisms

6

6.1 • Introduction and Comparative Anatomy

Digestive mechanisms provide the animal with a means of reducing complex dietary materials into forms suitable for absorption and utilization by the body. Mammals have highly specialized *alimentary tracts* that vary a little from species to species, depending on the dietary habit of the particular animal. The differences in diet establish the need for selective processing of the ingesta. Some features of digestion are common to all animals and are extensively discussed in this chapter. However, the modifications that have evolved in herbivores, both ruminants and nonruminants, are of considerable importance and will receive special attention.

There is a reasonable correspondence between the structure of various segments of the alimentary tract and the digestion of specific kinds of feed. It is therefore no surprise that the overall structure of the tract, and the proportion of the whole comprised by any given part, varies considerably among *carnivores* (meat-eating animals), *herbivores* (plant-eating animals), and *omnivores* (those that are indifferent). Figure 6–1 compares the alimentary tracts in a selection of species. Some generalizations are possible.

The gut of a rabbit is typical of nonruminant herbivores. The stomach and small intestine are relatively small. There is a highly developed cecum, branching off from the distal part of the small intestine. The cecum is a blind-ended sac-like structure that serves as a reservoir for fibrous material undergoing microbial digestion. A large cecum is a characteristic feature of the herbivores, particularly nonruminants. The large intestine, or colon, of rabbits is unremarkable and is characteristically filled with fecal pellets.

Figure 6–1. Anatomy of digestive tracts. The diagrams show the relative dimensions of the stomach, small intestine, cecum, and large intestine for species representing strikingly different dietary habits. (Collage is assembled and reproduced by permission of the publisher. From Stevens, C.E.: *Comparative Physiology of the Digestive System*, in Swenson, M.J., ed.: *Duke's Physiology of Domestic Animals*, 9th edition, Ithaca, NY: Comstock Publishing Company, Inc., 1977.)

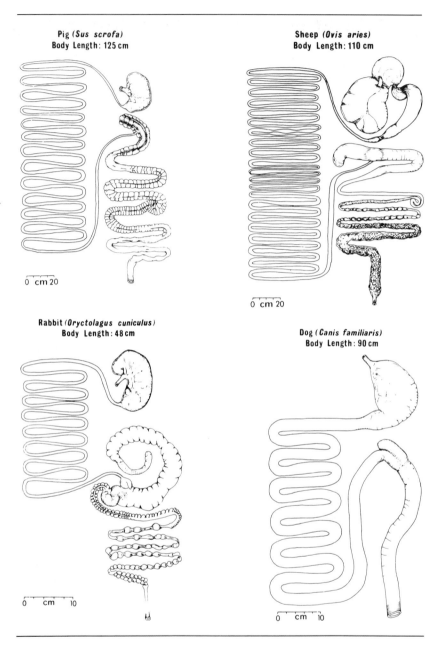

The sheep, a typical ruminant, has the complex stomach noted earlier in the introduction to splanchnology (see Figures 1–43 and 1–44 for diagrams of gut structures in situ). The stomach will be described in detail in Section 6.5. The ruminant's small intestine is proportionately very long, the cecum is of moderate size, and the colon is reasonably large. In sheep and goats, the colon usually contains aggregates of fecal pellets. These are not found in cattle.

The dog's stomach is typical of carnivores. The most striking feature is the apparent simplicity of the gut. The small intestine is short and has a wide luminal diameter. The cecum is poorly developed and the colon is unremarkable, appearing to be almost an elongated rectum. In view of the bulky fecal mass passed by dogs, the anatomic structure of the lower gut is quite consistent with its simple reservoir function.

The gut of a pig is shown as an example of an omnivore's gut. The dietary habit of an omnivore is intermediate between that of a carnivore and that of a nonruminant herbivore, and the gross anatomy of the gut is similarly intermediate. The large intestine assumes part of the function usually provided by the cecum in herbivores, and is a site of microbial digestion. The organ is therefore suited for extensive mixing and absorption, and so is relatively large and structured.

Earlier in this book we noted that living structures possess considerable complexity and that energy is consumed in assembling, from simple building units, the complex molecules that make up animals. The major components of the diets of most animals are complex polymeric substances that are synthesized by the living organisms making up the diet, whether plants or other animals. Of the multitude of compounds present in a "natural" diet, the *proteins*, *carbohydrates*, and *lipids* are quantitatively the most important. Their nature and their digestion will be described in some detail. *Vitamins* and *minerals*, qualitatively of great importance, contribute enormously to the well-being and normal development of animals. Some aspects of their digestion and assimilation will be noted, but the treatment will be superficial.

Many additional components such as the extracomplex plant structural polymers—for example, the lignins, molecules that are capable of eliciting pharmacologic responses in the consumer (e.g., alkaloids, poisons, and phytohormones, or plant-derived hormone-like compounds)—are of more specialized interest and are beyond the scope of an introductory text.

Mechanisms of Digestion

In the broadest sense, digestion includes the events from *ingestion* of feed, to chemical and physical *reduction* to simple products, to *absorption* from the digestive tract, to *elimination* of residues by defecation. The processes involved are highly regulated by combinations of voluntary and involuntary mechanisms, and neural and endocrine mechanisms. The trends and overlaps in these control mechanisms are the most important issues to take from the discussion in the remainder of this chapter.

For convenience, the digestive processes will be separated, on the basis of both anatomic and functional aspects, into three major segments:

- Ingestion and the processes leading to swallowing;

- Gastric processes, including the specializations of the ruminant;

- Intestinal processes and the nature of absorptive mechanisms.

6.2 • The Chemical Nature of Feeds

To understand the mechanisms employed by animals to liberate simple nutritive units for absorption, the reader must have some knowledge of dietary polymers. The material is treated more completely in Appendix B.

Lipids

The lipids of major energetic (caloric) consequence are *triglycerides,* or the triacyl esters of glycerol. The *fatty acids* are combined with *glycerol* by means of ester bonds involving each of the three hydroxyl groups of the glycerol (Figure 6–2). The fatty acid composition varies considerably, depending on the dietary source, but some generalization is possible. Plant lipids are usually enriched in *unsaturated* fatty acids, or those containing multiple olefinic, or $-C=C-$ bonds. Such triglycerides assume complex shapes (Figure 6–3) and do not readily solidify; they are called *oils.* A notable exception is palm oil, which contains much palmitic acid ($C_{16:0}$) and myristic acid ($C_{14:0}$). Palm oil has a transition temperature between solid and oil that approximates room temperature. The various oils tend to have relatively long fatty acids (C_{16}, C_{18}, and some C_{20}) and a high degree of unsaturation. The lipids of aquatic animals contain large quantities of C_{18}, C_{20}, C_{22}, and C_{24} fatty acids, also unsaturated. These have some importance because they remain fluid or oily despite the low environmental temperatures and often low body temperatures with which the animals survive.

The lipids of all animals reflect, in part, the nature of the dietary fatty acids, but also the mode of digestion. In omnivores, fatty acids of dietary origin may be liberated from the triglycerides, absorbed, then utilized for body fat accumulation, without any chemical change to the

fatty acid. The properties of the depot fats then partly reflect the properties of the dietary fat. It is well known that some fatty acids are less stable than others and readily oxidize to highly flavored or odoriferous products. Fat from animals that are fed large quantities of fish meal has a "fishy" odor. This trend is exaggerated if poor storage conditions of the feed mixture result in excessive oxidative change to the lipids before they are consumed.

Ruminants are able to modify dietary fatty acids prior to absorption, mainly by *hydrogenation* of the unsaturated plant lipids. This con-

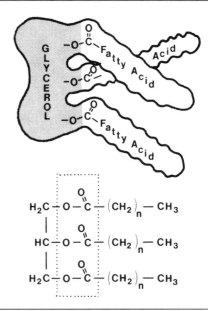

Figure 6–2. Triglyceride structure. Triglycerides are triacyl esters of glycerol. The upper figure depicts the overall structure with fatty acyl chains occupying a three-dimensional space. In the lower portion, the carboxyl groups of three fatty acids, shown with generic formulas, combine with each of the three hydroxyl groups of the glycerol. The dotted portion encloses the three ester bonds.

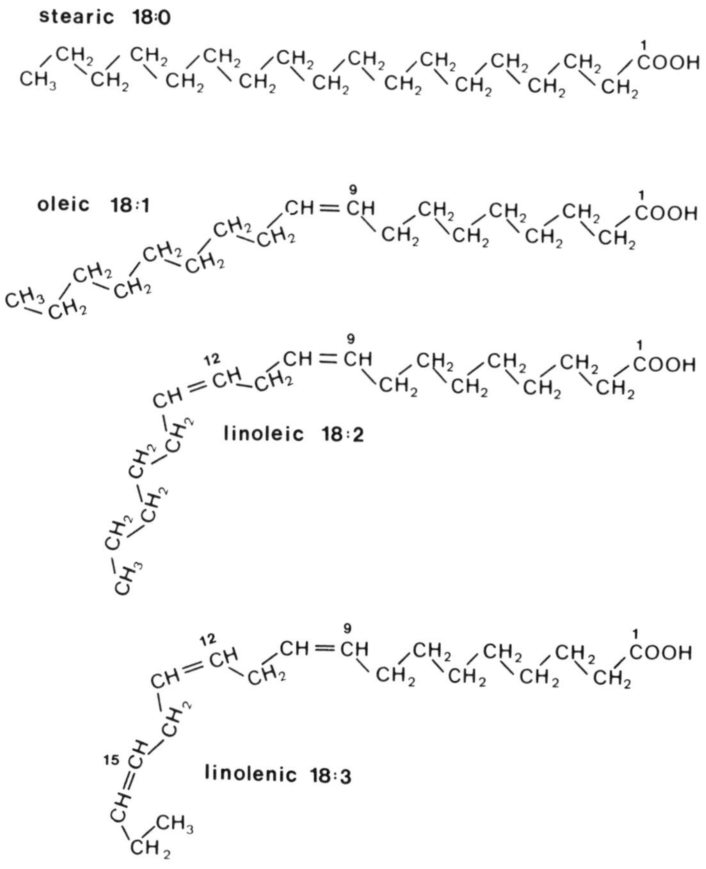

Figure 6–3. *Complex shapes of 18-carbon fatty acids.* In comparison to stearic acid (C$_{18:0}$), the *cis*-unsaturated acids are bent at each olefinic bond. The dienes (C$_{18:2}$) and trienes (C$_{18:3}$) are bent in multiple planes. Triglycerides containing these acids can pack together only loosely and so have low melting point temperatures. They are usually oils rather than solids. Plant lipids contain an abundance of unsaturated fatty acids and thus, when refined, these lipids are oils.

version of $-C=C-$ bonds to $-C-C-$, by incorporation of hydrogen, is called *reduction*. The environment established within the rumen is highly reductive and favors reactions of this kind. Ruminant depot lipid has a characteristic firmness, a reflection of its higher melting point, because the degree of unsaturation is much less than that of the dietary lipids. This hydrogenation phenomenon will be discussed later in relation to the symbiosis established between the host animal and its ruminal population of microbes.

Milk fat, an important caloric source, has unique properties that are of advantage to the digestive processes of the young animal. Milk fat triglycerides contain a wide spectrum of fatty acids (C$_{4:0}$ to C$_{18:3}$, or longer in some species).

The triglyceride molecules are unique because each contains one very short chain acid (C$_{4:0}$ or C$_{6:0}$) along with medium (C$_{8:0}$ to C$_{12:0}$) and long chain (C$_{14:0}$ or longer) acids. In Chapter 11 an explanation will be given for the synthesis of these components of milk fat by the specialized biosynthetic cells in the mammary glands.

Of less caloric importance are the nontriglyceride dietary lipids. Complex *polar lipids* such as the phospholipids (described in Chapter 2 in relation to membrane structure) are present in various feedstuffs. Many apolar substances, such as the fat-soluble vitamins, are closely associated with the dietary lipids. Their hydrophobic character could prevent normal processing in the watery environment of the gut lumen, so "tagging along" with the lipids provides them with a means of gaining access to the intestinal absorptive surfaces. Similarly, while they are of no great caloric significance, certain of the fatty acids, the so-called *essential fatty acids,* are nevertheless of critical importance to the well-being of terrestrial animals. These fatty acids, including linoleic ($C_{18:2}$) and linolenic ($C_{18:3}$) acid, are not synthesized by animals. They must be obtained from the diet. However, if provided with linoleic acid, animals can generate arachidonic acid ($C_{20:4}$), a key fatty acid that serves as the substrate for prostaglandin synthesis. Of considerable interest for human nutrition is the presence of *cholesterol* in many animal-derived foods. It is not an essential dietary component because animals, including man, are able to synthesize all that they need.

Proteins

Proteins are extremely heterogeneous polymers of *amino acids.* The monomeric units are combined by means of peptide, or amide, bonds between the amine of one acid and the carboxyl moiety of another (Figure 6–4).

Secondary linkages are possible, such as dithiol, or –S–S–, bonds that are established between available –SH side branches, as in the case of two cysteine residues being oxidatively com-

bined as cystine (Figure 6–5; see also Figure 4–15 for –S–S– bonds within peptide structures).

Small polymers, or polypeptides, are not major constituents of the diet, although they are formed by partial digestion of intermediate-sized oligopeptides and larger proteins.

The dietary proteins of animal origin vary in composition, depending on their anatomic origin. Because the structure of proteins is genetically coded, with only minor variants due to mutations, the amino acid composition and sequence in particular proteins are quite constant. For example, casein, a major protein constituent of milk, has a characteristic amino acid composition. Casein is a good example of a phosphoprotein in which many of the hydroxyl groups of the serine amino acid residues are phosphorylated. The abundant content of phosphates favors the tight association of casein with calcium. This is of considerable nutritional significance for actively growing young that have a substantial calcium requirement. It is also important as a way of providing calcium to adult humans, especially older individuals, many of whom exhibit excessive loss of bone calcium if their dietary intake is inadequate.

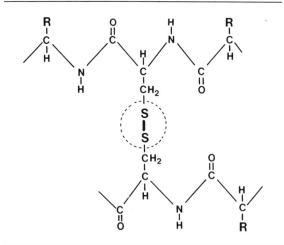

Figure 6–5. The dithiol bond. Protein chains can be folded on themselves; separate chains (see Figure 4–20 for insulin) may be linked by dithiol or disulfydryl bonds (dotted) between–SH groups on different amino acids.

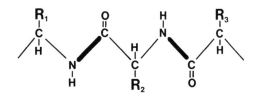

Figure 6–4. The peptide bond. Amino acids are combined covalently be means of amide or peptide bonds formed between the carboxyl group of one amino acid and the primary amine of another. In this short peptide sequence, R_1, R_2, and R_3 represent three distinct amino acid side groups (see Appendix B for specific examples).

The same constancy of amino acid composition is seen in the collagens, the specialized structural proteins of connective tissue (see Figure 1–11). A large proportion of the amino acids in collagens consists of proline and hydroxyproline.

It is important to recognize that different proteins—and there are thousands of them—are quite distinct in their amino acid composition and therefore in a number of other properties. The amino acid sequence, or primary structure, determines possibilities for higher order structure. A protein may be globular or almost spherical, or it may be quite asymmetric in shape, as described for fibrinogen in Chapter 5. The protein may possess rigidly defined helical regions, or other portions that assume random conformations. These structural features and the monomeric compositions dictate the solubility properties of proteins, and therefore their susceptibility to hydrolytic attack by enzymes operating in the aqueous milieu of the gut lumen.

The hydrolytic reactions are directed toward the amide bonds located either within the protein molecule or connecting the terminal amino acids. Different enzymes have different specificities for the site of amide hydrolysis. For example, *trypsin,* the powerful proteolytic enzyme of the small intestine, only hydrolyzes peptide bonds adjacent to basic amino acids such as lysine and arginine. Other enzymes act on bonds adjacent to aromatic amino acids, and so on. It is not difficult to imagine that marked differences exist in the ease of digestion of, say, milk proteins compared to the proteins of keratinized tissues such as skin. A carnivore that consumes prey nondiscriminately obtains a wide array of proteins, including pelage proteins such as those in hair or wool, which are essentially indigestible.

Even if the proteins can be readily digested, there is still an important consideration in the nature of the amino acids made available for absorption. Collagen-derived protein, such as gelatin, provides a poor balance of amino acids when compared to the amino acid mix available from casein. These differences in *protein quality* that seem so obvious for animal-derived food

are more difficult to appreciate in the case of plant proteins. In the past, much attention was given to differences in total protein content of various feedstuffs. For example, it has long been known that legumes have higher protein contents than nonleguminous plants. More recently, interest has focused on differences in the physicochemical properties of plant proteins that determine the ease of their digestion. The ease of digestion of plant proteins in the rumen of ruminants is now an important consideration in the formulation of animal rations.

Protein quality is an important aspect of nutritional physiology because the use of amino acids for anabolism within the animal requires that no particular amino acid becomes limiting, or protein synthesis will be arrested. At least half of the 20 or so amino acids commonly found in animal protein can be synthesized within the animal as needed, to balance their use in protein anabolism. This subject will be addressed in more detail in Chapter 7.

Plant amino acids are more diverse than animal amino acids, and some of the monomers cannot be synthesized by animals yet are essential for normal growth and functioning of the animal. These *essential amino acids* must be obtained from the diet. Protein quality has traditionally been evaluated by determining the adequacy of a particular protein for the support of growth of young animals. Even though a complete compositional analysis of the amino acids can be performed routinely, the prediction of a most suitable balance of the 20 or so individual monomers for a given animal's needs is still very inexact.

Biologic testing of protein quality using young growing animals usually employs casein as a ''reference'' or ''standard'' protein because it provides an optimal balance of amino acids. In a test of the *biologic value* of a protein, it might be found that the basic source protein needs to be supplemented with more of a certain amino acid to achieve growth performance in test animals equal to that obtained using the casein standard. That particular amino acid would therefore be considered to be limiting in the source diet. For example, a diet based on corn meal as a source of protein would probably need to be supplemented with the amino acid lysine to achieve optimal growth. The biologic values of the protein available from most commonly used feeds are well known and are carefully considered when mixed rations are formulated. Plant breeders have incorporated the findings of nutritionists into their selection schemes for improved strains of forage and grain plants. It is now possible to grow *high lysine corn* to provide a product with protein of higher biologic quality.

The situation is much more complex in ruminants, because the microbial population of the rumen may drastically alter the balance of amino acids that prevailed in the diet. The microorganisms synthesize protein of their own and, as the microbes pass into the remainder of the digestive tract, they then serve as a nutrient source for the host animal. From this it is clear that the biologic value of the proteins leaving the rumen, be they dietary or microbial, is the important issue to the animal. This end point is also of concern to animal scientists and it is studied in a variety of ways. It is possible to simulate certain aspects of rumen function in simple culture experiments in the laboratory. It is also possible to prepare animals surgically so that repeated sampling of the contents of the digestive tract, at any of a variety of locations, can be done without trauma to the animal.

Carbohydrates

The complex sugars are polymers of ether-linked (–C–O–C–) monosaccharides. The major animal-derived polysaccharide is *glycogen*, a storage form of glucose monomers, that is present in large amounts in liver and muscle. Glycogen turnover, or synthesis (glycogenesis) and breakdown (glycogenolysis), are important aspects of metabolism and will be considered in detail in Chapter 7. For the present, it is sufficient to note that glycogen is made up exclusively from glucose, linked by $\alpha_{[1-4]}$ glucosidic bonds (Figure 6–6), with some branching via $\alpha_{[1-6]}$ bonds. The

nature of the bonds determines which enzymes are capable of hydrolyzing the polymer to yield smaller units, eventually producing the monosaccharides suitable for absorption.

A substantial amount of animal carbohydrate exists as structural material rather than in the storage form represented by glycogen. The "ground substance", or intercellular solids, of many tissues contains polysaccharides made from amino sugars and sulfated sugars. These substances are termed *mucopolysaccharides*, mucoids, or, more correctly, *glycosaminoglycans*. Some examples of these materials are mucus in saliva, and the rubbery, shock-absorbing, lubricating material found on the articulating surfaces in joints. It has already been noted that many proteins are extensively glycosylated, and are called glycoproteins or mucoproteins. Several hormones, many plasma proteins, and many membrane proteins may be about 50% carbohydrate by weight. The well-known blood group substances of erythrocytes that provide the basis for different blood types are mucoproteins.

Plant and microbial polysaccharides are far more diverse than animal polysaccharides. The best-known plant polysaccharide of caloric significance to humans is *starch*, a mixture of two polymers, each of which is made up exclusively from glucose units. Starch is insoluble in water and is found as granules in plant cells. The major constituent is amylose, a linear $\alpha_{[1-4]}$ polymer, and the minor constituent, which accounts for just a small percentage of the total, is the highly branched $\alpha_{[1-4]}$ and $\alpha_{[1-6]}$ amylopectin.

Quantitatively of great importance, because it represents the major structural constituent of forages, is *cellulose* (Figure 6–7). Higher animals are unable to digest cellulose without the assistance of microbial populations harbored within their digestive tracts. Herbivores have developed various structural and functional specializations of their alimentary canals to facilitate the *symbiosis* established with their microbes. Omnivores, and less obviously carnivores, provide only a primitive environment in their large intestines for the microbial population, and most dietary cellulose is not digested but merely provides *bulk* to the digesta and feces. There is substantial interest in the apparently deleterious

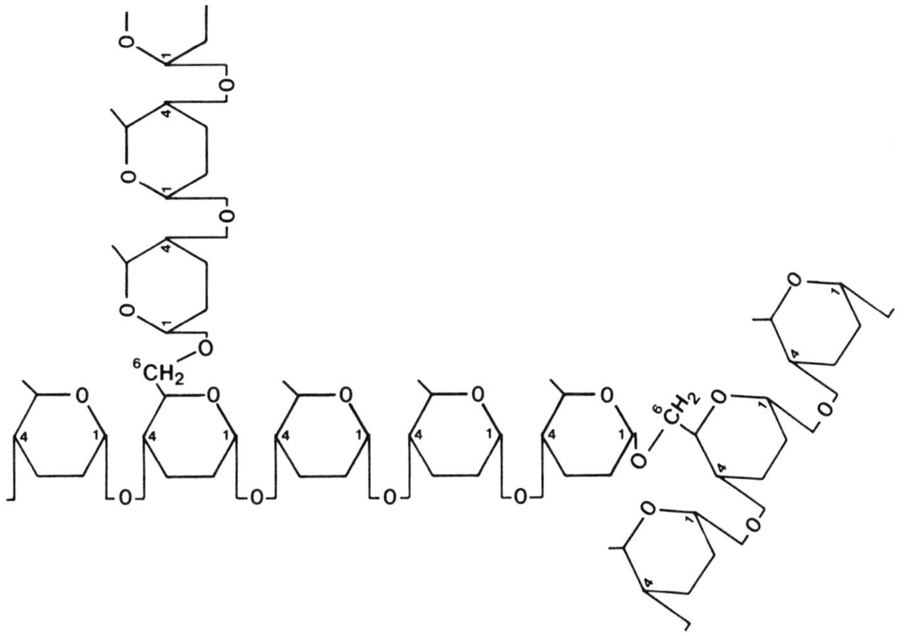

Figure 6–6. The chain structure of glycogen. Glycogen, the principal storage carbohydrate of animals, consists of thousands of glycosyl groups forming linear polymers linked α_{1-4} along with branching that begins with α_{1-6} bonds. The glucosyl moieties are shown schematically with carbons 1, 4, and 6 indicated.

health consequences of "overrefined" diets, or those lacking a high content of cellulose, or *fiber*.

Cellulose and hemicellulose are insoluble plant structural components of major dietary significance to herbivores, both ruminants and

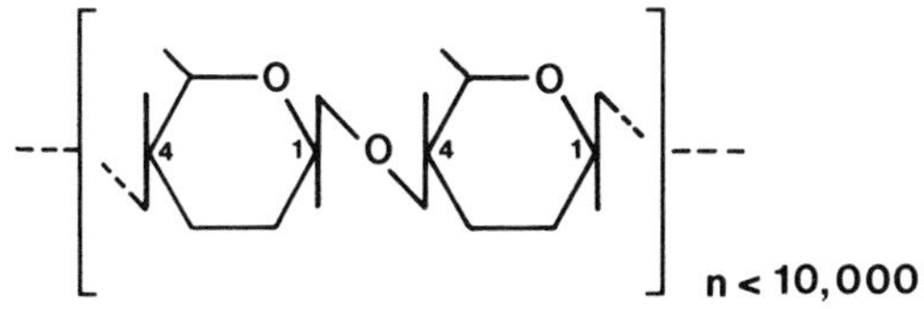

Figure 6–7. The chain structure of cellulose. Cellulose, the major structural carbohydrate polymer found in plant walls, is also assembled from glucosyl units but the ether linkages are β_{1-4} bonds that cannot be hydrolyzed by mammalian amylases. Animals can derive nutrients for absorption from cellulose only with the participation of the microbes inhabiting the gut.

nonruminants. The digestible components for fermentation systems include the *pectins*, but more complex substances, such as the *lignins*, are not fermented. Despite the great diversity of monomeric units and polymeric structure, the polysaccharides can all be reduced to a rather simple mixture of small organic acids, carbon dioxide (CO_2), water, hydrogen, and methane. The acids are volatile in steam and are commonly called *volatile fatty acids*. The straight chain acids (Figure 6–8) consist of acetic (C_2), propionic (C_3), butyric (C_4), valeric (C_5), and small amounts of caproic (C_6) acids.

Branched chain acids are also present. Their names are prefixed with *iso-*, as described in Appendix B. The reader should become familiar with the names and structures of the volatile fatty acids.

Simpler sugars are also important components of the diet, and animals, including man, may select among diets to increase the intake of

CH$_3$ COOH	acetic
CH$_3$ CH$_2$ COOH	propionic
CH$_3$ CH$_2$ CH$_2$ COOH	butyric
CH$_3$ CH$_2$ CH COOH CH$_3$	2-methylbutyric

Figure 6–8. Volatile fatty acids. Acetic, propionic, and butyric acids (2C, 3C, and 4C) are the major short chain products of rumen fermentation. In addition, 2-methylbutyric acid is shown as one example of a branched chain volatile acid.

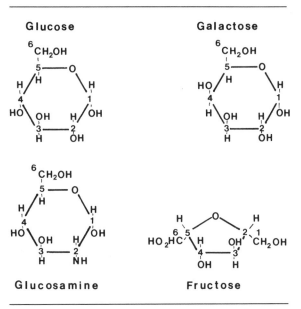

Glucose   Galactose

Glucosamine   Fructose

Figure 6–9. Monosaccharides. This selection of simple sugars includes three hexoses—glucose, galactose, and fructose—and one amino sugar—glucosamine (note the amine substitution on C_2). The parent monosaccharides have generic formulas of $C_n(H_2O)_n$. Hexoses have 6 carbons (n = 6) and pentoses have 5 carbons (n = 5). Note that glucose and galactose have identical elemental composition, but that the hydroxyl groups on C_4 are shown with different orientations. Galactose is an *epimer* of glucose.

these simple sugars. The reader will be most familiar with *sucrose*, a disaccharide of glucose and fructose (Figure 6–9), and with *lactose,* or milk sugar, a disaccharide of glucose and galactose. Many soluble saccharides are present in the cell sap of lush forages. These sugars can be released as a result of mastication, and they are very rapidly fermented by ruminal microbes, but in nonruminants they may be digested then absorbed to contribute substantially to total caloric needs.

6.3 • Ingestion and Swallowing

The desire to eat, the selection of feed, and its ingestion are all *voluntary* events, controlled by higher centers in the brain. The control of *appetite* has a substantial autonomic or involuntary component and is heavily influenced by chemoreception of a variety of signals. Most of the key nutrients that circulate in blood, such as glucose, nonesterified fatty acids, amino acids, and so forth, are continually monitored, and when their concentrations in the extracellular fluids fall below setpoints established for each, a drive to consume food is established. In ruminants, where volatile fatty acids are the most important energy substrates derived from digestion in the rumen, chemoreceptors specific for the volatile fatty acids provide input to the appetite centers in the brain. There are some highly selective appetite drives, such as a desire to consume salt. A salt-deficient animal may select a ration containing salt and refuse another ration that lacks this component. Physical factors such as distension of the gut from its content of bulky feeds, or feeds of very low dry matter content, such as lush pasture, may also provide input for appetite regulation.

Although appetite is the force behind the desire to consume feed, the drive is manifested in the *selection* and *ingestion* of feed.

Ingestion

Ingestive mechanisms vary substantially between animals, reflecting dietary habit, rate of eating, and anatomic structures of the head. The distribution and types of teeth on the upper and lower gums, the surface structures on the tongue, the size of the jaw, and the shape and mobility of the lips all influence how animals eat. For domestic herbivores, differences in the form of the upper lip dictate whether an animal is a "nibbler," such as sheep and goats, or whether the animal ingests feed by sweeping it back into its mouth using the tongue, as cattle do.

Sheep and goats *bite* with the incisors on the lower jaw against a toothless pad of gum. The integrity of these teeth is important for the nutritional well-being of these animals when they are grazing or eating browse-type feeds. Tooth wear can occur, particularly as a result of grazing sparse pastures, when substantial amounts of soil, grit, and sand may be taken in along with the forage.

Cattle tend to tear growing forage by tongue action rather than by biting. Cattle have some difficulty in consuming short forage, because the upper lip is not split and the animal has little ability to nibble. As shown in Figure 6–10, the bovine tongue is covered with *papillae* which are oriented backward, not unlike small barbs. These aid in grasping forage so that it can be pulled back and torn.

Mastication

The ingesta is mechanically reduced to smaller particles by grinding between the flat broad molars toward the rear of the buccal cavity. In foragers, the jaw is particularly mobile laterally (from side to side), and the tongue is bulky, particularly near its base. This facilitates moving the mouthful of ingesta back and forth over the molars. The work of biting, chewing, and swallowing is a considerable overhead energy cost to foraging animals. Depending on the species and the nature of the feed, there may be up to 50,000 jaw movements per day!

During mastication, or chewing, *saliva* is added to the ingesta while it remains in the buccal cavity. Saliva serves numerous functions in aid of digestion. In Chapter 3, the control of salivation was described as an example of secretomotor integration of reflex afferents from the buccal cavity, along with higher inputs (see Figure 3–37).

Saliva is produced by several pairs of salivary glands and the composition varies considerably between these glands. Some saliva is copious in volume and seems to be important in providing buffering salts, mainly $NaHCO_3$, to the digestive tract. For example, the parotid glands of cattle secrete 100 to 200 L/day of what is essentially a dilute solution of sodium bicarbonate. A variety of other ions and simple organic molecules are delivered into the digestive tract in saliva, and these are of special significance for the microbial population of the ruminant stomach. Other salivary glands produce smaller volumes of thick viscous secretion that seems to be important for structuring the ingesta into a bolus, then lubricating its surface to aid in swallowing.

The solvent properties of saliva are likely to

Figure 6–10. The bovine tongue. A view of the dorsal surface of the tongue shows the flattened papillae toward the rear and the rasp-like papillae near the tip (see enlargement). The latter are directed backward and they aid in prehensile, or feed gathering, activity. (Photograph courtesy of Dr. Pamela Livesay–Wilkins, New York State College of Veterinary Medicine, Cornell University.)

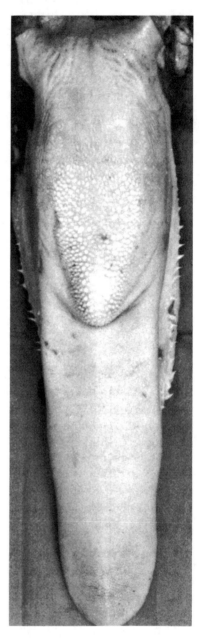

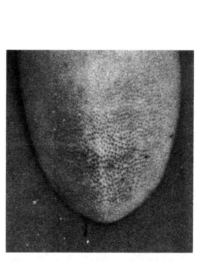

be important for distributing chemicals released from the feed to chemoreceptors, which in this case are called *taste receptors*. The mucus may serve in a protective role for the oral mucosa, particularly during ingestion of dry, brittle feed materials such as chaff, coarse hay, or cracked grains, which might be abrasive. A few species have enzymes and bacteriostatic components in saliva, though they are either not present or not important to digestive mechanisms in domestic animals. Some animals depend on copious salivation as a component of their thermoregulatory strategies. These special functions are described in Chapter 9.

Swallowing

At the rear of the buccal cavity, the digestive tract communicates with the respiratory tract in the *pharynx* (see Figure 1–21). These tracts are temporarily separated by reflex mechanisms during swallowing. The initial events in swallowing are, however, voluntary, or at least they can be voluntarily held in check. The muscle of the anterior tongue is striated and is contracted voluntarily to elevate the tongue against the hard palate. The ingesta is moved posteriorly to pass over tactile receptors that activate a reflex contraction of the base of the tongue. A *swallowing center* in the medulla oblongata coordinates swallowing in between respiratory movements.

The larynx elevates and the glottis closes to direct the bolus back into the *esophagus*.

The esophagus provides communication between the buccal cavity and the anterior, or cranial, portion of the stomach. Some variation exists in the muscular nature of the esophageal wall; in some species only the caudal portion is smooth muscle and the remainder is striated, while in others the bulk of the organ is made up of smooth muscle. The esophagus is located dorsad to the trachea in the neck region; it traverses the thoracic cavity then passes through the diaphragm to reach the stomach.

Movement of the bolus of ingesta in the esophagus is reflexly controlled and, in some species, may involve *peristalsis*. Peristalsis is a specialized propagational activity of the walls of some tubular structures. It requires that a region of contraction be preceded by a region of relaxation, so contents of the lumen can be propelled along. A more detailed explanation of this phenomenon is provided in Section 6.8. There is usually a further volume of saliva produced and swallowed after the buccal cavity has been cleaned of ingesta.

6.4 • Digestion in the Stomach

Digestion in the stomach involves three major aspects of gastric function: *reservoir function, mechanical reduction of feed,* and *hydrolytic or chemical digestion*. These aspects reflect the anatomic and functional organization of the stomach. In addition, the stomach serves several minor functions: a limited *absorptive function, an endocrine function, production of intrinsic factor,* and a *protective function,* by providing for vomiting.

In monogastric animals, the stomach is best considered as made up of three portions: the *cardia* (near the esophageal entrance), the *fundus* (body of the stomach), and the *antrum* (near the pylorus, or aboral exit) (Figure 6–11).

The stomach is a highly distensible muscular organ, effectively valved at both the entrance and exit. It is highly vascularized and has a specialized secretory mucous lining. The nature of the secretions varies over the three major zones, as described below. Knowledge of some of the properties of the stomach has been exploited by mankind for years. It has served as a container

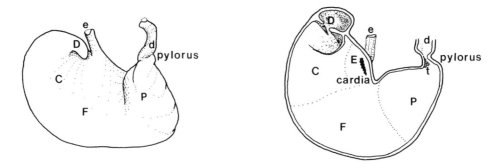

Figure 6–11. *The monogastric stomach of the pig.* The simple stomach is best considered functionally as being made up of the cardiac (C), fundic (F), and pyloric (P) regions. In pigs, the stomach is slightly more complex. There is an aglandular esophageal region (E) immediately adjacent to the cardia, the opening from the esophagus (e), and the cardiac region includes an incompletely separated blind sac (diverticulum, D). The pylorus is somewhat constricted by a fatty swelling called the torus (t); the pylorus provides communication from the stomach to the duodenum (d).

for fluids; the secretions have been used to brighten copper and bronze; and secretions have been used to clot milk to produce junket.

Systematic investigation of gastric function was first conducted by the physician William Beaumont in a human subject who had suffered a gunshot wound that healed to leave a permanent *gastric fistula.* A fistula is an opening established between the lumen of an internal organ and the exterior of the body. Surgical fistulation in experimental animals has been the most important experimental technique used to explore the control of secretory function. Beaumont's studies on his fistulated patient represent a classic series of investigations that established some general values for the volume and superficial characteristics of gastric juice in the human.

The next series of major discoveries were made by Pavlov, using dogs prepared with esophageal and gastric fistulas. The esophageal fistula can be temporarily opened so that all food that is swallowed passes out through the fistula and does not reach the stomach. Pavlov determined that there was a *cephalic* component to gastric secretion and that this consisted of a *psychic* and several *reflex* parts. Anticipation of ingestion, ingestion itself, and then swallowing

are all potent stimuli for gastric secretion. The control is achieved through *parasympathetic secretomotor innervation* of the stomach via the vagus nerve.

The gastric mucosa contains several types of secretory glands. Those in the cardia and pyloric regions produce mucus, while the fundic glands, located in the body of the stomach, are more specialized and have distinct secretions. Fundic glands (Figure 6–12) may include *chief* cells and *parietal* (oxyntic) cells.

The chief cells are the source of enzymes present in gastric juice. The most important is *pepsinogen,* the *zymogen,* or precursor form, of the endopeptidase *pepsin.* An endopeptidase is an enzyme capable of hydrolyzing amide bonds within the structure of a protein. The zymogen is not active as a proteolytic agent, so the cells producing it are not vulnerable to autodigestion. This represents a vital protective mechanism for the stomach. The active form, pepsin, is produced as a result of the action of hydrochloric acid, a normal component of gastric juice, on the pepsinogen molecule. Minor amylolytic and lipolytic activities may also be present in gastric juice. In general, however, starches and lipids are not subjected to extensive digestion in the monogastric stomach.

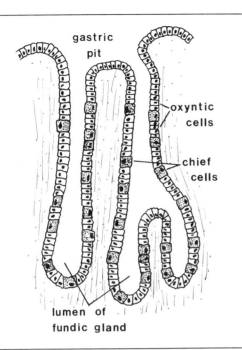

Figure 6–12. Glands of the fundic mucosa. The mucosal lining of the fundic region of the stomach is thrown into folds. Gastric pits overlie fundic glands that produce the enzymes and hydrochloric acid of the gastric secretion. Chief cells produce pepsinogen, the precursor to pepsin; oxyntic (parietal) cells are the source of the HCl. Additional mucus producing glands are found in the cardia and, less abundantly, in the fundus.

The parietal cells are specialized to secrete hydrochloric acid and *intrinsic factor,* a protein that serves as a carrier for the intestinal absorption of vitamin B_{12}. The secretion of HCl is quite impressive, as the pH of gastric contents is maintained at a value less than pH 1. A typical concentration of the HCl is about 0.15M. The exocrine secretion of H^+ ions is accompanied by active secretion of Cl^- ions. The parietal cell obtains the Cl^- from the interstitial fluid in exchange for HCO_3- passing from the cell to the interstitium (Figure 6–13). The bicarbonate is produced from CO_2 and H_2O via carbonic acid. The CO_2 may be produced within the cell from the very substantial metabolism that is required to support the active secretory mechanism, or it

may be taken up from the plasma or interstitial fluid. The elaboration of HCl by the parietal cell is yet another example of the application of the fundamental carbonate-bicarbonate buffering system that was described earlier. It is emphasized that gastric secretion is *voluminous, acidic, and contains enzymes.*

The cells of the stomach are protected from the strong acid by *mucus* secreted by the surface layer of cells. This layer is called a *mucous membrane,* and if it becomes damaged, the epithelium can be exposed to the acid with quite serious sequelae. Some largely nonionized, or very weak, acids, and particularly those that are hydrophobic, are able to pass across the gastric mucosal barrier and cause focal cell death, which leads to ulceration. The volatile fatty acids (acetic, propionic, and butyric) and the drug aspirin in acid solution, alcohol, and detergents such as the bile acids and lysolecithin all cause this type of damage.

In young ruminants, the *abomasum,* the glandular equivalent of the monogastric stomach, secretes *rennin,* an enzyme capable of clotting the casein present in ingested milk. It is believed that the clot causes prolonged gastric retention and thereby aids more complete digestion of the milk proteins by gastric pepsin, before the stomach contents pass on to the intestines.

Control of Gastric Secretion

The cephalic component of control of gastric secretion initiates secretory activity within the stomach, presumably in preparation for the arrival of swallowed ingesta. Two additional components of control over the stomach are important. These are the *gastric* and *intestinal* components. This subject needs elaboration, because there is quite clearly a gastric, or local, component of control over gastric function. It is quite apparent that the presence of digesta in the stomach is itself a potent source of stimulation for gastric secretion. A combination of chemical and physical stimuli initiates reflex- and

Figure 6–13. Secretion of gastric hydrochloric acid. Carbonic acid, generated from CO_2 and H_2O, dissociates into HCO_3^- and H^+ in the parietal cell. The HCO_3^- is recovered into the interstitium in exchange for Cl^- taken up by the cell. The H^+ is actively secreted into the lumen of the fundic gland, along with Cl^- providing electrochemical balance.

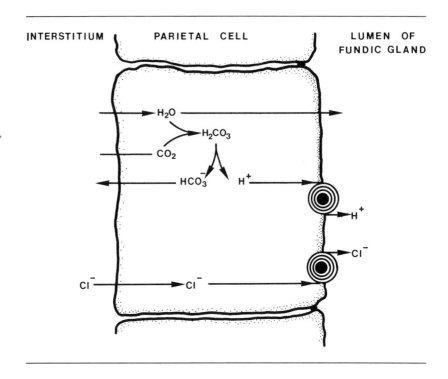

hormone-mediated gastric responses. The reflexes are *vagovagal*. That is, neurons in the vagus nerve conduct afferent impulses to the medulla oblongata, and other vagal neurons carry efferent (motor) traffic back to the stomach. As the typical parasympathetic effector agent, acetylcholine serves as the neurotransmitter, and the effector responses can be annulled by atropine. The medullary *gastric center* is also sensitive to factors involved in appetite control, particularly by the plasma concentration of glucose.

Vagal efferents exert major control over both gastric motility and the secretion of enzymes, but only minor control over acid secretion.

The major control on acid secretion is achieved by the hormone *gastrin*, a peptide hormone secreted by mucosal cells in the pyloric antral region. This is the more aboral portion of the stomach, near the exit to the small intestines. Gastrin acts on cells of the fundic glands, especially the acid-secreting parietal cells. Gastrin appears to act in part via the local production of histamine, which also serves to vasodilate blood vessels in the vicinity of the fundic glands. Histamine is a potent local vasodilatory agent. This

mediation by histamine is a good example of physiologic coordination, because the local increase in blood perfusion rate supports the increased metabolic needs of the cells during active, or energy-consuming, secretory episodes. Excessive acid production may create a milieu that favors the development of ulcers, and excessive acid aggravates the clinical discomfort associated with existing ulcers (Box 6–1).

The humoral mechanism, mediated via gastrin, was initially studied using completely *denervated* gastric fundic pouches. These pouches are surgically constructed from a portion of the fundic wall after complete isolation from the nerve supply to the fundus. They are prepared with a fistula opening to the exterior to permit collection of secretions. Secretory activity can therefore be monitored when stimuli are delivered to the remainder of the stomach that is repaired and still in communication with the esophagus and intestines.

The third component of control over gastric digestion, in this case an inhibitory control, is provided by the small intestine. It is well known that the mucosa of the first part of the small intestine, the duodenum, produces a blood-borne substance that exerts *inhibitory* control on the stomach. The influence is greatest when intact fats are present in the duodenal lumen, but the presence of any type of gastric content, such as acid, is an effective stimulus for the secretion of this inhibitor. In such circumstances, there is a reduction in gastric acid secretion, diminished gastric motility, and hence less frequent gastric emptying. Recently it has become apparent that the duodenal peptide called pancreozymin-cholecystokinin (PZ-CCK) is fully capable of exerting the actions described above. This peptide will be shown to have other important actions, the nature of which can be deduced from its name.

In addition to this hormonal inhibitor, there exists a mechanism called the *enterogastric reflex* that involves neurons of the *myenteric plexus,* a plexus of nerves usually found within the wall of the gut. The same kind of stimuli that activate the endocrine mechanism just described also seem to activate this neural mechanism. In addition, simple distension of the duodenum is effective (Figure 6–14).

Gastric Motility

Movements of the muscular wall of the stomach serve to churn and mix the contents, aiding in the mechanical reduction of the digesta. Elsewhere in the digestive tract, movements are important in presenting digestive end products to the absorptive surface, but this is of less importance in the stomach. The exception is in the ruminant stomachs where absorption of volatile acids, water, and gases are critical digestive processes.

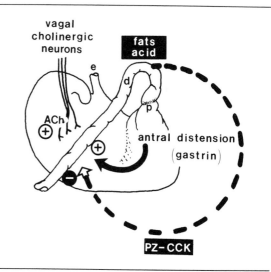

Figure 6–14. Control of gastric emptying. Cholinergic motor neurons from the vagus nerve exert a stimulatory influence on gastric motility and secretion. Distension of the pyloric antral region provokes secretion into blood of the hormone gastrin, which is also stimulatory on gastric function, as described in the text. Inhibitory neural pathways from the duodenum and inhibitory endocrine influences mediated by PZ-CCK and possibly other duodenal hormones balance the stimulatory controls. The presence of gastric contents such as acid and intact fats in the duodenum is especially important in constraining gastric emptying.

The result of gastric digestion, involving both mechanical and hydrolytic aspects, is the conversion of ingesta into *chyme*, an acid pulp. Gastric emptying delivers the chyme through the pyloric sphincter into the duodenum. The initial stimulus for emptying the stomach stems from distension of the antral wall by material of appropriate consistency. The extent of emptying is controlled by the interplay of facilitory and inhibitory controls, much the same as those controlling gastric secretory activity.

The control of gastric function then depends on an excitatory vagal innervation coupled with a stimulatory humoral component provided by gastrin. Opposing these facilitory influences are inhibitory influences arising from the duodenum. One is humoral and seems to be due to PZ-CCK. The other component is neural, the enterogastric reflex of the myenteric plexus. These paired control mechanisms—for example that of the vagus and that provided by gastrin—are cooperative. If the vagi are sectioned, the gastric response to gastrin is diminished. On the other hand, if the pyloric antral region is removed by partial gastrectomy, thereby removing the source of gastrin, the secretomotor potency of vagal efferent signals is similarly weakened.

Summary of Gastric Function

- There are three components of control of gastric function: cephalic, gastric, and intestinal.

- Neural and humoral mechanisms are cooperative.

- Gastric digestion is probably initiated by the cephalic mechanisms, sustained by the gastric component, then terminated by the intestinal component.

6.5 • The Ruminant Specialization

Anatomy of the Ruminant Stomach

The regional anatomy of the visceral organs of ruminants was described briefly in Chapter 1. The four component chambers of the stomach, the *reticulum*, the *rumen*, the *omasum*, and the *abomasum* (Figure 6–15), have characteristic features and functions. The reticulum and rumen are incompletely separated by a heavy fold of tissue that is oriented ventrodorsally. At the dorsal extremity, the two portions of the stomach are in free communication. The *reticulorumen* is the part of the stomach that provides the favorable ecosystem for the microbial population.

The reticulorumen lies to the left of the midline and, on the left and cranial aspects, is closely approximated to the diaphragm. The esophagus enters the craniodorsal portion of the rumen by means of a slitlike opening. The opening and the general region of the ruminal wall are called the *cardia*. Extending ventrally from the cardia, the right wall is thrown into two parallel folds that define the *esophageal groove*. This structure can be reflexly closed in young ruminants to provide a tubelike bypass between the cardia

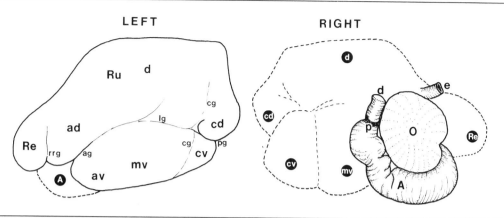

Figure 6–15. The ruminant stomach. The gross anatomy of the stomach can be deduced from these views. *Left:* The reticulorumen's distinct morphology results from its partial separation into sacs by folds or pillars in the wall. These correspond to grooves that are evident on the outer surface. Structures identified include the reticulum (Re); rumen (Ru); anterior dorsal sac (ad); dorsal rumen (d), caudodorsal sac (cd); anterior ventral sac (av); main ventral rumen (mv); caudoventral sac (cv); reticuloruminal groove (rrg); anterior groove (ag); left groove (lg); cardiac groove (cg); posterior groove (pg); and abomasum (A). *Right:* Best viewed from the right side are the esophagus (e), omasum (O), and abomasum (A), communicating with the duodenum (d) via the pylorus (p).

and the point of exit from the reticulorumen. Communication between the reticulorumen and the omasum is through the *omasal orifice.* The reticulum derives its name from the honeycomb-like pattern of raised folds (Figure 6–16) on the inner surface.

The lining of the reticulorumen is an epithelium of the keratinized, stratified squamous type. This type of epithelium is nonsecretory and so contains no glands. It is a protective surface but does have significant absorptive function in certain regions. The adult form is acquired after birth and indeed after the animal makes the transition to fibrous feeds.

The ruminal surface is specialized with *papillae,* rather than the honeycomb structures of the reticulum. In the dorsal region there is a transition from one form to the other. The rumen is partially divided into compartments by a series of massive folds, or *pillars.* These partially separate the dorsal and ventral portions and define the regions of the *cranial sac,* the *dorsal sac,* the *caudodorsal blind sac,* the *caudoventral blind sac,*

and the *main ventral sac.* The size and appearance of the papillae vary considerably between these regions of the rumen.

The wall of the reticulorumen is made up of smooth muscle with an epithelial lining. The organ is innervated primarily by branches of the vagus nerve which carry both sensory and motor neurons. The wall is richly vascularized from two ruminal arteries and venous drainage is collected into ruminal veins, then into a gastric vein, which delivers blood into the portal vein and thence to the liver.

The omasum has a characteristic lining of sizable *leaflike* folds of epithelium. These provide an enormous absorptive surface within a relatively small volume. Digesta reaching the omasum from the reticulum passes between the omasal folds on its way to the abomasum. The omasum lies to the right of the reticuloruminal fold and craniad to the abomasum. It receives arterial blood from branches of the omasoabomasal artery and its venous drainage is into the gastric vein.

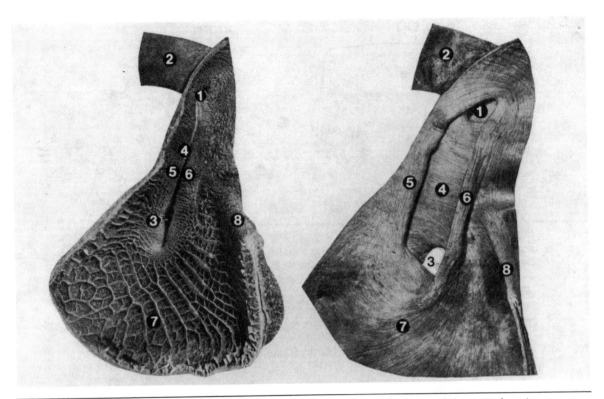

Figure 6–16. *The reticulum with the esophageal groove.* The epithelium of the reticulum is thrown up in regular folds giving a reticular (honeycomb-like) appearance. This is most obvious ventrally (7) and less so dorsally where a transition occurs to the papillae of the rumen. Note the esophageal groove between the cardia (1), the opening from the esophagus (2), and the reticulo-omasal orifice (3). The groove (4) is closed into a tube-like bypass by contraction of muscles in the lips on either side (5 and 6). The reticuloruminal fold (8) provides a partial separation of these two portions of the ruminant stomach. The photograph on the right was taken after removal of the epithelium; the lips have been spread somewhat to show the floor of the groove. (Reproduced by permission of the publisher. From Sisson, S. and Grossman, J.D.: *The Anatomy of Domestic Animals*, 3rd edition, Philadelphia, PA: W.B. Saunders Company, 1938.)

The last of the stomach chambers is the abomasum, the one portion that has a glandular, and hence secretory, mucosal lining. The largest part is the fundus, or body, which seems to be functionally analogous to the monogastric stomach. The caudal portion is the pyloric antrum and it communicates, via the pyloric sphincter, to the cranial portion of the small intestine. The abomasum shares a vascular supply and drainage with the omasum.

Motility of the Ruminant Stomach

Methods used to investigate rumen motility have included examinations via fistulas, permanent openings of the organ to the outside. Additionally, the placement of pressure-sensitive balloons and electromyographic sensors into the rumen wall has yielded information on the intact organ.

Extensive removal of the rumen wall required for preparation of fistulas can create abnormalities from the necessary denervation. Pressure sensors detect the net consequences of contractile activity in the muscular wall by virtue of the Laplace relationship (see Box 2–1). Electromyography detects biopotentials, including action potentials, in the smooth muscle of the wall. Radiography has been used to examine how the rumen contents are moved about, and motility of the rumen wall can be monitored if x-ray–opaque markers are surgically implanted onto the *serosal*, or peritoneal, surface of the wall and the animal is monitored by *fluoroscopy*. Fluoroscopy is a real-time radiographic modality in which an intensifying screen is used.

More recently, chronic surgical preparations have been devised in which a partial exteriorization, or herniation, of the rumen wall is created. A skin incision is made and a circle of abdominal wall is completely removed. The rumen wall is brought up into the hole so created and sutured around its periphery. The intact rumen wall is thus anchored to the cut edge of the abdominal musculature. The skin is then sutured down onto the rumen, rather than to its original attachment on the abdominal wall. For anterior rumen and reticular sites, a portion of the rib cage may be resected. After complete recovery and healing, the distending effect of the rumen contents pushes the hernia out as a small swelling. During contraction of that region of the rumen wall, the hernia is drawn in; then, during relaxation, it is pushed out again. Animals can be prepared with several such partial exteriorizations and the contractions at these locations can be recorded simultaneously by means of any suitable recording device. The sequence of contractions shown in Figure 6–17 is typical of multisite recording from animals prepared in the manner just described.

Major Motility Sequences

The A, or mixing, sequence has a characteristic Z-like pattern of propagation across the reticu-

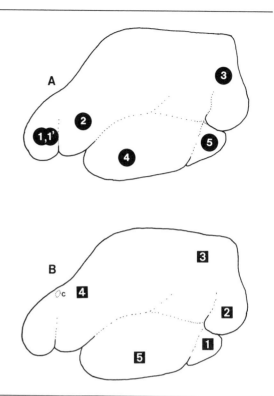

Figure 6–17. The "A" and "B" sequences. The pattern of the most important sequential, regional contractions of the wall of the reticulo-rumen are shown. *A:* Steps 1 to 5 show the typical sequence of contractions ("A" sequence), responsible for mixing the contents of the rumen. Note that this begins with a double (or biphasic) contraction of the reticulum (1 and 1'). The contraction is next evident in the anterior dorsal sac (2) of the rumen, the caudal region (3), the main ventral rumen (4), and finally in the caudoventral sac (5). *B:* The eructation—or "B"—sequence starts in the caudoventral blind sac (1), sweeps forward across the dorsum (2 and 3) to reach the vicinity (4) of the cardia (c), then is completed with contraction of the main ventral rumen (5).

lorumen. As illustrated in Figure 6–17, the **A** sequence begins with a biphasic contraction of the reticulum, followed by a contraction wave that sweeps back over the dorsal rumen to the caudodorsal area. The wave propagates through the anterior ventral, the main ventral, and finally the caudoventral region. A sequences provide for extensive mixing of rumen contents and for disturbing the layering effects that prevail during quiet (noncontractile) periods. The layering takes the form of a gas phase under the dorsal rumen wall, then a layer of coarse solids floating on the upper surface of the rumen fluid. Under the coarse, fibrous material is a layer of fine particles in suspension, then most ventrally a layer of rumen fluid that is virtually free of feed ingesta particles.

Animals that have grazed very sparse pasture or freshly sprouted grass may ingest substantial quantities of soil and sand, and these accumulate in the most ventral region of the reticulum and rumen, along with miscellaneous pieces of metal that may have been consumed inadvertently. Pieces of wire, nails, fencing staples, nuts and bolts, and even tines from haymaking equipment have been recovered from the reticulum. Any sharp object has the potential for rupturing the wall, especially since the reticulum engages in vigorous contractions. A common cause of *peritonitis* in ruminants results from the leaking of reticular contents through such punctures and into the peritoneal cavity. This is known as *hardware disease*.

Rumen fermentation results in the production of large quantities of gas. Distension of the dorsal rumen by this gas triggers an *eructation*, or B, sequence. The B sequence is initiated in the caudoventral blind sac and is followed by contraction of the caudodorsal blind sac, the dorsal rumen, and the craniodorsal area, or cardia. The gas "bubble" is pressed against the cardia and the esophageal opening and is forcibly ejected by a contraction of the main ventral rumen. This crescendo contraction pushes the liquid and semisolid contents dorsally and cranially until the gas pressure is sufficient to overcome the resistance of the cardia. The gas then escapes into the esophagus under pressure. Box 6–2 describes a condition in which this mechanism is unable to operate and gas accumulates within the reticulorumen.

The best-known motility sequence is that of *rumination*, a process of controlled regurgitation that enables further mastication of partially digested rumen contents. Rumination involves a coordinated series of events that employs the respiratory muscles, the larynx, the pharynx, the esophagus, the buccal apparatus, and the reticulum. In contrast to the biphasic contraction that

---

Box 6–2   Bloat

The normal process of gas elimination, described in relation to the B sequence, is markedly disturbed during *bloat*. A heavy, stable foam may be produced by a variety of plant components, particularly from legumes, and the foam interferes with the normal operation of a B sequence. The foamy gas phase resists being moved in the craniodorsal fashion, and continued rumen distension results initially in bloating and discomfort, then may progress to cause death of the animal. Bloated animals have difficulty breathing (*dyspnea*). The diaphragm is unable to flatten out as completely as normally because the distended rumen pushes forward.

A similar difficulty results if an animal is restrained, or accidentally becomes lodged after falling, and remains on its back or high on its right side. Gas cannot press against the cardia and so cannot escape from the rumen. Gas formation also continues for a while in a freshly dead animal. Because there is no means for the gas to escape, the dead animal becomes bloated.

starts an A sequence, rumination is initiated by a discrete single contraction of the reticulum. At the height of the reticular contraction there is an inspiratory effort, but this occurs when the glottis is closed and hence no air is permitted to flow into the lungs. As might be predicted, inspiration against a closed glottis generates great negative pressure in the thorax. This negativity is transmitted to the thoracic portion of the esophagus. The partial vacuum sucks up a bolus of reticular contents through the cardia, and a proc-

ess of reverse peristalsis rapidly lifts the bolus into the buccal cavity. This is immediately followed by a discrete swallowing event which serves to remove the liquid portion of the bolus and returns it to the rumen. The residue is then chewed again, has more saliva added to it, then is again swallowed. A full rumination sequence, as described, is usually followed by one or more A sequences, then additional ruminations. The reflex control of the rumination sequence is described in some detail in Box 6–3.

Box 6–3   Reflex Control of Rumination

Rumination does not occur after complete vagotomy, but can still take place in intact animals that have been treated with atropine. This indicates that the efferent, or motor neurons, in the vagus nerve are not necessary, whereas the afferent, or sensory neurons, are required. The important sensory areas for initiating rumination include the surface of the reticulum and rumen near the cardia and the cranial pillar. This is the partial wall that separates the craniodorsal from the cranioventral regions of the rumen. All components of the rumination process occur in decerebrate animals. In these experimental animals, the brain stem is surgically sectioned anterior to the pons, so that there are no functional cerebral cortices. There is thus no requirement for voluntary control.

Specific sites in the hypothalamus, when stimulated, can initiate rumination. Because several reflexes are involved in coordinating the rumination process, and many of these are regulated by medullary centers, it is convenient to consider the overall system as orchestrated from a *rumination center*. The various efferent limbs of these reflexes are as follows:

Reticular contraction—Vagus n.

Esophagus—Vagus n.

Diaphragm—Phrenic n.

Salivation—Cranial nerves

Mastication, swallowing—Cranial nerves

The A sequence, described in the text, is also subject to control via a *vagovagal* reflex. The reflex depends on both sensory and motor neurons within the vagal trunk. Additional afferents arise from sensory receptors located in the buccal cavity and esophagus. Most sensory receptors for A sequences are stretch receptors, but there is some simple tactile (touch) input, and some receptors that are best described as being chemical. For example, excessive abomasal acidity can initiate the A sequence. The most potent stimulus for a B sequence is simply gaseous distension of the dorsal rumen wall.

6.6 • Microbial Digestion

Although there are important differences in function, the overall processes of microbial digestion in the rumen, cecum, and colon have major features in common. The evolution of the ruminant has allowed improved function of the microbial system by the more favorable environment that is provided. The fermentation site is readily buffered by continuous input of serous, or watery, bicarbonate-rich saliva. Certain nutrients, for example urea and mineral ions, are also furnished from the host animal to the microbial population in this way. The rumen also has ready communication with the buccal cavity for remastication and removal of gas. The disadvantage of a prepeptic location is that all feeds are potentially subject to fermentation changes before regular gastric and intestinal processes can occur. This is the basis for the statement that "it is the rumen and the microbes that are fed, and not the animal."

Carbohydrate Digestion in the Rumen

Of major interest is the ability of the microbial population to effect degradation of cellulose, the essentially insoluble carbohydrate polymer that constitutes a major part of plant cell walls, and thus is a major dietary component for herbivores. The rumen population is mixed (10^{10} bacteria/mL; 10^6 protozoa/mL) and changes dynamically with alterations in diet. At birth, the rumen must be microbe free because the fetus has come from a sterile environment. The rumen population is established by *inoculation* during postnatal life. The population is mainly anaerobic, although some *facultative aerobes* are present to consume the oxygen that enters with every bolus of feed. The microbial population requires a protected environment in order to perform optimally. This is achieved in several ways:

- Frequent additions of substrate, or feed;

- Continuous provision of base in serous saliva to buffer the acids produced as fermentation end products;

- Continuous removal of fermentation products by absorption, eructation, and passage to the omasum;

- Relatively constant temperature;

- Stable osmotic environment achieved by additions of water;

- Control of redox potential by processes that consume hydrogen.

Gross disturbances in these parameters can alter the balance of microbial species making up the population and thereby alter the pattern of fermentation. For example, excess acidity may generate a lactic acid–producing fermentation with subsequent depression of appetite. Excess redox potential may reduce sulfate ions to hydrogen sulfide, as a means of consuming hydrogen. Alternatively, hydrogen can be consumed by excessive ammonification of nitrogenous substrates. It will be noted later that hydrogen is incorporated into unsaturated fatty acids.

Of the variety of functions of the microbes, four are especially important:

- Digestion to transform and solubilize otherwise insoluble dietary components such as cellulose;

- Incorporation of feed materials into constituents of the *microbial biomass*, including the synthesis of amino acids from organic ketoacids and free ammonia, then subsequent assembly of microbial protein;

- Size reduction of fibrous feed to permit passage through the reticulo-omasal orifice and into the remainder of the gut;

- Production of volatile fatty acids, capable of providing up to 70% of the energy requirements of the host animal.

Fermentation of carbohydrates can be considered in two stages: *Primary fermentation* is the production of small molecular weight intermediaries such as lactate, fumarate, succinate (Figure 6–18). *Secondary fermentation* provides for further conversion of the primary products to volatile fatty acids such as acetate, propionate, butyrate, plus minor constituents such as valerate (C_5) and some branched chain C_5 acids. These volatile fatty acids were illustrated in Figure 6–8.

Different bacterial classes function to ferment insoluble carbohydrates, such as cellulose and hemicellulose, and soluble components, such as starches and simple sugars. The latter compounds are liberated when the plant cells are opened. Protozoa may ingest very small food particles, such as starch granules, or they may consume bacteria. With changes in diet formulation, there are changes in both the microbial population and the resulting products of fer-

mentation. The causes of these alterations may be quite complex. For example, with lush pasture diets, mastication may release up to 70% of the plant cell contents, yielding soluble material for rapid fermentation. In contrast, a more fibrous feed, such as poor quality hay, may yield only trivial amounts of readily solubilized components. This difference alone could result in a major species change in the microbial population.

Related to the normal balance established between diet composition and microbial population, any sudden major change in the diet may produce abnormal fermentations, with potential digestive dysfunction, malaise, or even severe metabolic and or health problems for the host animal. Certain feed constituents may result in altered proportions of the major volatile fatty acids. For example, addition of corn starch will increase the production of propionic acid, a major *glucogenic* substrate for the ruminant animal. Glucogenic is the term applied to nutrients or substrates that can be converted within the animal into glucose. These compounds are very important to ruminants, and they will be discussed in detail in Chapter 7.

Protein Digestion in the Rumen

The microbial population is also responsible for protein degradation in the rumen. In part this is achieved by the secretion of microbial proteolytic enzymes and in part it is due to the engulfing of particulate material by protozoa. Like carbohydrates, dietary protein is present in various forms. In general, cytoplasmic proteins, or those of the plant cell sap, are soluble, while cell wall, or solid phase, proteins may be quite insoluble. Very soluble protein is almost completely degraded in the rumen. For example, less than 3% of casein added experimentally to an otherwise typical diet is likely to escape rumen processes and so remains to pass on to the hind gut. Less soluble or insoluble proteins may be

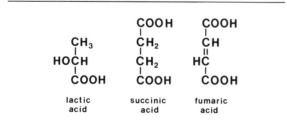

Figure 6–18. Fermentation intermediates. The organic three carbon and four carbon intermediates—lactate, fumarate, and succinate—are shown. These are products of primary fermentation and are usually processed further to the volatile fatty acids (shown in Figure 6–8) by secondary fermentation.

protected in part from the microbes, and they pass on with the microbes as the rumen contents are washed out into the rest of the gut. They are then subjected to peptic and intestinal digestion in the usual fashion.

Diets can be formulated to increase the insoluble protein component, or proteins can be "protected" and added to the diet as a supplement. Early experimental work used casein, treated with formaldehyde or glutaraldehyde, to render it virtually insoluble until passed on to the acidic environment of the abomasum. This approach established the principle of *protected proteins* and prompted the search for naturally "protected" protein sources in feedstuffs. It is now quite clear that some feeds contain protein that is more likely to pass through the rumen without substantial microbial degradation.

Microbial synthesis of protein in the ruminal environment is important to the host animal. This is because the microbial protein is made available to the animal following peptic and tryptic, or intestinal, digestion of the microbes that inevitably pass out of the rumen. Microbial protein synthesis may use amino acids generated from proteolysis of soluble dietary proteins in the rumen.

Amino acids may be synthesized de novo from ammonia and organic acids and bases, liberated in the course of primary fermentation. This ability to use nitrogen that need not be derived from protein sources can be commercially important in animal production. A number of industrially produced nitrogenous compounds that are easily synthesized, such as urea and biuret, can be carefully added to the diet to partly substitute for dietary protein. In extreme examples of this strategy, animals can be fed purified cellulose, or even newsprint, supplemented with urea, to provide a totally artificial diet. In the ruminant, this ability of the microbes to use nonprotein nitrogen provides a valuable measure of nitrogen economy because urea, which is secreted into the gut as a normal constituent of saliva, is recycled through the rumen rather than simply excreted in urine and therefore lost to the animal. This cycle will be described further in Chapter 7.

Lipid Digestion in the Rumen

Dietary lipids are hydrolyzed by ester cleavage by lipases produced by the microbes. The glycerol is fermented to yield propionic acid, and the fatty acids liberated from the triglyceride undergo modification. Plant fatty acids are highly unsaturated. The highly reducing conditions that generally prevail in the rumen result in hydrogen being incorporated into the olefinic, or unsaturated, bonds in the fatty acids, thereby producing more saturated fatty acids. Another major fate for the hydrogen generated in the rumen is incorporation into *methane*, another fermentation product that is either absorbed from the rumen for eventual respiratory removal or eructated with the CO_2.

The hydrogenation of dietary lipids by the rumen population is responsible for the relatively firm fat of ruminant animals (that is, higher melting point), compared to the "oily" consistency of most plant lipids (for example, corn oil). If the oil is incorporated as droplets in a protein emulsion, then "protected" by treatment with formaldehyde, it can escape rumen hydrogenation. The oil is then presented to the hind gut in its native, polyunsaturated form. The formaldehyde-treated particles break down in the abomasum and the fat droplets are released to pass on to the small intestine. Animals fed such diets have softer carcass fat, and milk fat that is capable of being transformed to a butter that remains soft and spreadable, even at refrigerator temperatures! Rations containing protected lipids have also been formulated as a means of providing animals with a diet of higher caloric density. Unfortunately, excessive fat entering the small intestine activates the PZ-CCK feedback on abomasal function and interferes with gastric emptying. This may result in inappetance.

The products of microbial digestion have various fates:

1. Fermentation gases may be absorbed, ejected by eructation, subjected to synthetic processes in the rumen, or passed out of the rumen in solution to the hind gut.

2. Organic acids of low molecular weight may be absorbed through the rumen wall, incorporated into the microbial biomass, or passed out of the rumen to the remainder of the gut.

3. Long chain fatty acids derived from dietary lipids form water-soluble salts, or soaps, and pass on for absorption in the hind gut.

4. The microbial biomass is continually washed out, along with particles of digesta that have been reduced in size so that they can pass through the orifice to the omasum. This material is then subjected to digestion by the host in the remainder of the digestive tract.

During passage through the omasum, digesta is concentrated by water absorption, and further absorption of the volatile fatty acids occurs. The omasum is structurally well suited for this function. The inner surface is thrown into leaflike folds over which the digesta passes on its way to the abomasum. This process of concentration also aids abomasal digestion, the near equivalent of nonruminant gastric digestion, because it reduces water loading of the acid environment that is required for efficient peptic proteolysis. A reduced volume of digesta in the abomasum means that less acid must be secreted to achieve adequate reduction in pH.

Although the abomasal contents still contain substantial amounts of nonsoluble carbohydrates, such as cellulose and lignin, they are not dissimilar to the gastric contents of monogastric animals. The physiologic mechanisms underlying the digestive processes occurring beyond the stomach are essentially the same for ruminants and nonruminants. However, the nonruminant herbivores have a highly developed intestinal and cecal fermentation system that may require some specialized control.

6.7 • Accessory Digestive Organs

Intestinal digestion depends on precise control of the pH of the luminal contents, the secretions of the intestinal mucosa, and most important, secretions of accessory digestive organs. Refer to the introductory description of the abdominal viscera in Chapter 1 for the location of the gallbladder and pancreas in relation to the liver, stomach, and small intestine. These relations are shown schematically in Figure 6–19.

The small intestine is made up of three portions. The first, beginning at the pylorus and extending to form a loop enclosing the pancreas on its mesentery, is the *duodenum*. The second portion is the *jejunum*. The terminal segment is the *ileum*. The general organization of the intestine can be deduced from an examination of Figure 1–17, which shows the relationship between the suspensory ligament, the outer longitudinal muscle layer, an inner circular layer, and an internal mucosal lining. The gut is suspended from the abdominal wall on a mesothelium called the *mesentery*. This is covered on both sides with *peritoneum* and carries nerves, blood vessels, and lymphatics to and from the gut.

The liver and pancreas are the most important accessory organs of digestion. Their secretions are added to the contents of the small intestine under controls that originate from the gut wall. Chyme entering the duodenum, after passage through the pylorus, is quite acidic; it is

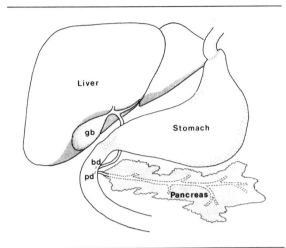

Figure 6–19. Accessory digestive organs. This diagram shows the relative locations of the liver, stomach, gall bladder, and pancreas. The gall bladder (gb) lies on the visceral surface of the liver where it collects hepatic bile. Upon contraction of the gall bladder, bile is delivered through a duct (bd) into the upper portion of the duodenum. The duct may be common with the duct draining the exocrine portion of the pancreas (pd). The ducts may also be separate, as shown here.

quickly neutralized and made slightly alkaline to suit the pH optima of the enzymes that function in the intestine. Base is added by way of bile, derived from the liver, along with the serous secretions of the pancreas.

Bile

Bile is a secretory product of the liver that collects in a series of *canaliculi,* or channels within the tissue of the liver. These come together before they exit from the body of the liver, and in some species they supply the hepatic secretion to a secondary storage and processing organ called the *gallbladder.* Most mammals possess gallbladders, but the horse, rat, and deer do not. In the gallbladder the biliary secretions are concentrated by reabsorption of water. Limited fur-

ther secretion of constituents may also occur. In species that lack gallbladders, the ducts from the liver lead directly into a *bile duct* that empties into the duodenum. Bile ducts may or may not fuse with pancreatic ducts before reaching the intestine. In either situation the secretions are added to the intestinal contents in the proximal portion of the duodenum.

There are no enzymes in bile. The major constituents are bile *salts,* bile *acids,* and bile *pigments.* The salts are a combination of organic and inorganic acids with attendant alkali metal cations, mainly Na^+. The liver is the principal organ of detoxification in the body and most of this activity is achieved by conjugating toxins and certain metabolic wastes with carriers such as glucuronic acid. These detoxified glucuronide derivatives have high water solubility and they pass into the bile.

The major bile salts are metabolites of cholesterol and, along with lysolecithin, they serve as important *emulsifying* or detergent agents within the small intestine. Lysolecithin is the product of phospholipase action on lecithin and so is the phospholipid that has lost one fatty acid. These emulsifying agents disperse fat droplets into minute microdroplets, called micelles, and in so doing the surface area per unit volume of the "particle" is enormously increased. Detergents are specialized surface-active molecules. They confer a *hydrophilic coat* to an otherwise *hydrophobic droplet.* In the earlier description of surface tension, emphasis was placed on the surfaces between liquid and air. Similar forces operate on surfaces between hydrophobic substances and aqueous solutions. The enzymes that hydrolyze the lipids in the digesta act in the aqueous phase, or exclusively at the surface of the lipid droplets. The dietary lipids are therefore broken down into a fine emulsion of large total surface area, and the bile components confer on them a hydrophilic shell to permit access for the lipases that hydrolyze the lipids.

Extremely small droplets of dietary lipid, converted into micelles as described, may be absorbed from the intestinal lumen with only partial prior hydrolysis, as described in Section 6.8.

The other major constituent of bile is the pigmented material, or bile pigments. The origin and fate of these are described in Box 6–4.

Substances that stimulate hepatic secretion of bile are called *choleretics*. The most potent choleretic stimulus is the presence, in the cells of the liver, of the bile constituents themselves. It is likely that the enterohepatic circulation, with the continued delivery of reabsorbed bile components back to the liver, is the most efficient way of providing a constant stimulus to the liver. This would ensure continued secretion of bile and therefore an ongoing means of providing elimination of detoxified substances into the digestive tract.

Not all bile constituents that reach the gut lumen are reabsorbed, so efficient elimination of these substances can occur. On the other hand, some bile constituents may be efficiently conserved by this mechanism for reuse. The detergents and emulsifying constituents are needed in the gut lumen only until the fats and oils have been digested and absorbed, so it may be quite appropriate to recover these digestive aids and recycle them for future use.

The gallbladder serves as a reservoir and acts to concentrate hepatic bile about tenfold. Bile is delivered to the intestine only when it is needed, and this is of importance in minimizing reflux of potentially damaging detergents back into the stomach. Reference was made earlier to the effect of these components on the integrity of the gastric mucosal barrier (see Section 6.4).

Agents that cause contraction of the smooth muscle of the gallbladder, and cause ejection of gallbladder bile through the bile duct and into the duodenum, are called *cholecystagogues*. The most important stimuli for gallbladder contraction are PZ-CCK and cholinergic vagal influences. The word cholecystokinin actually means stimulator *(kinin)* of the gall *(chole)* bladder *(cyst)*.

The intestinal hormone PZ-CCK is a peptide that is structurally related to glucagon. PZ-CCK is the likely endocrine mediator of the reflex control by the intestine over gastric function. The hormone is secreted in response to the presence of fats in the duodenum and, by delivering bile into the lumen, it serves to aid in fat digestion. Further emptying of the stomach is prevented by the action on gastric motility so that duodenal

---

Box 6–4   Bile Pigments

The bile pigments are degradation products of *heme,* the iron-containing nonpeptide moiety of hemoglobin, and many oxidative enzymes in the body. These pigments are toxic if accumulated in the body and they cause whole-body coloration, as in *jaundice.* Impaired liver function, such as in *hepatitis,* is often signalled by specific symptoms that include jaundice. Two major heme derivatives are *biliverdin* and *bilirubin.* The former is greenish in color *(-verdin)* and the latter is reddish *(-rubin).* Together, they give rise to the green-brown color of bile and ultimately the brownish color of feces.

Bile components may be reabsorbed from the intestines into the portal blood system, which drains the digestive tract, and they are carried back to the liver for extraction and resecretion. This is called the *enterohepatic circulation.* There is a net loss of constituents in each cycle, probably of the order of 10% to 15%, and this seemingly futile cycling suggests that some advantage must accrue from it, or it is very inefficient indeed. Intestinal conversion of the primary pigments to *urobilinogen,* followed by partial reabsorption, produces the pigment that is excreted in urine, giving the latter its characteristic color.

digestive mechanisms are not overwhelmed. Another function of PZ-CCK will be noted in relation to pancreatic function in the next section of this chapter. The importance of the vagal component of gallbladder contraction is not well known, although it is quite consistent with the general pattern of overlap in control of the gut that is provided by neural and endocrine mechanisms.

Pancreatic Secretions

The other major accessory digestive organ is the pancreas, a mixed function tissue that is located in the mesentery, usually in the first loop of the duodenum. The pancreas is both an important endocrine gland and an exocrine secretory gland. Pancreatic juice passes to the small intestine through one or more pancreatic ducts. As noted earlier, in some species these ducts fuse with the bile duct before they reach the intestinal lumen.

The exocrine function of the pancreas is controlled by at least two hormones produced by the duodenal mucosa. Secretin, the original hormone to be named, produces a copious serous secretion from the pancreas. It is essentially a dilute solution of sodium bicarbonate that is slightly alkaline (pH 8 to 8.3). The addition of pancreatic enzymes to this dilute salt solution results from either vagal secretomotor innervation or, more important, as a result of the action of PZ-CCK.

A diverse array of pancreatic enzymes is known, and these enzymes are responsible for the final hydrolytic processing of the digesta into units capable of being absorbed. Each of the three major nutrient classes—carbohydrates, lipids, and proteins—are processed. Many minor constituents are hydrolyzed for absorption exclusively by the pancreatic enzymes. All of these enzymes have pH optima at or above neutrality. Such conditions are provided by the alkaline secretions of the pancreas and to a lesser degree by the bile. Thus, the serous secretions controlled by secretin neutralize and buffer the pH, while the enzymic component, controlled by PZ-CCK, is responsible for the hydrolytic activity. The enzymes and their actions are described systematically in the next section. In addition, some hydrolytic changes, for example the cleavage of triglycerides to glycerol and free fatty acids, may occur spontaneously at a pH of 8 or above. This is because the ester bonds are labile in alkali, and it is the basis for the manufacturing of soaps from animal or plant lipids by heating them with alkali.

6.8 • Intestinal Digestion and Absorption

Intestinal Digestion

Intestinal digestion starts with the entry of chyme into the duodenum and terminates with expulsion of residuum during defecation. With the exception of defecation, all processes are involuntary, but they depend on a combination of neural and endocrine controls. The major processes are chemical reduction of the digesta to the final forms suited for absorption, the continued propulsion of digesta along the tract, and the absorptive process itself. The main emphasis of the first portion of this section is on the chemical mechanisms resulting in the final digestive products. The latter portion will describe the absorptive mechanisms.

Lipid Digestion

Pancreatic lipase preferentially hydrolyzes triglycerides at the 1 or 3 position of the glycerol molecule. Phospholipids may also be hydrolyzed by lipase, but only the fatty acid at the 1 carbon position is removed. The products are free fatty acids, 2-monoglycerides, and 2-lysolecithin, respectively. It was noted earlier that certain bile constituents act as emulsifying agents; they are far more effective in the presence of 2-monoglycerides and lysolecithin. It is rather intriguing that the products of lipid digestion are themselves able to aid further lipid digestion. Lipid digestion presents some special problems because of the hydrophobic character of the substrates and products. The materials aggregate as micelles, the structure of which is shown in Figure 6–20.

Bile acids and monoglycerides spontaneously form micelles within the intestinal lumen. The micelles then take up free fatty acids that have been liberated by lipases from lipids in the digesta. This is an example of "like dissolves in like." The micelles that are in proximity to the mucosal lining of the intestine yield the fatty acids and monoglycerides for absorption. Any products of lipid digestion that are adequately water soluble need not use the micelle transporting mechanism just described.

Carbohydrate Digestion

Pancreatic amylases reduce polymeric carbohydrates, such as starch and glycogen, into much smaller, or oligomeric, portions. In many cases digestion will proceed completely through to disaccharide units, the most common of which is maltose, or glucosyl-glucose. It should be recalled that the ether linkages in cellulose and related carbohydrates with $\beta_{[1-4]}$ glycosidic bonds cannot be hydrolyzed by amylases. Amylase hydrolysis is effective only on polymers such as

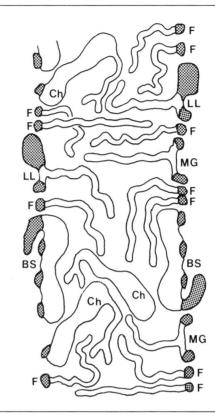

Figure 6–20. Organization of micelles. Micelles form by the association of an outer coat of bile salts (BS) with the polar regions of other amphipatic molecules, particularly lysolecithin (LL) and 2'-monoglycerides (MG), enclosing a lipid interior in which free fatty acids (F) and cholesterol (Ch) are found in abundance. The polar or hydrophilic regions (shaded) face outward to contact the aqueous phase of the intestinal contents. The inner, or hydrophobic, region provides the environment suited for dissolving other lipid products of digestion.

animal-derived glycogen and plant-derived starch, and their partially digested products.

Final hydrolysis to monosaccharides, by enzymes of the intestinal mucosa or those in the intestinal juice, precedes absorption. The intestinal juice, or *succus entericus,* is a secretory product of the intestinal mucosa itself. It contains a number of enzymes and mucus. The epithelial lining of the intestine is very dynamic and cells are continually shed into the lumen; they are also continually replenished so that the integrity of the epithelial lining is preserved. This shedding of epithelial cells continues throughout life and is known as *desquamation*. The process is energetically very expensive to the animal, second only to the energy cost of the Na^+-K^+-ATPase pump, that has been noted before.

Some of the enzymes may be liberated from these cells when the latter break down after being released from the intestinal wall. Of the numerous enzymes present, of great importance for digestion of the major classes of nutrients would be those providing the final hydrolysis of disaccharides and the small peptides. *Maltase* hydrolyzes maltose (glucose · glucose); *lactase* hydrolyzes lactose, or milk sugar (galactose · glucose); *sucrase* hydrolyzes sucrose (glucose · fructose); and so forth.

Protein Digestion

Pancreatic juice contains an inactive precursor, or zymogen, of the powerful proteolytic enzyme, *trypsin*. The zymogen is trypsinogen, and its activation is due to action of *enterokinase*, an enzyme secreted by the intestinal mucosal glands. Trypsin hydrolyzes peptide bonds adjacent to the basic amino acids, lysine and arginine, to produce small peptide products. Other peptidases are present both in pancreatic juice and in other intestinal secretions. These further reduce the oligopeptides to dipeptides and eventually to individual amino acids.

The intestinal juice also contains exopeptidases, which remove terminal amino acids from small peptides, one at a time. For example, carboxypeptidase removes the C-terminal amino acid, exposes a new C-terminal, then releases that, over and over, until the molecule is completely hydrolyzed. Similarly, aminopeptidases remove amino acids, one at a time, from the amino terminal end.

There is some suggestion for an endocrine control of the secretion of intestinal juice by yet another hormonal factor that can be extracted from duodenal mucosa, called *enterocrinin*.

Intestinal Motility

Movements of the wall of the lower alimentary tract serve a number of functions:

- Mechanical mixing of the contents of the gut lumen;

- Transport of digesta down the tract;

- Presentation of soluble nutrients to the absorptive surface.

Most movements involve isotonic muscular activity in the form of lengthening and shortening of the smooth muscle of the gut wall while maintaining a relatively constant tension.

The muscle typically has inherent rhythmicity that is *myogenic*, or arises in the muscle cells themselves independently of any neural control. In addition, a nerve net, the *intrinsic plexus*, is included in much of the gut wall to coordinate cycles of contraction and relaxation at different points along the length of the gut. Finally, there is some overall control exerted by an *extrinsic neural supply*, derived from the autonomic nervous system. As emphasized elsewhere, this neural input is relatively more important in the anterior portions and somewhat less important further along the digestive tract.

There are three distinct types of movement observed in the gut: peristalsis, pendulum movements, and segmental movements.

Peristalsis involves both the circular and longitudinal muscle layers and consists of a propagated sequence of contraction, preceded by a relaxation. These coordinated activities serve to squeeze digesta along the gut. Pendulum movements are rhythmic cycles of shortening and lengthening of the longitudinal muscle layers which provide for mixing of the luminal contents. Additional local mixing is achieved by segmental movements that involve exclusively the circular muscle layer and take the form of phasic constrictions of the wall.

Peristalsis is controlled in large part by the

intrinsic plexuses. One of these, *Auerbach's plexus,* lies between the longitudinal and circular layers of the muscle. The other, *Meissner's plexus,* is located between the circular muscle layer and the mucosa lining the gut lumen. As with many smooth muscle systems, innervation is provided to bundles of cells rather than individual cells, but the latter are coupled electrically by gap junctions and therefore the cells function as an electrical syncytium. Such muscle was described in Chapter 3 as a *single unit* smooth muscle. Because of this arrangement, it is convenient to consider each layer, the longitudinal and circular muscles, as functional effector units rather than as a series of individual cells. The mechanism providing for coordination of contraction and relaxation, as needed to satisfy the definition of peristalsis, is outlined in Box 6–5.

The movement of digesta in the lower gut involves the series of motile sequences described above. Movement between different portions of the whole gut is under control of a series of reflexes. The *gastroileal* and *gastrocolic* reflexes account for the synchronized movement of luminal contents. They are most obvious in very young animals, in which defecation occurs shortly after each feeding. These reflexes ensure that no portion of the tract becomes overloaded, and they serve to synchronize movement of the intestinal contents to gastric events.

Only one phase of the overall postesophageal process is subject to voluntary control, and that is *defecation.* Distension of the rectum reflexly contracts the internal anal sphincter, thereby opening it. The external sphincter, a striated muscle that is tonically contracted, must be relaxed under voluntary control before defecation can occur. Striated muscle cannot be neurally signalled to relax, except by integration at the dendrites of the motor nerves. This vol-

---

Box 6–5   Peristalsis

The longitudinal muscle receives an excitatory cholinergic innervation from Auerbach's plexus (Figure 6–21). Circular muscle receives both excitatory and inhibitory innervations. As noted earlier, smooth muscle can be subjected to inhibitory influences by some neurotransmitters. The inhibitory neurons are arranged so that they release transmitter 1 to 2 cm aborally, or in the direction away from the mouth, to the location of the cell body. The inhibitory effect is achieved by an abrupt increase in membrane potential that renders the smooth muscle cell less excitable, or more refractory to stimulation by agonists.

The prime input stimulus for peristalsis is radial stretch of the intestinal wall caused by a distending effect of the digesta in the lumen. This input activates two descending, or aboral, neural pathways. First, the inhibitory fibers cause focal relaxation 1 to 3 cm ahead of the stretch. This is followed by excitatory discharge causing contraction of the circular layer and then the longitudinal layer. Thus, the whole sequence, which propagates aborally along the gut, consists of relaxation followed by contraction, and propulsion of luminal contents from the contracted into the relaxed segments.

These events involve polysynaptic connections between the afferent neurons from stretch receptors and the effector neurons with their functional effector units of bundles of smooth muscle. This constitutes a reflex, even though all components lie within the gut wall. The receptors and afferent cell bodies lie in Meissner's plexus; the efferents and sites of release of transmitters are associated with Auerbach's plexus.

Figure 6–21. Neural control of peristalsis. This section of the intestinal wall is oriented with the serosal, or peritoneal, surface uppermost and the mucosal surface, lining the lumen, below. Note the opportunity for local reflexes, originating from stretch receptors, to control both the circular and the longitudinal smooth muscle of the gut wall. The influences are projected ahead of the site of stretch; any afferent input supplies an excitatory efferent pathway that simultaneously activates the circular and longitudinal muscle. The two descending neurons, one inhibitory (DIN) and one excitatory (DEN), originated from a site to the left of the stretch receptor shown. The inhibition is projected onto the circular muscle (−) slightly ahead of the excitatory influence (+). (Simplified figure is based on Fig. 1 from Hirst, G.D.S.: Mechanisms of Peristalsis. Brit. Med. Bull. 1979; 35: 263–268.)

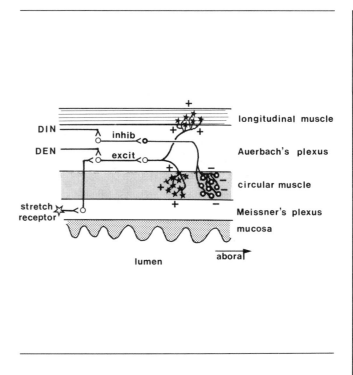

untary act is mediated by descending nerve tracts that impinge on the motor nerves in the spinal column.

The expulsion of rectal contents is achieved by expiration against a closed glottis, contraction of the abdominal muscles, transmission of intraabdominal pressure into the pelvic cavity, and relaxation of the external anal sphincter. In animals, these events are coordinated with elevation of the tail and sometimes with flexion of the spine, which also helps generate intraabdominal pressure.

Absorption of Digestive End Products

Specialized mechanisms are provided in different parts of the alimentary tract for the selective assimilation of nutrients that have been liberated by the digestive process. The major site, though by no means the only one, is the intestinal wall.

Irrespective of where absorption takes place, three major requirements must be satisfied for absorption to proceed:

- Nutrients must be in an appropriate chemical form for transport across epithelial barriers;

- A sufficiently large absorptive surface must be available;

- Sufficient time must be allowed.

Some minor absorption occurs in the buccal cavity if the appropriate chemical form is present in the ingesta. Normally, the contact time before swallowing is insufficient for significant absorption and the absorptive surface is too small for this process to be very efficient. The stomach is usually not an important site of absorption, except in the ruminants where structural modifications, such as the rumen papillae and the leaves of the omasum, provide a very large absorptive surface, and the major fermentation products (volatile fatty acids) are readily absorbed. Ammonia is also absorbed in the gas phase along with methane. In some species, alcohol and glucose can be absorbed across the stomach wall. Most absorption occurs in the small intestine, especially in the terminal portion, the ileum.

Various specialized mechanisms are used to actively absorb the products of digestion. These use metabolic energy to transport solutes against concentration gradients and into the blood circulatory system of the gut. In some cases carrier molecules in the epithelial cell surface membrane may be used as pumps. These carriers discriminate between even closely related chemical structures. For example, the transport of monosaccharides and small organic acids may be quite stereospecific. Active transport has directionality so the absorptive process is also unidirectional, from the gut lumen toward the bloodstream.

Absorptive processes for even the most simple nutrients are subject to a wide array of controlling and permissive factors. For example, glucose absorption requires the presence of several ions including Na^+, K^+, Ca^{2+}, and a minimal level of some vitamins. It is also sensitive to thyroid and adrenal cortex hormones, and can be blocked by structural analogues of glucose. This type of information has been obtained from surgically prepared intestinal loops, isolated from the remainder of the intestines and accessible from outside the abdominal wall via fistulas at either end. Segments of gut can also be studied in vitro by forming sealed sacs of excised intestine, or by placing part of the gut wall over a tube, like a dialysis membrane, and examining the movement of radioactively labeled molecules across this tissue barrier.

The most complicated absorptive mechanism involves pinocytosis and it is used to absorb macromolecules such as the globulin antibodies in new-born ruminants. Pinocytosis involves invagination of the lumen surface membrane and the pinching off, into the cell cytoplasm, of vesicles containing material from the gut lumen. Once in the cell, the intact droplet may move across the cell to the surface adjacent to the capillaries and then release its contents into the interstitial space. Alternatively, the droplet may be broken down within the epithelial cell so that its contents enter the solution phase of the cytoplasm. Final movement may then occur across the opposite membrane adjacent to the capillary.

Most soluble components are absorbed into blood capillaries in the gut wall. The less soluble components absorbed from the digestive tract move into the lymphatic system. Each intestinal villus is supplied with a blind-ended capillary-like structure termed a lacteal. A very leaky basement membrane supporting the endothelial cells allows facile movement of tissue fluid into the lacteal vessels and from there into the lymph vessels. Lymphatic absorption is particularly important for lipids. Lipids, after partial or complete hydrolysis to fatty acids and monoglycerides in the gut lumen, are taken up from the micelles by the intestinal epithelium. Within the mucosal cells, they are recombined as triglycerides and packaged with cholesterol and phospholipids to form chylomicra. The chylomicra are released from the mucosal cells and taken up by the lymphatics. Although they are particulate and not solutes, the chylomicra present no problems to the circulatory system, access to which is gained by the lymph vessels draining into the jugular vein and subclavian vein in the upper thorax.

Lymph vessels are loaded with chylomicra some hours after an animal is fed lipid such as a large cream meal, and with suitable lighting, the lipid droplets can be seen in the blood vessels in the eye.

The lymphatic system is present in most tissues of the body, and its function in absorption from the gut is a mere specialization of the overall system. As noted briefly in Chapter 5, lymph moves in much the same way as venous blood. In the villi, some pumping of lymph occurs by the action of smooth muscle cells within the villus. These are supposedly under the control of an intestinal hormone called villikinin. Movement in the large lymph vessels, which are equipped with flaplike valves, is due to abdominal and thoracic pumping during respiratory activity. It will be recalled that negative thoracic pressure is transmitted to vessels such as the great veins and lymph ducts with each inspiration. This provides a "drawing" force for fluids such as blood and lymph contained within the vessels. A key factor determining lymph flow is the actual rate of formation of the lymph. This will be described in some detail in the next section.

The major site for absorption of nutrients is in the small intestine, although the stomach is particularly important in ruminants. In monogastrics (such as hamsters) that have large ceca, absorption of volatile fatty acids may occur in the large intestine, and other products of fermentation such as CO_2 and methane may be absorbed or passed out of the tract in the gas phase as *flatus*. Water absorption occurs in the omasum, ileum, and colon.

Fecal residues comprise undigested fiber, debris from desquamated or sloughed-off intestinal epithelium, some excreted products derived from bile (e.g., pigments), intestinal bacteria, and mucus.

6.9 • The Enterohepatic Catchment

The blood vascular system of the digestive tract, along with a rich lymphatic drainage system, is particularly important because of its involvement in absorptive mechanisms. The blood system is atypical when compared to the general statements made in Chapter 5 because venous blood, collected up from the digestive tract, is carried to the liver before being returned to the right side of the heart. In this section the arterial, venous, and lymphatic systems of the gut and liver are described in some detail.

Arterial System

The major arteries supplying the digestive tract branch off from the *abdominal aorta* in the lumbar region (Figure 6–22). Immediately upon exiting from the thorax through the dorsal limit of the diaphragm (see Figure 1–41), the *celiac artery* arises. This major vessel is about 10 cm long in cattle and it branches further to give rise to the *hepatic artery*, the left and right *ruminal arteries*, the *omasoabomasal artery*, and the *splenic artery*. The hepatic artery supplies the liver; the other vessels are also named on the basis of the structures they supply.

Caudal to the site of origin of the celiac artery, the next major vessel is the *anterior mesenteric artery*. This vessel branches to supply most of the intestines. There are several intermediate-sized arteries that branch further and finally run as small vessels within the mesentery supporting the digestive tract.

After the renal arteries leave the aorta, the *posterior mesenteric artery* branches off to supply the terminal portion of the large intestine and the rectum.

Venous System

With the exception of the venous drainage from the wall of the rectum, blood from all of the gut beyond the esophagus is collected into the *portal vein* for transport to the liver. The portal vein

Figure 6–22. Visceral blood circulation. The major arterial supplies (shaded) and the tributaries of venous drainage from the gut are depicted in this schematic diagram. The abdominal aorta (aa) supplies three major branches: celiac (c), anterior mesenteric (a), and posterior mesenteric (p) arteries. The celiac then gives rise to lesser branches: hepatic (h), from which the gall bladder (G) and pancreas (P) are supplied; the splenic (s), supplying the spleen (Sp); right ruminal (rr), supplying the majority of the reticulo-rumen (Re-Ru); and the left ruminal (lr) and omasal-abomasal (oa), supplying the remainder of the stomach. The intestines are supplied primarily by the anterior mesenteric artery with a lesser contribution by the posterior mesenteric artery. With the exception of a very minor portion of the venous effluent from the rectum passing directly to the vena cava, all venous drainage collects into the portal vein (pv) to be delivered to the liver before finally joining the vena cava (vc) through the hepatic veins (hv). Most portal blood is obtained from the mesenteric vein (m); the remainder is collected from the gastrosplenic vein (gs).

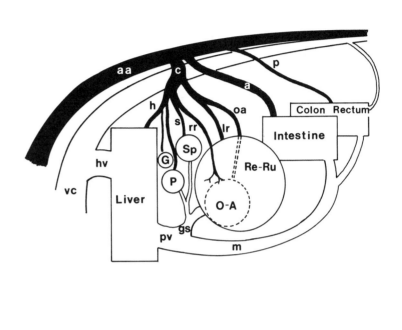

collects from two main tributaries, the *gastric vein* and the *mesenteric vein*. The gastric vein in turn collects blood from the rumen and other stomach structures, the spleen, and the pancreas. A small portion of duodenal venous flow also collects into the gastric vein. The remainder of the intestine drains into the mesenteric vein. The combined drainage from the digestive tract reaches the liver via the portal vein. The flow of blood is substantial, particularly after feeding, and represents about 25% to 30% of cardiac output.

The anatomic arrangement whereby blood collected from the gut is necessarily delivered to the liver before gaining access to the general circulation has important nutritive and metabolic consequences. The liver is by far the most important organ in the body for metabolic transformations, as will be detailed in Chapter 7. The portal system ensures that the liver has first opportunity to take up nutrients that are absorbed directly into the bloodstream. Equally significant is the collection of pancreatic venous blood via the gastric veins and its delivery to the liver through the portal vein. The pancreatic hormones insulin and glucagon have their most important actions on the liver. More will be said of these roles in the next chapter.

The liver receives blood from two distinct sources. The hepatic artery supplies oxygenated blood under central arterial pressure in the typical fashion for the perfusion of any tissue. The portal blood has already perfused one set of capillaries and has the general properties of venous blood when it reaches the liver. It is atypical of most venous blood in that it contains high concentrations of nutrients, and because of water absorbed from the gut, it is somewhat diluted.

The two sources of blood reaching the liver can be handled differently because of the internal structure of the liver, but there is a single effluent from the liver. The *hepatic veins*, several in number, drain into the abdominal vena cava as the latter passes over the dorsal surface of the liver, just before it enters the thorax. The veins are not evident as distinct structures outside of the liver.

Lymphatic System

Two major lymphatic vessels, one arising from the *gastric lymph gland* and the other from the *intestinal lymph gland*, come together within the abdominal cavity as the *intestinal lymph trunk.* This, along with the *lumbar lymphatic trunk,* runs into the *cisterna chyli,* located between the aorta and the dorsal abdominal wall in the vicinity of the last thoracic vertebra. Output from this organ travels by way of the *thoracic duct,* across the thorax, to drain into the anterior vena cava near the heart.

The origins of the lymphatics in the gut wall are the lacteals in the intestinal wall. These blind-ended endothelial structures pick up extracellular fluids along with chylomicra produced by the mucosal lining and collect into small lymphatics lying within the thickness of the mesentery. The lymphatics pass through a series of progressively larger lymph glands and eventually reach the major abdominal glands before emptying into the trunk lymphatics.

In contrast to the fate of blood collected from the gut, which must pass through the liver, the lymph is delivered directly into the general venous circulation without passing through the liver.

The formation of lymph in the gut wall is in part quite typical of lymph formation in any tissue, and in part quite different. As noted in connection with capillary function in Chapter 5, there is usually net loss of fluid from blood capillaries into the tissues, and this tissue fluid is, in approximation, an ultrafiltrate of serum. The principal factors influencing accumulation of tissue fluid are the Starling filtration forces, described in Chapter 5. The major variable, which changes in relation to events within the gut, is perfusion rate, because of the marked increases in blood flow that occur during digestion. In addition, the metabolic activity associated with motility and energy-consuming processes, such as secretion of digestive juice and active transport in absorption, all favor fluid transfer into the tissues from the capillaries. This activity causes hypoxemia and hypercapia, and both are potent contributory factors for capillary leakage. They therefore serve to promote lymph formation.

Much of the tissue fluid in parts of the gut obtains its volume from absorbed water. Water may pass through to the venous end of the capillaries and be carried away into the portal blood, or it may be collected into the lymphatics. Because the water will reduce colloid osmotic pressure in the capillaries, there is yet another driving force for continued formation of lymph.

Summary of Enterohepatic Catchment

- The circulatory mechanisms described in this section—the portal blood system and the abdominal lymphatic system—are the means by which absorbed nutrients are delivered to the body's tissues.

- Nutrients that are transported in the portal blood are first delivered to the liver for initial processing. The liver is provided with a direct arterial blood supply in addition to the portal blood.

- Digestive end products that are harvested by the lymphatics—and lipids are the most significant of these—bypass the liver and enter the general circulation.

6.10 • Digestion in the Chicken

The digestive mechanism in the chicken is considerably simpler than that for omnivorous and especially herbivorous mammals. The milieu within the gut tends to be predominantly acid at all locations. I will describe briefly the structure of the gut, which differs from that of mammals, before considering the functional aspects.

Anatomy

The overall length of the digestive tract is relatively short (expressed as a multiple of body length) when compared to the mammalian forms. The beak encloses a beak cavity that communicates with the sublingual cavity, analogous to the buccal cavity. Birds lack teeth but certain species are capable of mechanically reducing ingesta by virtue of sharp edges on the beak. In other species, the beak is merely prehensile. The tongue of the chicken is essentially inflexible and incapable of propagated contraction from front to rear as the first step toward swallowing as in mammals. In addition, the beak and nasal cavities are incompletely separated, there is no hard palate nor are there cheek muscles.

Salivary glands occur both in paired and single form and secrete an acid mucus into the sublingual cavity. Recall that mammalian saliva is either mucous or serous, the latter being a dilute buffer solution of slightly alkaline reaction.

The esophagus is a multilayered, striated muscle tube possessing a mucus-secreting epithelium. Distally, in the thoracic region and slightly offset to the right of the median plane, the esophagus is dilated into the *crop* (Figure 6–23), a storage and secretory organ that is filled with ingesta after the stomach is loaded. The stomach has two distinct compartments. Anteriorly, the *proventriculus,* which is thin-walled and highly glandular, secretes gastric juice consisting of hydrochloric acid and enzymes. The *ventriculus (gizzard)* is thick-walled, muscular, and keratinized. Its limited secretory function is mainly of mucus and is presumably protective to the epithelium. In its most distal area, called the *pylorus* as in mammals, the lining possesses villous folds with pyloric glands. There is no pyloric sphincter between the gizzard and the duodenum.

The intestine differs from that of mammals in the virtual lack of a colon (or large intestine). The duodenum loops to enclose multiple lobes of pancreatic tissue on the mesentery, and two pancreatic ducts and one bile duct enter the duodenum near the jejunum. The ileum terminates in a very short segment of colon from which two

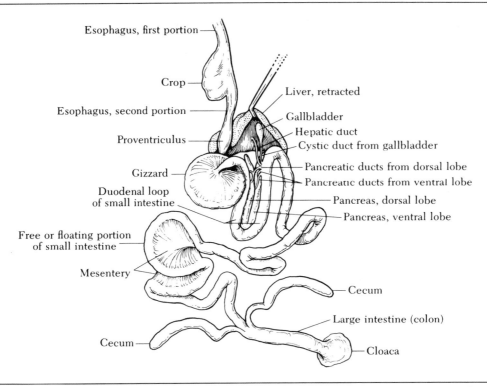

Figure 6–23. *Digestive tract of the chicken.* The gut of the chicken is shown here, partially dissected from its in situ organization to clarify the sequential relations along its length. (Reprinted by permission of the publisher. From Sturkie, P.D.: *Avian Physiology*, 2nd edition, Ithaca, NY: Cornell University Press, 1965.)

ceca arise, partially isolated by cecal valves. Many birds possess, in the distal portion of the small intestine, a lymphoid structure called Meckel's diverticulum, a remnant of the stalk of the yolk sac from embryonic life. The short rectum passes to the cloacal structure, consisting of three parts, each separated by annular folds. The proximal portion is a dilated ampulla, and the middle portion is glandular with the uretal openings, the vasa deferentia of the male reproductive tract (see Section 10.7) and the slit-like opening of the reproductive tract in females (Section 10.7). The distal portion is noteworthy because a lymphoid tissue unique to birds (the *Bursa of Fabricius*) is located dorsally. Finally, the cloaca leads to the anus *(vent)*, consisting of two sphincters, an inner smooth muscle, and outer striated muscle.

The liver exists as two lobes connected by an isthmus. The right lobe possesses a gallbladder supplied by a bile duct from the hepatic tissue. On the left side, the bile duct bypasses the gallbladder and directly supplies the intestine. Chicken bile is weakly acidic and possesses some amylolytic activity. Pancreatic juice is similar to that of mammals but is less basic. It was noted earlier that digestion in the chicken occurs without the distinctly alkaline intestinal phase characteristic of mammals.

Digestive Mechanisms

Ingesta entering the beak, the prehensile structure, and sublingual cavities is, in effect, crammed back toward the pharynx because there is little opportunity for any propagated muscular effort within these most proximal cavities. Passage down the esophagus is by slow peristalsis. Water intake poses special problems because the nasal passages are always open and there are no cheek muscles to create a vacuum for sucking. Drinking is achieved by scooping up water in the beak then elevating the head so the liquid simply flows by gravity into the esophagus.

During feeding the proventriculus and gizzard are first filled, then the crop is used to hold additional ingesta. Vagomotor controls regulate emptying of the crop contents into the stomach. Secretory function has both a cephalic and gastric component (as described for mammals in Section 6.4). The most important specialization stems from the powerful muscular contractions of the gizzard, which provide a crushing and grinding action on the gastric contents. When the tract is dissected, gritty mineral material is often found in the gizzard. Domestic birds, especially layers, are supplied with grit such as crushed shells and limestone as part of the diet. The strongly acidic conditions favor solubilization of calcium so much of the mineral residue is material other than calcium salts.

The ceca provide for microbial digestion of fiber and serve as a secondary site of absorption. The major location of absorption of digested nutrients is the epithelium of the ileum. The rectum has some capacity for water absorption. Fecal material is brownish in color, but is voided as a mixture with the whitish uric acid crystals from urinary excretion.

6.11 • Exercises

1. List four functions of saliva.

_____

_____

_____

_____

2. Identify the hormone that is most important in the control of the following digestive functions:

   Delivery of bile from the gallbladder.

   Secretion of serous pancreatic juice.

   Stimulation of gastric secretion.

   Addition of enzymes to pancreatic juice.

3. Which of the hormones identified in question 2 are produced by the duodenal mucosa?

_____   _____

What is the source of the other peptide?

_____

4. How many functions of the stomach can you list?

_____   _____

_____   _____

_____   _____

_____   _____

5. Sketch and label the general structures of a simple monogastric digestive tract. Locate the pancreas and gallbladder.

6. What single word describes the most important physicochemical change, resulting from an interaction between dietary fats and bile components, that aids lipid digestion?

_____

Where does this take place?

_____

What function is served by this modification?

_____

7. Name the most important volatile fatty acids

_____   _____   _____

8. Be sure to have a comprehensive and detailed understanding of the operation of at least one reflex that serves to aid digestive processes. You should understand the nature of the stimulus, the site of reception, the afferent and efferent pathways, the site of integration, the target, and the form of the response.

Metabolism

7

7.1 • Gross Energetics and Metabolism

Phases of Metabolism

Metabolism consists of two general phases, *catabolism* and *anabolism*. Catabolism involves the breakdown of substances toward their end products, usually with the release of energy that either is used immediately in other biochemical reactions, is stored, or is dissipated as heat (Figure 7–1). Heat production is not always wasteful. In Chapter 9 this subject will be developed in relation to themoregulatory mechanisms for homeotherms, animals that maintain relatively constant core temperatures. Anabolism involves the building of substances from different or less complex precursors into products that are more complex. This usually consumes energy, and the

stored products may be important as energy reserves, as in the case of fat stores in adipose tissue.

Many biochemical reactions or processes are reversible. The direction of the reaction depends on the relative concentrations of reacting substances, their energy relationships, and pH. If there are strong similarities between the precursor and product and if their energy levels are similar, reactions are often reversible. An example of a reversible reaction is the transfer of a high-energy phosphate group between adenosine triphosphate (ATP) and creatine in the case of muscle (see Chapter 3). Thus, different directions of the same reaction pathway can occur, namely formation or breakdown of creatine phosphate, though not concurrently. However, if the energy level and the reaction product are

Figure 7–1. Phases of metabolism. Nutrients entering the substrate pool are subjected to transformations that may be regarded as being anabolic or catabolic. The former lead to biosynthesis and a building up of chemical complexity, whereas catabolism is usually degradative and yields energy. Note, however, that some of the energy carriers are subsequently used for anabolic events.

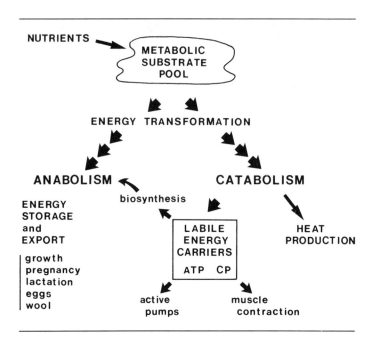

markedly different from their precursors, the reaction is often irreversible; then, in many cases a series of reactions is needed to bypass an energy-obstructed step.

Overall, the metabolic reactions of cells are the manifestations of life itself, and the basis for other vital phenomena such as reproduction, growth, and sensitivity to the environment. By far the largest part of intermediary metabolism goes toward making feed energy and products of digestion available to the body's cells. Metabolic cellular reactions are also the basis for the dynamic state of the body's constituents. The idea that body components are continually changing, some forming and some breaking down, was proposed by Schoenheimer in the early 1940s. Schoenheimer's model emphasized that nothing is static and that there is constant turnover and replacement of cellular components. Today, 40 years later, we take for granted the dynamic state of the body.

All of the energy-producing foods such as carbohydrates, fats, and proteins can be altered chemically. If they are oxidized and transformed to CO_2, H_2O, and other oxides, they can be made to release their energy. The energy is not released rapidly as in combustion because the desirable output of energy in the body is not only heat energy but the energy that drives muscular contraction, the secretion of glandular products, low-level chemical reactions, and maintenance of resting potentials in nerves, among other vital processes. The variety of biochemical mechanisms available to provide this gradual and controlled release of energy is largely beyond the scope of this introduction. Indeed, description of the products of digestion as energy sources and the useful forms of energy carriers within animals will be deferred until a more general overview of energetics has been considered.

Gross Energetics and Calorimetry

Energy has a very precise meaning in the physical sciences: it is the capacity for performing work. Although it is conceptually easier for biologists to grasp the notion of energy as expressed in *heating units* or *calories* (Box 7–1), in current usage energy is expressed in the formal units of *joules* (1 joule is the work done by a force of 1 newton acting over a distance of 1 meter; $m^2 \cdot kg \cdot sec^{-2}$). The various units of energy, and there are many of them, are readily interconverted (e.g., 1 cal = 4.187 joules [J] = 0.004 British Thermal Units [BTU]).

We glibly say that animals consume energy and use it to maintain themselves and to perform productive functions such as lactation, growth, reproduction, work (as in draft animals), and so on. Of course we understand that animals consume feedstuffs, not energy per se, and that digestive mechanisms liberate molecules that are more amenable to biochemical oxidation for the controlled release of energy in the animal. Some of the feed is indigestible and so cannot be assimilated by the animal. Of course, the digestibility varies with both the chemical nature of the feed component and the species of animal that consumes it. The age of the animal may be yet another source of variation, especially in ruminants, where the digestive tract is functionally quite different in young and adult animals.

The gross or total potential energy content of an oxidizable material is more readily determined than is its precise chemical nature. If a known quantity or mass of material is completely combusted in an oxygen atmosphere and the liberated heat is quantified, then the caloric content of that material can be determined. This methodology is called *calorimetry*, or measurement of energy. Standardized equipment and methods are widely used to *destructively* determine the energy content of feeds, human foods, animal products such as meat and milk, whole animal carcasses, feces, urine, etc. Other forms of calorimetry that are nondestructive are used to directly or indirectly measure heat production by living animals. These will be described later in relation to metabolism.

Ingested "energy" is measured by determining the energy content of the feed ration and the quantity of the ration that is consumed. Suitable precautions are taken to correct such measurements for errors due to feed spillage, selectivity in ingestion of nonhomogeneous diets, and the like when conducting what nutritionists call "feeding trials." The possible fates of the gross energy intake are outlined in Figure 7–2 and will be briefly described here. At least a portion of the ingested fibrous feed will not be digested by the animal and so will contribute to the energy content of the feces. The terms *digestible energy* and *digestibility* (the latter expressed as a fraction or percentage) are used as descriptors of a given feedstuff. The measurements are usually expressed on the basis of per-day consumption, in this case of *digestible energy*, though the determinations are usually made over 7 or more days, particularly in animals that have lengthy digestion times. Thus, the daily consumption of total energy minus the energy content of the feces is referred to as *apparent digestible energy*. The "apparent" is included because a portion of the energy content of feces arises from desquamated intestinal mucosa cells (see Chapter 6) and var-

---

Box 7–1   The Caloric System of Energy Units

The mass of data already obtained for domestic animals, feedstuffs, specific biochemical substances and reactions, and so forth was, in the past, presented in caloric units. A calorie is the amount of energy required to increase the temperature of 1 gm of water from 14.5 C to 15.5 C at a pressure of 1 atmosphere. The calorie should not be confused with the *kilocalorie* (kcal), which is 1,000 calories. Also important in animal energetics is the even larger *megacalorie* (Mcal = 1,000,000 calories).

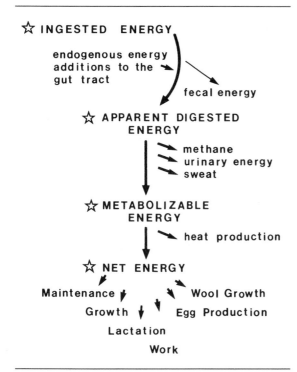

☆ INGESTED ENERGY

endogenous energy
additions to the
gut tract

fecal energy

☆ APPARENT DIGESTED
ENERGY

methane
urinary energy
sweat

☆ METABOLIZABLE
ENERGY

heat production

☆ NET ENERGY

Maintenance   Wool Growth

Growth   Egg Production

Lactation

Work

Figure 7–2. The processing of nutrient energy. This diagram depicts the fate of ingested energy and the losses that occur in the gut and during metabolism.

ious organic substances secreted or excreted into the intestinal tract. Because of these components, apparent digestible energy is usually a slight underestimate of true digestible energy. The latter may be viewed as the amount of energy that is removed from the ingesta as a result of digestive processes.

The next fraction of interest is *metabolizable energy.* This is the portion of the total energy consumed that is directly available for biochemical oxidation, be it for maintaining the integrity of the animal, for heat generation, or for more obvious productive processes. Metabolizable energy is less than digestible energy (ME~0.8 × DE) because some additional losses beyond those in the feces must be accounted for. Oxidizable substances are lost in the urine of all animals and in the gaseous products of gut fermentation, especially methane, in herbivores and omnivores.

Metabolizable energy is the quantity of energy entering the body in useful form. Metabolizable energy is used to fuel productive processes, to maintain or add to the tissue mass, to enable various forms of work to be performed, and to provide necessary heat to the body. Some of these functions are elaborated below.

The notion of the energy cost of *maintenance* of an animal is a convenient way of lumping together all of the processes that contribute to life support. Obviously, this energy is not directly "recovered" in any tangible product such as milk or eggs, or in activities such as locomotion. The energy cost of maintaining normal gradients of Na^+ and K^+ across the cell membrane, by driving the Na^+-K^+–ATPase pump, is a sizable burden to the animal. The staggering number of erythrocytes produced continuously through the life span and the daily turnover of intestinal mucosal cells are also energetically expensive. The vital life support systems described in Chapter 5 depend critically on energy provision, for example to power the circulation and distribution of blood, to contract the diaphragm, and to drive the active pumps of the kidney tubules. To these can be added the energy cost of assimilating the nutrients themselves—the work of ingestion, mastication, gut wall muscular activity, the generation of digestive secretions, the cost of the absorptive processes, and so on. All of these items, and others not specifically identified, constitute maintenance.

Although it is somewhat unrealistic, it is often stated that maintenance is the energy cost of preserving an adult animal under sedentary conditions without weight loss or gain while it is in a thermoneutral environment. In this situation an animal need not specifically expend energy to maintain its body temperature. Somewhat similar parameters are used in defining *basal metabolic rate*, a term applied particularly to humans. The basal metabolic rate is the energy consumption of a recumbent individual in a quiet, thermoneutral environment, in a postabsorptive state, usually 12 to 16 hours after consuming a meal.

Metabolic rate is usually determined by indirect calorimetry during which the rate of consumption of oxygen is measured and then converted into its energetic equivalent, expressed in joules. This is possible because the amount of oxygen required to completely oxidize the major food components—carbohydrate, fat, and protein—is known. If carbon dioxide production is measured simultaneously with oxygen consumption, the *respiratory quotient* (CO_2 produced divided by O_2 consumed) can be obtained and can be used to determine the approximate nature of the substrates being oxidized. *Direct calorimetry*, or the direct measurement of heat production, in large domestic animals requires elaborate, expensive installations, trained animals, and patient investigators. Few such calorimeters, or metabolism chambers, have been constructed and maintained anywhere in the world.

The final component of the total energy consumed by animals is termed *net energy*. Net energy is used both for maintenance and for productive purposes. It is the energy equivalent of the portion of metabolizable energy that is completely useful to the body for maintenance and production. Because energy transformations are not 100% efficient, heat production necessarily accompanies these activities. The amount of such heat varies with the level of feeding and the nature of the use of assimilated nutrients. For example, heat production is much greater in a dairy cow producing large yields of milk than in the same animal when it is held at maintenance. Two components of this *heat increment* are (1) heat produced as part of fermentation processes in the gut, and (2) heat produced during metabolic transformation, both anabolic and catabolic, of absorbed nutrients.

For convenience, net energy is usually determined indirectly, though all such methods of estimation are standardized to direct calorimetric procedures. For example, the caloric content of milk varies fairly closely with the fat content of the milk, and knowledge of the composition of the milk allows reasonably accurate estimation of its energy content. Similarly, during the fattening phase of animal growth, changes in live weight largely reflect changes in the extent of the fat depots, and these can be converted approximately into energy equivalents. For critical studies, animals would be killed and processed to enable a truly representative sample to be drawn; the samples would then be subjected to calorimetry. Obviously, this can be done only once with a particular animal; comparative slaughter studies are designed so that a sample of the animals is removed before and another sample is removed after the conduct of the study (perhaps a feeding study with a novel ration), and group comparisons of the two samples provide information on the change in carcass or whole body energy deposition. For studies of locomotion, treadmills or standardized traction machines, called *ergometric devices*, provide very accurate direct measures of work performed.

For metabolic and productive processes, it is possible to calculate efficiencies of the use of the energy. The *gross efficiency* is simply the energy content of the product expressed as a fraction, usually a percentage, of the total energy consumed in producing it. The gross efficiencies range from as low as about 10% for fattening a large mature animal to as high as 30% to 35% for growth in young animals such as broiler chickens and for milk production; the higher values apply particularly to smaller animals. Far more useful in assessing the nature of the biologic mechanisms underlying a productive process is the index *net efficiency*. This is the energy content of the product as a fraction of the metabolizable energy used in its production.

7.2 • Energy Sources for Metabolic Reactions

The most useful form of high energy, readily available within biologic molecules, is contained within ATP. ATP is a molecule containing three phosphate groups, the last two of which are connected by high-energy bonds (Figure 7–3). There are approximately 7,400 calories per mole contained within the terminal bond, and loss of this one phosphate group from a mole of ATP yields adenosine diphosphate (ADP) and releases the 7,400 calories of energy. There are, of course, other high-energy compounds such as creatine phosphate. The energy contained within creatine phosphate can be transferred to and from ATP by the reversible reaction:

$$ATP + Creatine \rightleftharpoons ADP + Creatine\ phosphate$$

The synthesis of ATP in most cells is the main function of the mitochondria. Within the mitochondria, the final stages of oxidation of energy carriers occurs and the small portions of energy released during oxidation are incorporated into the synthesis of ATP from ADP:

$$ADP + Phosphate + Energy \rightarrow ATP$$

The reactions leading to ATP synthesis are collectively known as *oxidative phosphorylation*, and water, the oxidation product of hydrogen, is formed as a byproduct. Central to the formation of ATP is the generation of reduced coenzymes by hundreds of individual steps in intermediary metabolism. The coenzymes of interest now are proton carriers, and they are recycled for further use by passing on their hydrogen ions to other carriers within the mitochondria, ultimately providing the hydrogen for water formation and the energy for ATP synthesis.

Figure 7–3. Adenosine triphosphate. ATP is the most important labile energy carrier; the terminal phosphate bond has a very large free energy of hydrolysis. The structure shows the constituent molecular relatives of ATP.

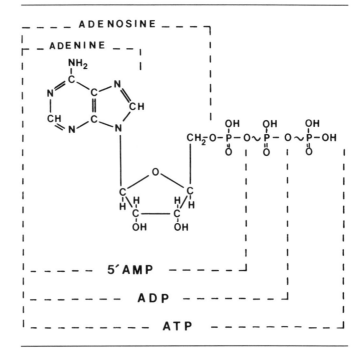

Compounds of widely differing chemical nature such as monosaccharides, amino acids, and fatty acids enter into the pathways of intermediary metabolism through unique initial reactions that will be described in the following sections. Some production of reduced coenzymes, and hence the potential for ATP synthesis, attends the preliminary hydrolytic processing of these various substrates. However, by far the most important steps in the final hydrolytic liberation of energy for ATP synthesis occur in the *tricarboxylic acid* (TCA) cycle, also known as the Krebs cycle. This linked series of reactions involves 2, 4, 5, and 6 carbon compounds and is illustrated in Figure 7–4. In the simplest form of operation, substrate input is by means of acetylcoenzyme A (acetyl-CoA), the coenzyme A–activated form of acetic acid. Acetyl-CoA condenses with the 4 carbon compound, oxaloacetate, to form citric acid, a 6 carbon tricarboxylic acid, hence the name given to the cycle.

The output products from a single cycle of acetyl-CoA processing are:

$$2 \; CO_2 + 1 \; ATP + 1 \; CoA + 8 \; H \quad \text{(as reduced}$$
$$\text{coenzymes—equivalent}$$
$$\text{to another 12 moles of ATP)}$$

The reduced coenzymes serve to carry energy liberated from the initial substrate, in this case acetyl-CoA, into the pathways of oxidative phosphorylation. Water and carbon dioxide are byproducts of the cycle. They leave the cell to join the general body pools of these substances and are eventually eliminated by mechanisms described earlier. The array of compounds constituting the intermediates of the cycle as shown in Figure 7–4 are involved in a multitude of reactions in addition to the direct processing of acetyl-CoA into its products. For example, several of the intermediates are the deaminated forms of certain amino acids and can be transformed to or from those amino acids by addition or removal of an amino group, as will be described in Section 7.3. Citric acid is a secretory product found in a number of body secretions,

Figure 7–4. Inputs and outputs of the tricarboxylic acid (TCA) cycle. This summary diagram of the TCA cycle shows the consumption of the two carbon compound acetyl CoA by condensation with oxaloacetate, to form citrate (a six carbon tricarboxylic compound) with the release of the CoA. During one round of processing, two molecules of carbon dioxide and eight protons—shown as H· to indicate that they are carried away on coenzymes (see later) and one ATP equivalent—are the output products. The eight protons are used in oxidative phosphorylation to generate a maximum of another twelve molecules of ATP.

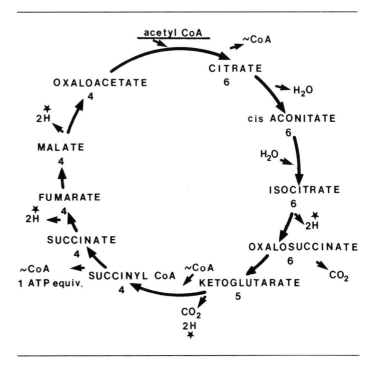

such as milk, and so has an alternate fate to being dehydrated to *cis*-aconitate.

The important fermentation product, propionic acid, noted before to be a key glucogenic substrate in ruminants, is processed by the TCA cycle in the manner indicated in Figure 7–5. This figure also shows that oxaloacetate, in addition to being the condensation acceptor for acetyl-CoA, can leave the intermediate pool of the TCA cycle and be processed to generate glucose. The reactions leading to glucose synthesis from non-

carbohydrate precursors constitute *gluconeogenesis*; this is a particularly important process by which animals obtain glucose and will be described in more detail later in this chapter.

Summary of the TCA Cycle

- The TCA cycle provides for the generation of 12 moles of ATP from the reduced coen-

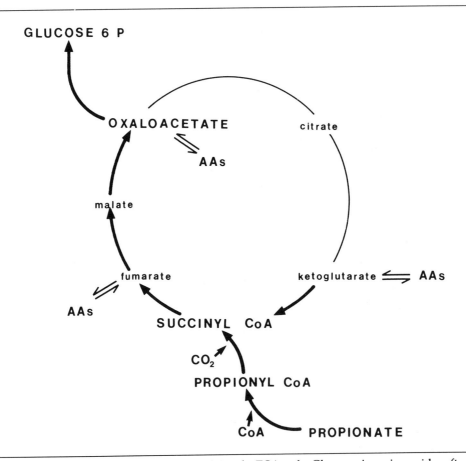

Figure 7–5. Gluconeogenic pathways involving the TCA cycle. Glucogenic amino acids, after deamination, can enter the cycle at several locations. Propionate, obtained from fermentation in the gut, is activated and subsequently carboxylated to form succinyl CoA. The key intermediate is oxaloacetate. If there is a surplus beyond that required to condense with acetyl CoA, oxaloacetate enters reverse glycolytic pathways to generate glucose-6-P. In the liver, glucose-6-P can be dephosphorylated to generate glucose for export to the rest of the body.

zymes produced from oxidation of 1 mole of acetyl-CoA.

- TCA cycle intermediates may be drawn off into alternate metabolic pathways for amino acid or glucose synthesis.

- Intermediates may be supplemented by inputs from other substrates such as propionic acid and selected amino acids.

It was noted earlier that reduced coenzymes may be produced by many reactions other than those of the TCA cycle. In Sections 7.4 and 7.5, which address aspects of lipid and carbohydrate metabolism, several such examples will be noted. Although the energy equivalents of these intermediary reactions are important, they are quantitatively minor compared to production within the TCA cycle. It must also be appreciated that the reduced coenzymes are required for anabolic reactions by contributing reducing equivalents for the saturation of olefinic bonds and the conversation of carbonyl groups into their reduced, or hydroxy-, forms (Figure 7–6). Reductive steps such as these are especially important in lipid synthesis. Thus, reduced coenzymes have important fates in addition to use in the generation of ATP. In many instances the relative abundance of the oxidized and reduced forms of a particular coenzyme is a prime determinant of the direction taken by a reversible reaction or series of reactions.

Before considering the types of anabolic and catabolic conversions undergone by the major classes of nutrient or substrate molecules, it is worthwhile to emphasize again that the ultimate source of the substrates from which energy can be harvested is from the diet. Digestive mechanisms provide merely the first phase of processing; the absorbed, or assimilated, nutrients enter body pools to serve as substrates for anabolism and the catabolic reactions that generate reducing equivalents and useful energy.

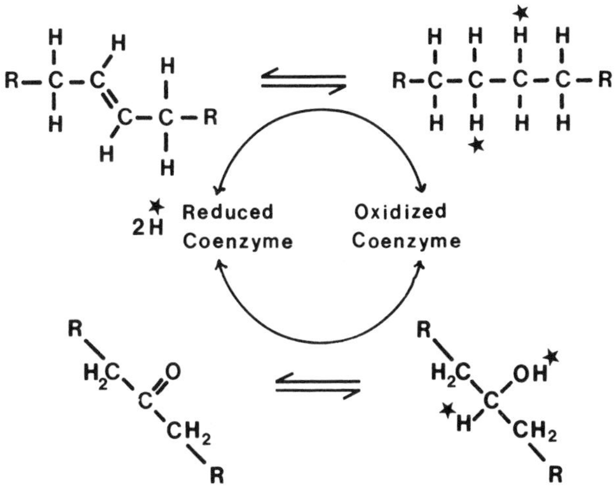

Figure 7–6. Uses of reducing equivalents. Protons carried in the form of reduced coenzymes are used to saturate olefinic bonds (upper reaction) and to reduce ketones to the corresponding hydroxy compounds (lower reaction). Such exchanges of reducing equivalents are often reversible. For example, the oxidation of a hydroxy compound to the ketone can be used to generate reduced coenzymes. The hydrogens transferred by these reactions are shown with stars.

7.3 • Metabolism of Nitrogenous Compounds: Proteins and Amino Acids

The proteins in the body are in a state of dynamic equilibrium. There is continuous breakdown and resynthesis of proteins throughout life. Again, this is catabolism and anabolism proceeding hand in hand. The amino acids formed by the breakdown of endogenous proteins are no different from amino acids that are obtained in the gut from the digestion of dietary protein. In an adult, nonpregnant, nonlactating animal, when protein breakdown equals protein buildup, the animal is said to be in *nitrogen balance.* Actually, because the balance is in terms of gram atoms of nitrogen rather than protein, that statement is an oversimplification. Nitrogen balance really means that the amount of nitrogen or nitrogenous compounds taken in in the feed is equal to the amount of nitrogen or nitrogenous compounds excreted. In a growing animal, anabolism normally exceeds catabolism, and the animal is said to be in a positive nitrogen balance, because there is a net accumulation of nitrogen in the body. If the animal is fasted over a prolonged period, it will be in negative nitrogen balance. The body constituents are broken down and nitrogenous compounds are eliminated faster than they are replaced. Thus, there is a net loss of nitrogen from the body.

The amino acids necessary for protein synthesis in the body's cells are taken from a pool of free amino acids in the extracellular fluids. This pool reflects the balance of amino acids utilized by the body and the input of amino acids resulting from breakdown of tissue protein, amino acids synthesized in the liver, and those absorbed from the gut. As a rough guide, the concentration of amino acids in plasma ranges between 45 and 60 mg/100 mL.

The synthesis of proteins is a fairly complicated process in which amino acids are linked together by a series of peptide, or amide, bonds in a constant sequence that varies with the specific protein being synthesized. The synthesis takes place in the cytoplasm of cells on the surface of ribosomes, where the sequence for the amino acids is coded by the bases that make up messenger ribonucleic acid (mRNA).

Protein synthesis is greater in young animals than in adults provided with the same diet. This demonstrates that protein synthesis is a function of the physiologic state of the animal and can be partly independent of the dietary availability of amino acids. Similarly, there is greater protein synthesis in animals during pregnancy and lactation. These are physiologic states in which anabolic processes are especially important. Of course, overriding any physiologic drive toward protein synthesis is the fact that the availability of amino acids as substrates will ultimately be limiting for the extent of protein synthesis.

Amino acids that are present in amounts in excess of those required for protein synthesis are not stored as such but are further catabolized to yield energy. The first step in the breakdown of amino acids involves the transfer, or simple removal, of amino groups (Figure 7–7). Once freed of its amino group, the residue may enter glycolytic or TCA pathways and can be oxidized to yield carbon dioxide and water. Energy that is released is collected and incorporated into ATP. In some cases the deaminated residue can be converted to glucose, and so it can be called a *glucogenic substrate.* Amino acids suited to this type of conversion are particularly important in ruminants because they provide a significant source of glucose to the animal. The other amino acids cannot result in the net synthesis of glucose but rather contribute to the pool of intermediates suited for oxidation. Acetyl-CoA is at the hub of such reactions, and because acetyl-CoA is in equilibrium with the 4C compounds

Figure 7–7. An example of oxidative deamination. One mechanism for removing the amino group of an amino acid consumes water and generates ammonia and protons, in the form of a reduced coenzyme (shown as H·). In this case, the amino acid glutamate is oxidized to the TCA cycle intermediate, ketoglutarate.

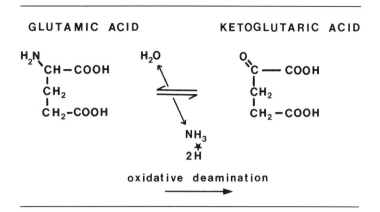

called ketone bodies (see Section 7.4), amino acids that are degraded in this fashion are called *ketogenic* rather than glucogenic.

The ammonia formed by deamination of the amino acids may be transferred to other organic acids to synthesize other amino acids, or the surplus ammonia may be converted to *urea* and excreted. Ammonia is toxic to cells when the concentrations exceed approximately 10^{-4} M. The ammonia may be directly converted to urea in the cell in which it is produced, or it may leave that cell and be converted into urea elsewhere. It will be recalled that free ammonia diffuses out of renal tubular cells to be reduced to the ammonium ion in the tubular fluid. More typically, an overall reaction takes place:

$$2 NH_3 + H_2CO_3 \rightarrow H_2N\text{–}CO\text{–}NH_2 + 2 H_2O$$

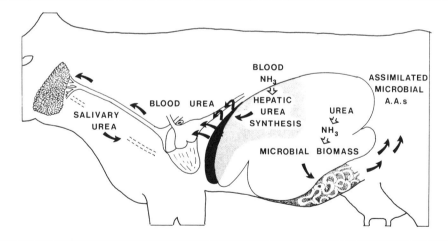

Figure 7–8. Urea cycling in ruminants. Ammonia is removed from the body after its conversion to urea, mainly in the liver. Blood urea is cleared by urinary excretion and, in ruminants, by its continued addition to saliva. Salivary urea reaches the rumen where it is hydrolyzed by the microbes; the free NH_3 so generated is then used by the bacteria for their own protein synthesis. Finally, microbial protein is subject to proteolytic digestion in the animal's gut. Some of the absorbed amino acids will actually contain $-NH_2$ groups that were initially waste products from the animal's own metabolism.

in which two molecules of ammonia are coupled with one molecule of carbonic acid to produce urea and two water molecules.

The actual reactions of the *urea cycle* are quite complex and occur primarily in the liver. This is known because surgical removal of the liver from animals results in relatively quick elimination of urea from the bloodstream. For many years, the formation of urea from ammonia was considered to be a critical life support process simply because it removed the otherwise toxic ammonia. Now, urea synthesis is considered to be of additional importance because it provides a direct means of eliminating carbonic acid from the body.

Urea is a normal constituent of saliva. In fact, in the ruminant animal, rather substantial amounts of urea pass from blood, via saliva, into the gastrointestinal tract every day. Within the rumen, the microbes are capable of breaking urea down to ammonia and carbon dioxide:

$$H_2N-CO-NH_2 + H_2O \rightarrow 2\,NH_3 + CO_2$$

and then are able to incorporate the free ammonia into the new synthesis of their own amino acids. These bacterial-derived amino acids are then subsequently reabsorbed and used by the animal after intestinal digestion (Figure 7–8). Therefore, urea, an excretion product in the first instance, can become a substrate for microbial synthesis of new amino acids, and then these can be cycled back into the animal's amino acid pool. This is an extremely important aspect of the nitrogen economy of ruminant animals.

7.4 • Metabolism of Lipids

The biologically important lipids are triglycerides, phospholipids, and sterols. The lipids in the animal body are in a dynamic state of constant catabolism and anabolism. Within cells they form two main types: *structural lipids*, mainly found in the cell membrane, and *neutral fat*, stored as energy reserves, particularly in adipose cells.

Blood plasma contains about 300 mg of lipids per 100 mL. About 50% of lipid exists as phospholipids, about 30% as triglycerides, and some 20% as cholesterol. Besides these major fractions, the plasma contains small amounts of *nonesterified* or *free fatty acids*. The nonesterified fatty acids have a very rapid turnover rate and represent the main form in which fatty acids are transferred from fat depots to the site of oxidation. Fatty acids are not oxidized within reg-

ular, or "white," adipose tissue. Thermogenic adipose tissue, also called *brown fat*, is quite different in form (see Figure 1–9) and function. The cytoplasm contains numerous small lipid droplets and the cells contain many mitochondria. Brown fat is a major source of heat for newborn animals. The oxidation of fat liberates huge quantities of heat, and this is used by the newborn for several hours to maintain thermal equilibrium until its digestive system is operational. This aspect of lipid metabolism will be described further in Chapter 9 in relation to thermoregulation.

The oxidation of fatty acids takes place in the mitochondria of the liver, muscle, and various other tissues by a process known as beta oxidation. In this process, the fatty acids are progressively broken down into the two-carbon units, acetyl-CoA (Figure 7–9). The CoA esters of fatty acids are the form in which virtually all lipid catabolism takes place. Acetyl-CoA may enter the TCA cycle and be oxidized to carbon dioxide and water, again with the transfer of released energy partly to be stored in ATP and partly released as heat. The 2C units may also be temporarily stored as ketone bodies, and this will be described below. Many tissues are capable of synthesizing fatty acids from these same 2C units. The pathway for fatty acid synthesis is not, however, simply a reverse of the pathway for fat oxidation, but details of the differences are beyond the scope of the present treatment. It is sufficient to state that fatty acid synthesis consumes acetyl-CoA, reducing equivalents in the form of reduced coenzymes, and requires energy from ATP hydrolysis. The consumption of energy is quite typical of anabolic processes.

Most of the absorbed fats from the gut are present in the form of *chylomicra*. These colloidal particles are complex mixtures of triglycerides, phospholipids, cholesterol, and proteins. They are formed primarily in the wall of the intestine but can be modified in various tissues. Somewhat similar lipoproteins are formed in the liver. About 25% to 35% of this complex mixture is protein. The precise composition of the lipoproteins varies with the species of animal and its diet. Lipoproteins provide a convenient means of transporting hydrophobic compounds, the lipids, within the watery medium of the blood plasma. The nonesterified or free fatty acids are also hydrophobic, and when they are released from adipose tissue into the circulation, they form a loose association with circulating plasma proteins, particularly serum albumin, and so their effective solubility in plasma is increased. This is an excellent example of hydrophobic interaction between the hydrophobic nonesterified

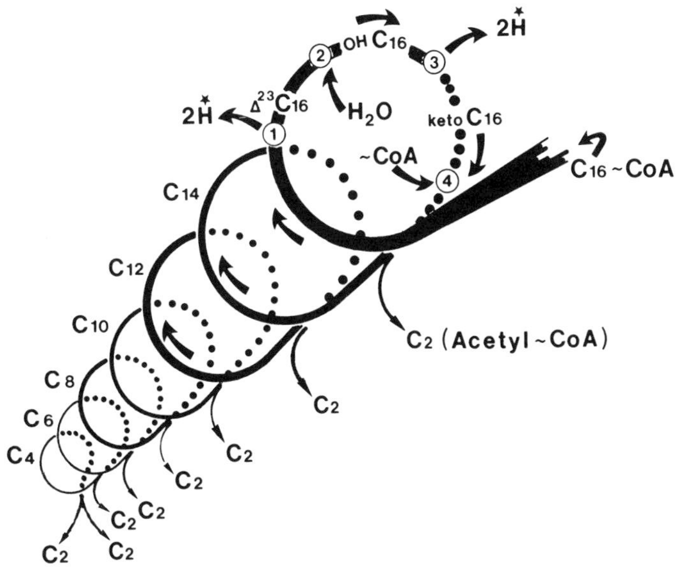

Figure 7–9. *Beta-oxidation of long chain fatty acids.* This unconventional diagram illustrates the cyclic nature of the catabolism of fatty acids. The input substrate is a fatty acid CoA ester, in this case palmityl CoA. One round of hydrolysis (and oxidation) involving steps 1 through 4 results in one acetyl CoA being split off along with four protons, carried off on coenzymes (H·). The original substrate has lost a two carbon segment and enters the next round as myristyl CoA ($C_{14:0}$). Beta oxidation proceeds in this fashion until the final round generates two molecules of acetyl CoA. In each round, the reactions involve: (1) desaturation between carbons 2 and 3 which yields the first pair of H·; (2) hydration of the delta 2–3 double bond to form a hydroxy-compound; (3) oxidation of the hydroxy- into a keto-derivative by removing the second pair of protons; and (4) cleavage of the two carbon fragment as acetyl CoA. Large amounts of reduced coenzymes are generated, and a molecule of CoA is consumed for each round of the cycle.

fatty acids and the hydrophobic domains on the serum albumin.

The lipids, carried in the form of lipoproteins, are transported to peripheral tissues. At some locations these lipoproteins are broken down to release constituent fatty acids, to be taken up by cells. This is a particularly important process within adipose tissue, the site of fat storage. The mechanism is intriguing. The inner surface of the capillaries within adipose tissue contains an enzyme called *lipoprotein lipase,* which hydrolyzes triglycerides to nonesterified fatty acids and glycerol. The glycerol is retained within the circulation and cycles back to the liver, but the nonesterified fatty acids in this instance are taken up by the adipocytes, where they are incorporated into triglycerides within the cell (Figure 7–10). The nonesterified fatty acids are activated by conversion into the CoA ester form and three fatty acyl CoA esters combine with an activated form of glycerol, alpha-glycerophosphate, which is produced in the adipocyte from glucose. The result is the formation of a new triglyceride molecule. This describes the most important mechanism of synthesis of depot fat. The newly formed triglycerides coalesce into existing microdroplets of fat and eventually into a single large fat droplet in a mature adipocyte. This occurs because of the biophysical forces operating at the interface between the lipid and aqueous phases of the cytoplasm.

Under catabolic conditions, for example during negative energy balance, the stored fats are subjected to hydrolysis by lipases present within the adipocyte, so that nonesterified fatty acids may be liberated from the storage form (Figure 7–10). The lipase found within the adipocyte is activated by hormones and so is called *hormone-sensitive lipase.* This process is called *lipolysis,* or fat mobilization, and is stimulated by a number of hormones. All of these lipolytic hormones act via the agency of the intracellular messenger, cyclic AMP (cAMP). The hormone causes activation of adenylate cyclase, the enzyme capable of amplifying the endocrine signal by producing quantities of cAMP from ATP. In turn, cAMP activates protein kinases responsible for regulating the activity of the lipases.

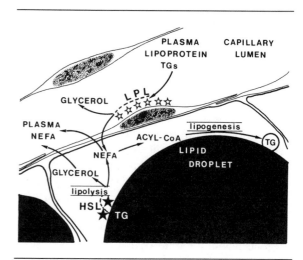

Figure 7–10. Lipid exchanges between the circulation and adipocyte. Plasma lipoproteins carry triglycerides within the circulation. These are subjected to hydrolysis by lipoprotein lipase (LPL), an enzyme located within the capillary lumen but attached to the endothelial cell. The fatty acids that are liberated are taken up into the adipocyte where they enter a pool of nonesterified fatty acids (NEFAs). The NEFAs may be activated into CoA esters (acyl CoA) and then used in triglyceride synthesis, finally to be incorporated into the lipid droplet. Glycerol, produced by the action of LPL, remains in the circulation and is used for glucose synthesis elsewhere. Triglycerides at the cytoplasmic interface of the lipid droplet are hydrolyzed by hormone sensitive lipase (HSL) by the process called lipolysis. Their products are released from the cell as glycerol and NEFAs. Some of the NEFAs may be reincorporated into the lipid droplet, but it is unlikely that HSL will be activated at the same time that lipogenesis is taking place.

The nonesterified fatty acids released into the circulation after lipolysis in adipose tissue travel in association with plasma proteins until they are taken up by liver and some other tissues, such as the heart, where they may serve as energy substrates. After being activated to the form of CoA esters, they are then broken down by beta oxidation to 2C units and further oxidized to carbon dioxide and water, as described earlier.

The amount of acetyl-CoA present in the cell

at a given time may be in excess of the amount that can be processed within the TCA cycle. It will be recalled that acetyl-CoA enters the TCA cycle by condensing with the 4C intermediate oxaloacetate, thereby forming citric acid. In order for acetyl-CoA to be processed, the availability of oxaloacetate must not be limiting. Now, because oxaloacetate can be drawn away, particularly for use in gluconeogenesis, situations can arise in which there is insufficient oxaloacetate present to handle the flux of excessive quantities of acetyl-CoA into the TCA cycle.

When acetyl-CoA concentrations are in excess, the acetyl-CoA condenses to form *ketone bodies*. The formation of ketone bodies (Figure 7–11) releases the CoA, enabling it to be used again to initiate metabolism of additional nonesterified fatty acids. This is a method of conserving CoA and is particularly important when animals are in negative energy balance. In such conditions, dietary energy sources are inadequate for the maintenance of body functions, or may be absent altogether. The animal will have already mobilized all readily available storage forms of carbohydrate and is now mobilizing body lipid stores. As the quantity of nonesterified fatty acids increases, fatty acid oxidation accelerates; but all this takes place at a time when any substrates capable of being converted to glucose are so consumed, with priority given to preserving glucose homeostasis. So acetyl-CoA accumulates because the capacity of the TCA

cycle is embarrassed, and the CoA is conserved by ketone body formation, or *ketogenesis.*

Of course, the excessive production of ketone bodies in this condition has serious consequences. The ketone bodies include *acetoacetic acid, beta-hydroxybutyric acid,* and *acetone.* The first two are interconvertible and may, in certain circumstances, be transformed back to acetyl-CoA. Alternatively, acetoacetic acid may be decarboxylated to acetone by an irreversible reaction. The two acids, acetoacetate and beta-hydroxybutyric acid, are sufficiently hydrophilic that high concentrations can build up in plasma. The acids, although weak relative to the more familiar mineral acids such as HCl and H_2SO_4, nevertheless dissociate and contribute a substantial excess of H^+ ions to the extracellular fluids.

There are normally small amounts of ketone bodies in the circulation of animals, and they are of no consequence. The concentrations are much greater during conditions of starvation, in early lactation, and sometimes in late pregnancy. In these situations the demand for nutrients exceeds the capabilities of dietary provision. Excessive amounts of acetoacetic acid are toxic to the body, in addition to the pronounced lowering of blood pH, or metabolic acidosis, caused by both acetoacetatic and beta-hydroxybutyric acids.

The production of acetone by decarboxylation is a detoxifying process of the body because the acetone is easily eliminated, either in expired

Figure 7–11. Ketogenesis. Amounts of acetyl CoA in excess of what can be processed by the TCA cycle enter ketogenesis, a mechanism for conserving coenzyme A. Two molecules of acetyl CoA condense into acetoacetyl CoA with the release of one CoA. The four carbon product is then de-esterified to release the other CoA. Acetoacetate may be reduced to beta-hydroxybutyrate, decarboxylated to acetone, or released directly from the cell.

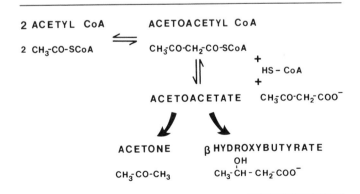

air or in the urine. A *ketotic* animal, one exhibiting the effects of excessive ketone body formation, can be readily detected by the distinct aroma of acetone on its breath and in its urine.

The process of ketogenesis will be mentioned again in relation to nutritional stress in Section 7.6, and in relation to the metabolic burden of lactation in Chapter 11.

7.5 • Carbohydrate Metabolism

Carbohydrate metabolism is fundamentally different in ruminant animals and in nonruminant animals. The two should really be considered separately. In this introduction, carbohydrate metabolism in nonruminant animals will be described as the general case, and specializations or distinctions in ruminants will be noted. In nonruminants, dietary carbohydrates are hydrolyzed within the gut to monosaccharides and absorbed in this form. Virtually all absorbed monosaccharides enter the portal blood circulation and are transported directly to the liver. Only minor amounts of carbohydrates are absorbed into the lymph.

At the liver, the monosaccharides are taken up from the portal blood and those that are not glucose are converted to either glucose or fructose within the liver cells. The uptake of monosaccharides is rather complete but it is nevertheless dependent on the presence of insulin. If the hepatic uptake of monosaccharides is incomplete, then they pass into the peripheral circulation and become available to the body tissues in general. Depending on the status of the glucose pool, or the balance between glucose input and glucose utilization, the liver may release glucose and make it available to peripheral tissues. During the *absorptive phase* of the digestive process, the liver serves as a net uptake site (Figure 7–12).

The glucose entering the liver (Figure 7–13) is either stored in the form of liver glycogen, or used to provide alpha-glycerophosphate for lipid synthesis, or hydrolyzed to form acetyl-CoA. The acetyl-CoA is then completely oxidized to water and carbon dioxide via the TCA cycle, or alternatively it may be used as a substrate for the synthesis of fatty acids, as noted in the previous section. In ruminant animals, this would be a wasteful use of scarce glucose supplies because there is an alternative source of 2C units to the animal in the form of acetic acid, the major volatile fatty acid from the rumen. *Ruminants do not generate acetyl-CoA from glucose. Instead, they directly activate acetate to acetyl-CoA.*

The conversion of glucose into the storage form as glycogen is called *glycogenesis*, terminology that is consistent with the conversion of any substance into triglycerides being referred to as *lipogenesis*. Both of these synthetic processes are anabolic in nature and consume energy; both are stimulated by insulin.

Carbohydrates are found in all tissues of the body, and the extracellular pool of glucose can be rapidly augmented from the diet or by mobilization of glycogen stored in the liver. The breakdown of glycogen into monosaccharides, either for release to the circulation or for use within the cell, is termed *glycogenolysis*. The other major storage form of carbohydrate is the gly-

Figure 7–12. Hepatic uptake and release of glucose. Net extraction of glucose (actually many nutrients) occurs from the portal circulation during the absorptive phase. The peripheral tissues still receive a supply of glucose but the liver buffers the excessive amounts that would otherwise be present during absorption from the gut. Later, during the postabsorptive phase, the gut may consume more glucose than it absorbs (see arrows) and the needs of peripheral tissues will be met by net release from the liver. The width of the bars representing the circulation provides an approximation of plasma concentrations of glucose in the various locations.

ABSORPTIVE – hepatic glycogenesis

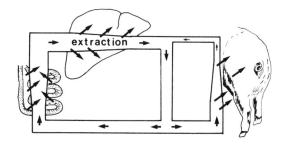

POST ABSORPTIVE – glycogenolysis

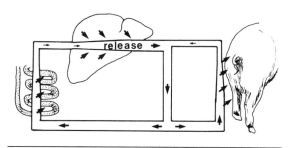

Figure 7–13. Fate of glucose taken up by the liver. After glucose is converted to glucose-6-P, it is either converted to its storage form as glycogen or subjected to hydrolysis to produce reducing equivalents and intermediates for use in protein synthesis and lipogenesis. Ruminants do not generate acetyl CoA by these reactions because it would be a wasteful use of scarce glucose.

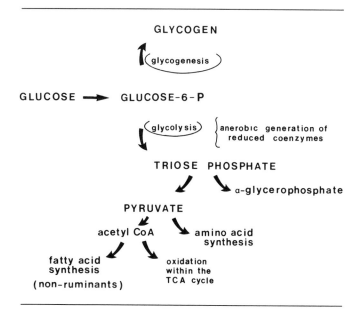

cogen deposited in muscle. In contrast to the glycogen in liver, muscle glycogen is not mobilized to provide a direct source of blood glucose. It is used exclusively as a fuel for muscle (Box 7–2). Alternatively, glucose can be produced from noncarbohydrate precursor molecules such as certain amino acids, and others to

be described below, by the process called *gluconeogenesis*. It is important to have a clear understanding of the meaning of these terms: glycogenesis (-*genesis*, to form), glycogenolysis (-*lysis*, to break down), and gluconeogenesis (-*neogenesis*, new formation).

Carbohydrate levels in blood, in the inter-

Box 7–2   Muscle Glycogen

The skeletal muscle system in a typical body represents about an 18-fold greater mass than the liver. Somewhat in excess of 50% of the total monosaccharide equivalent in a nonruminant animal is present in the form of muscle glycogen. Muscle glycogen is not a direct source of glucose that can be made available for blood transport because glycogenolysis in muscle produces a form of glucose (glucose-6-phosphate) that cannot leave the muscle cell. Instead, muscle glucose is used in glycolysis to yield energy for the muscle.

During the complete oxidation of glucose to carbon dioxide, water, and energy, 38 high-energy phosphate bonds are produced from one molecule of glucose. The overall reaction is:

$$C_6H_{12}O_6 + 6\ O_2 + 38\ ADP \rightarrow$$
$$6\ CO_2 + 6\ H_2O + 38\ ATP$$

This describes the complete breakdown of glucose in the presence of oxygen and is referred to as *aerobic glycolysis*. However, muscles are often required to perform when oxygen availability is a limiting factor, and an alternative form of metabolism occurs. With reference to the biochemical pathways shown in Figure 7–14, glucose is broken down only as far as pyruvic acid. The pyruvic acid, a 3C intermediate, instead of being converted to acetyl-CoA and then entering the TCA cycle, accumulates and is largely converted to lactic acid, another 3C compound. The conversion of 1

mole of glucose to 2 moles of pyruvate consumes no oxygen yet provides a net yield of 2 moles of ATP. The conversion of pyruvate to lactate serves to regenerate oxidized coenzymes to enable glycolytic processing of additional glucose.

Lactic acid can accumulate in skeletal muscle during anaerobic metabolism and it gives rise to the sensation of fatigue. More usually, the lactate is released from the cell and enters the bloodstream. These products of glycolysis, particularly lactic acid, are transported to the liver, taken up there, and resynthesized into glucose. The glucose can then either be stored as liver glycogen or released to contribute to the circulating glucose pool. The glucose finds its way back to muscle, is taken up again, and is either subjected directly to glycolysis as above, or if the muscle is no longer active, stored as glycogen. This whole process of cycling glucose products between muscle and the liver is known as the *Cori cycle*.

The advantage of independence from oxygen supply must be balanced against the marked loss in efficiency of ATP generation from anaerobic glycolysis of glucose to lactate (about 25% as ATP, 75% as heat). This is equivalent to an immediate recovery of a mere 2% of the caloric content of glucose in the form of ATP. When complete oxidative degradation, involving glycolysis and the TCA cycle, is possible, the recovery of calories from glucose in the 38 ATPs represents an overall efficiency of some 40%, with the remainder being released as heat.

Figure 7–14. The Cori cycle. Muscles in nonruminant animals are fueled primarily by the glycolytic processing of glucose-6-P obtained from the breakdown of glycogen or from the direct uptake of blood glucose. When operating under aerobic conditions, two molecules of pyruvate, formed from glucose-6-P, are decarboxylated to acetyl CoA and the two carbon units are oxidized within the TCA cycle, as described earlier. When the oxygen supply becomes limiting (hypoxia), oxidative phosphorylation is arrested, acetyl CoA cannot be processed, and pyruvate is converted to lactate and leaves the cell. This "shunting" device permits continued glycolytic processing without need for oxygen, yet still enables the generation of some ATP for muscle function. The lactate returns to the liver, is converted back to glucose-6-phosphate, and then either released as free glucose or stored as hepatic glycogen. The counter-clockwise cycling of lactate and glucose, known as the Cori cycle, enables muscles to continue to function despite a lack of local oxygen.

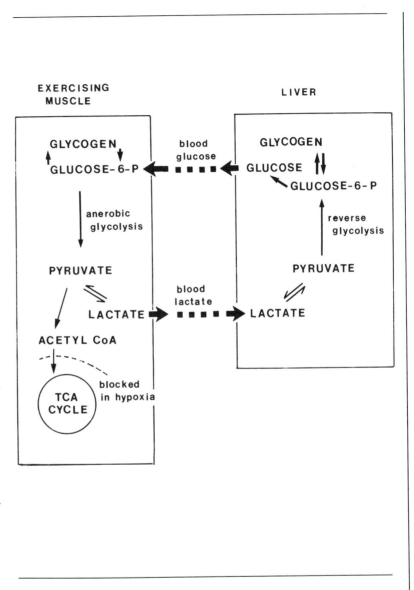

stitial fluid, and in solid tissues vary with the diet and in relation to the time after eating. Immediately after a monogastric animal consumes a meal, blood levels of glucose are high and there may also be substantial concentrations of other monosaccharides, such as fructose and galactose. However, it is reasonable to consider glucose as the most important circulating monosaccharide. Normal blood concentrations of glucose in a nonruminant, some hours after a meal, will be approximately 90 mg/100 ml. In the case of diabetics lacking insulin, blood glucose may be considerably higher, and a figure of 200 mg/100 ml is not unreasonable: in diabetics, tissue use of glucose is suboptimal so blood concentrations of glucose remain elevated. If the concentrations exceed a value of approximately 170 to 180 mg/100 ml, there is incomplete recovery of glucose that has been filtered in the kidney, and glucosuria will result. This is because there is a threshold concentration of glucose in the renal filtrate beyond which glucose cannot be recovered by active transport.

Carbohydrates are depleted from blood by oxidation within the cells, by storage as muscle or liver glycogen, or by conversion into fat within the liver and adipose tissue. Several hours after a meal in nonruminant animals, the animal is said to be in the *postabsorptive phase*. Glucose utilization at this stage far outstrips the entry of glucose from the intestines so equilibrium of the glucose pool is achieved by mobilization, primarily of liver glycogen. Glycogen reserves are broken down by the process of glycogenolysis, under the control of hormones such as glucagon from the pancreas or catecholamines from the adrenal medulla.

Many tissues can switch between glucose and other substrates, depending on their relative availability. Glucose sparing in this fashion reduces the overall rate of glucose utilization and favors the requirements of critical tissues, such as a pregnant uterus or the brain, that depend on the continuous availability of at least some glucose.

As noted earlier, the utilization of scarce glucose or its glycolytic product within the cell, pyruvic acid, to form acetyl-CoA is inefficient for ruminants. These animals have a readily available supply of acetic acid absorbed from the rumen. The acetic acid can be activated to acetyl-CoA and then pass into fatty acid synthesis or into ketogenesis (the production of ketone bodies), or the acetyl-CoA can be completely oxidized to carbon dioxide and water within the TCA cycle.

This represents a very important method of glucose conservation, and considering that very little glucose is absorbed directly from the gut of ruminants, this has survival advantages.

The major problem facing the ruminant animal is how the individual obtains the glucose it needs for the variety of processes critically dependent on glucose.

Most of the glucose in the glucose pool of a ruminant animal has been produced within the animal from noncarbohydrate precursors (Figure 7–15). Some of the absorbed digestive products serve as substrates for glucose synthesis. Some endogenous compounds such as glycerol, lactic acid, and selected amino acids are also converted to glucose. These gluconeogenic processes appear to be dependent on glucocorticoid hormones from the adrenal cortex for their normal operation.

The major substrate available to the ruminant for gluconeogenesis is propionic acid, absorbed from the rumen. This three-carbon carboxylic acid is taken up by the liver, activated into a CoA ester, then carboxylated and enters the TCA cycle (see Figure 7–5), only to leave it promptly thereafter to enter a pathway of reverse glycolysis, resulting in the production of glucose-6-phosphate. The glucose-6-phosphate may then enter the pathways of glycogenesis, as noted before. In liver cells, the phosphate can be removed to produce free glucose and the latter can be released into the bloodstream.

The organic acids that were produced by

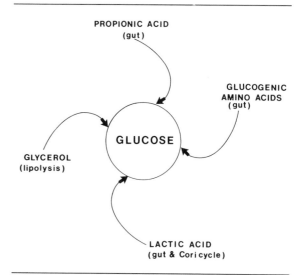

Figure 7–15. Glucogenic precursors. The major substrates used for gluconeogenesis include glucogenic amino acids, lactate, and glycerol. In ruminants, propionic acid from rumen fermentation is the most important glucogenic substrate, as illustrated earlier in Figure 7–5.

deamination of amino acids (see Section 7.3) may provide the appropriate form of intermediaries to enter reverse glycolysis. Lactic acid and pyruvic acid released from exercising muscle can be converted to glucose (see Box 7–2). Finally, the glycerol liberated into the circulation as a result of lipolysis of triglycerides in peripheral tissues (see Figure 7–10) may be taken up by the liver and converted back to glucose. Substrates that are capable of being converted to glucose by the mechanisms just outlined can be called glucogenic substrates. Others that can only generate acetyl-CoA are called ketogenic substrates. For example, the small amounts of butyric acid that are absorbed from the rumen are considered to be ketogenic because they either directly enter the reactions involved in ketone body synthesis or the butyric acid can be activated and converted to acetyl-CoA and then used for all of the typical reactions in which acetyl-CoA is used: fatty acid synthesis, ketogenesis, and oxidation to carbon dioxide and water.

7.6 • Pathophysiology of Metabolism

The preceding five sections briefly examined the major aspects of intermediary metabolism that provide for energy generation, interconversion of types of substrates, and the basic elements of anabolism and catabolism. Anabolic reactions build up molecular complexity, consuming substrate and energy, and result in the formation of glycogen, proteins, and storage lipids. Catabolism breaks down complex compounds into those that are simpler and, if taken to completion, produces a variety of oxides—carbon dioxide, water, and others—and results in the release of useful amounts of energy. These two phases of metabolism, anabolism and catabolism, are very closely regulated on a minute-by-minute basis with most of the regulation at a whole-body level being achieved by hormone action. To generalize, insulin is an anabolic hormone and favors anabolic reactions. Glucagon, catecholamines, and to a lesser extent the adrenal glucocorticoid hormones are all catabolic hormones. The ultimate input to metabolic pathways comes from the substrates and products of digestion. On the output side, energy is produced or energy may be consumed in building up complexity as part of anabolism.

In animal production, anabolic processes are of prime interest because they underlie animal growth and the processes of pregnancy and lactation. The extent to which these take place, as seen in rate of growth or development of the fetus, or level of milk production, reflects the availability of substrates provided by metabolic pathways.

In part, there are physiologic drives to each of these processes such that substrate consumption, for example in support of pregnancy, may outstrip the ability of metabolism to meet the needs for anabolism. Normally, this would trigger increased appetite and therefore increased input into the metabolic pathways, but that is not always possible: feed availability may be the limiting factor, especially under range conditions. In such cases the animal will adjust its metabolism according to physiologic priorities, with quite striking consequences. For example, a pregnant animal seems to be committed to supporting the anabolic needs of the conceptus.

The changes in maternal metabolism required to support those needs may in fact compromise the well-being of the mother. This is well illustrated in pregnant sheep that are carrying multiple fetuses if the level of nutrition is inadequate to meet the needs of the pregnancy. The adjustment in metabolism results in mobilization of stored body reserves of carbohydrate, protein, and finally fat. The animal loses condition, or shows a decrease in body weight, as a result of these catabolic events. The metabolic pathways may be flooded with products of catabolism, excessive amounts of acetyl-CoA are produced, and ketone bodies accumulate and may eventually result in malaise of the mother.

Animals are surprisingly tolerant of changes in the overall direction of metabolism and, normally, adaptive mechanisms come into play to ensure maintenance of homeostasis. It should be recognized, however, that the animal is operating at the limits of its comfort ranges for many critical variables, and relatively minor additional burdens placed on the animal will result in stress. In the case of the sheep in late pregnancy supporting the needs of multiple fetuses, the metabolic well-being of the animal can be quite easily tipped over the edge and a disease state created. In this particular case, the condition is called *pregnancy toxemia*. The symptoms of toxemia in pregnant sheep result from excessive concentrations of acetoacetic acid and inadequate concentrations of glucose in the blood. These result in neurologic disturbances, including body twitching, yet a general lack of activity. For the latter reason, the disease is referred to commonly as sleepy sickness.

In its advanced stages in pregnant sheep, little can be done to cure pregnancy toxemia. The animal, of course, has no flexibility in decreasing the requirements of the conceptus. The animal cannot elect to terminate the pregnancy. It is difficult to correct the advanced stages of this condition by dietary manipulation, though the administration, usually intravenously, of glucose or glucogenic substrates may provide some relief. Far more satisfactory is the adoption of a nutritional regimen that fully meets the requirements of the pregnant animal, thereby avoiding the metabolic pressures that might precipitate the disorder.

A closely related metabolic disorder involving excessive glucose utilization and ketogenesis is *lactation ketosis*, seen in cattle very early in lactation. This will be described further, in relation to the metabolic burden of lactation, in Chapter 11. In early lactation, most high-performing cattle are in negative energy balance. This means that the caloric content of the milk being produced, along with the needs for maintenance, exceeds the caloric intake of the animal. The difference is made up by mobilization of body reserves, with characteristic and very obvious weight loss. Typically, it is not until about 6 to 8 weeks into lactation before the intake of dietary energy balances the animal's needs. During this time, the animal mobilizes large quantities of body fat in an attempt to meet the deficit, and a very similar metabolic picture prevails as that described in the sheep in late pregnancy. Excessive production of ketone bodies results in clinical ketosis. Ketotic cows exhibit many of the symptoms described earlier for the sheep, but while the condition is equally life-threatening, it is somewhat easier to remedy. The cow attempts to adjust its level of milk production to reduce the demand for substrates. Even so, the condition of ketosis is a major limiting factor for milk production in intensive dairying operations.

Pathogenesis

The examples just provided of the demands of anabolic processes outstripping the ability of the diet or the animal's reserves to maintain homeostasis, have pathologic consequences. Clearly, these are not diseases with an infectious etiology; there is no microorganism provoking the disease. Rather, the disturbance to the animal results from a critical physiologic variable, perhaps low blood glucose or high blood ketones, grossly exceeding the comfort range for those variables.

Minor excursions beyond the comfort range are accommodated and handled by homeostatic mechanisms.

Major deviations from the comfort zone impose stress on the animal. This will be discussed further in Chapter 9.

These stresses manifest as disease states, so they should be analyzed with reference to the term pathogenesis.

It should be clear from these descriptions that preventing these conditions from occurring is much more likely to be successful than trying to cure them once they have occurred. Understanding the cause of these pathophysiologic conditions is the first step toward prevention. Additionally, the symptoms of these diseases usually do not appear suddenly. With a reasonable understanding of the mechanisms underlying the problems, it is possible to detect the conditions in their early stages, when corrective measures are much more likely to be effective. The whole notion of homeostasis and comfort zone, stress, and pathogenesis will be addressed in further detail in Chapter 9.

7.7 • Exercises

1. Distinguish *direct* from *indirect* calorimetry.

2. Why is propionic acid called a glucogenic substrate when acetic acid is called ketogenic?

3. What is the major determinant of whether or not acetyl-CoA is completely oxidized to CO_2 and H_2O?

4. Based on what you know to be the main stimulus for secretion of insulin and its most obvious action in liver, would you expect gluconeogenesis to be *stimulated* or *suppressed* under the influence of this hormone?

5. Define *energy balance*.

If a fat animal is deprived of sufficient feed to meet its needs, it may mobilize huge quantities of its lipid stores and may be prone to a metabolic disorder.

What is this condition?

What biochemical events are responsible?

How can the condition be diagnosed?

Why is acetoacetate decarboxylated?

6. Identify two good reasons why ruminant animals do not form acetyl-CoA from pyruvate.

7. Distinguish *glycogenesis* from *glycogenolysis*.

Which process occurs when an athlete is "sugar-loaded" just before an endurance event?

Which process is activated during the exercise?

What is the main reason for glycogenesis and glycogenolysis taking place in monogastric animals offered large infrequent meals?

8. What is the source of the glyceryl "backbone" of storage lipid, and what is its fate after complete lipolysis has occurred?

9. Briefly describe the nitrogen conservation strategy that is unique to ruminant animals.

10. Outline what you understand of the term *pathogenesis*.

11. Indicate the quantitatively most important glucogenic precursor for an adult ruminant animal:

      lactate   glycerol   propionate

12. Identify four uses of *net energy*.

Growth and Development

8

The everyday notions about growth will be quite familiar to the reader but the specific biologic details are complex and their analysis can be confusing. The growth of animals from conception to maturity is at the heart of animal production. It is the most obvious form in which anabolic mechanisms are expressed. Operationally, growth is any increase in metabolically active protoplasm; hence the term can be applied to the dynamics of a single cell as it passes through its life cycle. Aspects of growth at the cellular level will be described below. More typically, growth in multicellular organisms is considered at the grossest possible level, that of the whole individual. Thus growth manifests as an overall increase in size, weight, any linear dimension, or more complex geometric index that reflects increased mass. The reader is familiar with comparisons like "animal A is *heavier* than animal B," "this individual is *taller* than that individual," "one animal is *fatter* than another," and so on.

It requires little analysis to appreciate that what is observed at the whole-body level is the integration of a host of growth processes taking place in the multitude of organ systems making up that individual. In turn, events at the organ level inevitably reflect the dynamics of the tissues and cells comprising them.

Growth of all of these tissues, in all but the very simplest of life forms, is asynchronic. Tissues do not all grow at the same time or at the same rate. Indeed, the progressive changes in body shape, introduced earlier as morphology, and familiar to everyone as correlates of aging, result from internal structural changes in an animal's body. Structural changes in turn usually relate to physiologic maturation. One organ or organ system may begin accelerated growth at a time when the growth of some other system may be decelerating or may even have ceased. Differential growth, along the lines of these examples, is called *development*.

The first section of this chapter is concerned

with the mechanisms influencing growth of cells. The second will describe the growth and development of major tissue types and organ systems:

bone, muscle, and **adipose tissue**. Finally, patterns of growth at the whole-body level will be described.

8.1 • The Cell Biology of Growth

General Terminology

Growth is defined as any increase in metabolically active protoplasm. Two fundamental components are the increase in cell number, or *proliferation,* and the increase in size of individual cells. The proliferation, or multiplication, of cells is technically described as *hyperplasia.* The antonym is *hypoplasia,* and cessation of proliferation is *aplasia.* Increased size, irrespective of proliferation, is called *hypertrophy;* the antonym is *atrophy,* or regression. Proliferation is always evidenced by significant numbers of the cells undergoing cell division and others that are actively synthesizing deoxyribonucleic acid (DNA). These are important aspects of the *cell cycle,* to be described in detail below.

A localized, abnormal increase in the number of cells, actively dividing and possibly having escaped normal control mechanisms, is called a *tumor.* Tumorigenesis, the process by which seemingly normal cells are transformed into cells that have escaped control, is a partly understood phenomenon and is of particular importance, not just because it helps explain aspects of cancer biology, but because it sheds light on control mechanisms that can be expected to underlie the normal growth process.

Mitosis and the Cell Cycle

Unless they have undergone specific *differentiation,* or specialization for a particular function that often coincidently limits their capacity for further division, cells can be regarded as potentially immortal. In other words, the nondescript cell can multiply repeatedly by a cycle of cell growth and cell division.

In the absence of extrinsic influences that might affect the genetic material, called *mutagens,* or that might trigger differentiation, every generation or crop of daughter cells is an exact copy of the original parent cell. Of course, the original cell ages and will deteriorate because the life support systems within that cell cannot preserve it indefinitely. The cell will progress through its life cycle and eventually die. Similarly, a group of nondifferentiated cells in a multicellular organism can survive no longer than the host animal, because the latter provides life support through virtually all of the mechanisms described in earlier chapters of this book. Even when such cells are removed from the complexity of the animal's body and maintained in cell culture in the laboratory, normal cells do not express the immortality noted above. Eventually under even ideal culture conditions the rate of multiplication dwindles, then ceases altogether. *Transformed* cells, on the other hand, can proliferate with ease. The **HeLa** cell lines are all ultimately derived from a human tumor taken from a patient some 40 years ago, and subsets of HeLa cells are used all over the world. The cells are also in frozen storage in countless laboratories and will probably be used in cell biology research indefinitely.

In the absence of a commitment to differentiation, the newly produced daughter cell enters the cell cycle as an interphase cell, depicted in Figure 8–1, in the **G₁,** or first gap phase. Certain growth factors influence the cell at this stage, prompting it to enter the **S** phase, or synthetic phase. The **S** phase is when most obvious growth of the cell occurs, and, more importantly, when DNA synthesis takes place to produce a dou-

bling of the initial complement of DNA in preparation for subsequent mitosis.

After another transient spell in **G₂,** the second gap phase, the mature cell proceeds into mitosis, or cell division. Mitosis occupies some 10% to 15% of the duration of the cell cycle and the whole cycle might recur as frequently as every few hours or as infrequently as once every several days or even weeks. In differentiated cells, the cell cycle may be interrupted almost totally, so mitoses may not be evident or may occur only very infrequently. In this case, at any one time only a very minor proportion of all cells might be engaged in mitotic events.

The individual stages of mitosis are readily classified as *prophase, metaphase, anaphase,* and *telophase* (see Figure 8–1) and are frequently subclassified into early, intermediate, and late por-

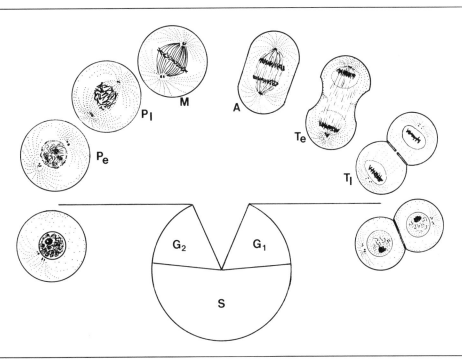

Figure 8–1. The cell cycle. Mitosis occupies a relatively small segment of the cell cycle. The stages of mitosis depicted here (described in detail in the text) begin with early prophase (P_e), and proceed through late prophase (P_l), metaphase (M), anaphase (A), early telophase (T_e), and late telophase (T_l), immediately before cytokinesis produces two daughter cells.

tions thereof. This finest level of description is not critical for present purposes.

The cell that is not presently engaged in mitosis is called *interphase*. Its activity during the **S** phase is highly anabolic, with DNA and protein being synthesized and organelle growth taking place. In **G₂** it is metabolically active, although anabolic and catabolic events are probably essentially in balance.

The interphase cell has a distinct nucleus bounded by a nuclear membrane, or envelope, described earlier as being a specialized portion of the endoplasmic reticulum. The nuclear contents include a *nucleolus* (plural, nucleoli) and indistinct *chromosomes* dispersed in the nucleoplasm. Peripheral to the nuclear membrane, one particular organelle of significance in mitosis is the *centrosome*, consisting of two *centrioles*. The remainder of the cytoplasm was described in Chapters 1 and 2 and needs no further description here.

Prophase is characterized by longitudinally doubled chromosomes, each pair of *chromatids* being joined at the *centromere*. During prophase, the two pairs of centrioles migrate toward opposite poles of the cell, and from each set is organized an *aster*, a radiating pattern of delicate intracellular fibers. In the diagram, prophase is shown at both an early to intermediate stage and then at the late stage. Earlier, the nucleolus disappears and the nuclear membrane disintegrates and is taken into the endoplasmic reticulum. The chromosomes are still partially indistinct. In late prophase, the pairs of chromosomes are quite obvious and are organized on another set of fibers forming between the two centrosomes. This structure is called the *spindle*. Each fiber is a microtubule made up of polymerized tubulin, noted earlier in relation to the cytoskeleton.

In metaphase, the chromosomes are still joined in pairs by their centromeres and are organized equatorially while still attached to the now very distinct spindle fibers.

During anaphase, the centromeres holding the pairs of chromatids together break down so that individual chromatids are free to separate as daughter chromosomes, each still firmly attached to a spindle fiber. The fibers draw the daughter chromosomes toward the centrosomes at either pole. Anaphase proceeds until the movement and polarization of the chromosomes is complete.

Telophase marks the beginning of a new nuclear envelope forming around each completely polarized set of chromosomes. The highly organized spindle disappears, although aster fibers are still apparent extending between the two centrosomes. Later, in telophase, nuclear morphology is more distinct, the chromosomes begin to uncoil, and nucleoli appear within the now completely formed nuclear envelope. The plasmalemma forms a deep furrow into the cytoplasm between the two nuclei and will eventually section the telophase cell into two daughter cells.

The term *karyokinesis* describes nuclear division, while *cytokinesis* describes the final division of the cell. There are occasional instances in which karyokinesis can occur without attendant cytokinesis, thus creating a binucleate condition: a *diplokaryocyte*. Such cells in the placenta of ruminant animals are known to be the source of placental lactogen (see Chapter 4).

The daughter cells resulting from normal cytokinesis contain equal amounts of nuclear material, one half of the total DNA complement present when the parent cell left **G₂** and entered prophase. Because the chromosomes are uncoiled and indistinct in the daughter cells, the fact that each is a single strand is not obvious. The material is replicated during the subsequent **S** phase. Each daughter cell has approximately one half of the cytoplasm and is approximately 0.7 to 0.8 of the diameter of the parent cell.

Control of Mitosis

The control of mitosis is really the control of cellular events during **G₁** when the daughter cell is either made competent to progress to the **S** phase to begin DNA synthesis or is committed to differentiation. The dogma that cell differentiation and cell proliferation are mutually exclusive processes is, however, oversimplistic because some differentiated cells are quite capable of further divisions. The nature of the trigger for differentiation is known in only very few instances, but in most of these cases, it involves exposure of the G_1 cell to one or more of the hormones described in Chapter 4. In addition, some nonhormonal regulators play a role. In the development of epithelium, for example, exposure to vitamin A at the appropriate stage of the cell cycle determines whether the cells differentiate to the keratinized form, as in skin, or become mucous epithelium.

The control that leads to a normal, nontransformed G_1 cell moving on to the S phase is less well understood. It now seems likely that several humoral signals are required and at least some of these regulators include the growth factors that were briefly mentioned in Chapter 4. One very important factor is called platelet-derived growth factor **(PDGF)**. Others, such as insulin-like growth factor I **(IGF-I)**, epidermal growth factor **(EGF)**, and other less well characterized factors, play critical roles before the cell can progress to the S phase of the cell cycle. Many of these regulators may be autocrines and may actually be produced by the same cells that will serve as targets for the growth factors.

The proliferation of many cell types under culture conditions is very sensitive to cell population density. At low densities, replication may be slow or nonexistent, while relatively high cell densities may be required for rapid growth. Growth factors produced by the cells themselves will be present in higher concentrations in the culture medium of high-density cultures. Addition of various growth factors to the medium used to culture cells at low density can cause a marked acceleration of proliferation.

Certain transformed cells seem to be less dependent on availability of these growth factors in the culture medium. In some cases these cells are known to produce abnormally large quantities of growth factors as a result of the transformation. In other cases, for example in some virus-infected cells, the viral genes are capable of coding the synthesis of the growth factors. Some tumorous cells proliferate rapidly because a portion of their DNA, called *oncogenes*, which are not expressed in normal cells but are in neoplastic cells, likewise code synthesis of these growth factors.

The discovery and detailed study of the growth factors has been aided enormously by the methods of cell biology, and this discipline has a very useful place in probing the mechanisms of growth. Equally important, and far more challenging, is the task of taking the information obtained by cell biologists and integrating it into the milieu of the whole animal.

8.2 • Growth of Bone, Muscle, and Adipose Tissue

Bone

Bone is a tissue that undergoes continual turnover by the combined processes of anabolism and catabolism. Anabolism, in the case of bone, is also called *apposition*, while the term *resorption* is applied to the catabolic events. Bone formation is the function of cells called *osteoblasts*. These cells secrete the organic matrix *osteoid* in various locations, and this matrix, consisting of glycosaminoglycans, collagens, and citric and ascorbic acids, is subsequently mineralized by deposition of salts, primarily calcium phosphate. Bone apposition occurs on surfaces such as already extant bone, under the periosteum, and in the cartilaginous matrix in the primary spongiosa of developing bones. The deposition of calcium apatite, the form of calcium phosphate in bone, occurs very promptly to quite a great extent and then continues very slowly until the process is completed. As the bone mineralizes, the osteoblasts become surrounded by mineral deposits and are then known as *osteocytes*.

The resorption of bone involves mobilization of both the mineral and organic components and occurs by means of two mechanisms. The less important process is called *osteoclasia* and is due to the action of specialized phagocytic cells with more than one nucleus, called *osteoclasts*. These cells are found mainly on surfaces, including partially modified bone at fracture locations. Far more important is the process called *osteolysis,* one of the functions of the osteocytes once they are deep within mineralized tissue. These cells serve to resorb mineral as part of the body's strategy for maintaining calcium homeostasis (Box 8–1), they cause changes in the complex carbohydrates of the matrix, and they can cause degradation of the collagen. It is emphasized that osteolysis occurs deep within formed

---

Box 8–1   Bone and Calcium Homeostasis

Bone is the depot tissue for the storage of calcium in the body and calcium homeostasis is intimately dependent on movement of calcium out of and into the mineralized tissues, to and from the extracellular fluids.

Parathyroid hormone and calcitonin provide most of the control of calcium fluxes between the depot and the plasma. The mechanisms were described in Chapter 4. To give the reader some idea of the magnitude of these fluxes, the values in Figure 8–2 indicate that for a mature cow with a skeletal reserve of about 7,000 gm of calcium, only about 8 to 9 gm is readily available in the extracellular fluids. When the animals are fed to maintain equilibrium conditions, approximately 1 gm/hour of Ca^{2+} could be absorbed from the gut, but this is virtually balanced by about 1 gm/hour moving in the opposite direction to leave in the feces. Fluxes to and from bone are also each about 1 gm/hour. In late pregnancy, the net accumulation in the fetus requires about 0.2 gm/hour, so minor changes in the efficiency of uptake from the gut or a small shift in the apposition-resorption equilibrium can easily accommodate this need. During lactation, however, the net additional requirement for milk synthesis is relatively enormous, of the order of 1 gm/hour. More substantial changes in calcium uptake from the gut or resorption from bone are needed or the readily available pool would be rapidly depleted.

The physiologic comfort range of calcium concentrations in the extracellular fluid is relatively narrow and even marginal hypocalcemia may cause neuromuscular disorders. The frequency of *parturient paresis,* or *milk fever,* a serious clinical condition due to severe hypocalcemia at or shortly after the initiation of milk secretion, attests to the difficulty of highly productive dairy animals having to suddenly make drastic changes in their calcium metabolism.

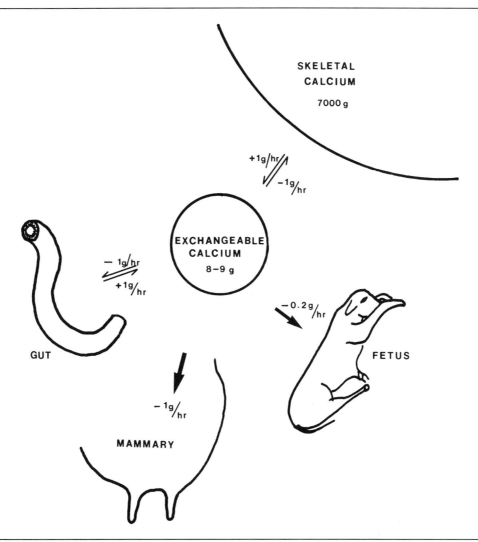

Figure 8–2. *Calcium fluxes in cattle.* A tiny proportion of the total calcium reserve of a mature animal is readily exchangeable. This represents the ionic form of calcium found in the fluid compartments. Of course, the exchangeable pool is buffered by bone apposition and resorption, and is subject to inputs and ouputs as shown here.

bone and is a totally normal process enabling bones to exhibit dynamic changes in structure and composition.

Bone Formation and the Growth of Bones

The processes of apposition and resorption underlie the formation of all bones, despite characteristic differences in bone form. In very immature states, such as during the first part of fetal life, there is no mineralized *(ossified)* tissue, and blocks of mesenchymal and connective tissue initially provide the supportive function. These nonossified structures may include cartilaginous rods, plates, and disks.

The rod-shaped cartilages will serve as *models*

for subsequent formation of long bones, such as those of the limbs. The disks are found along the dorsum of the fetus and will give rise to vertebrae. The structures visible in Figure 8–3 are cartilaginous models, with the very beginnings of ossification in sheep fetuses, in the first third of gestation.

The timing of ossification of the various bone models in the immature skeleton is a characteristic of development that varies remarkably little within a given species. The presence of mineral is detected by x-rays, and radiographic examination of a fetus can be used to age it with the precision of a day or so.

The growth and development of a long bone from its cartilaginous model involve *endochondral ossification*. The following description applies to a long bone, the mature form of which has a shaft region, or *diaphysis*, and head regions, or *epiphyses*, at either end (Figure 8–4). Mineralization is first evident in the central region of the solid cartilaginous model and proceeds centripetally from the peripheral surface until a solid core of bone is established (Figure 8–5). Ossification then occurs on either side of the core and gradually proceeds toward each end of the model. While this is taking place, the model itself is still growing because chondrocytes continue to proliferate and secrete cartilage matrix. In most instances, chondrocytes at either end of the ossified core and those located peripherally, between the core and the superficial periosteum, are dividing.

Secondary loci of ossification appear within the epiphyses and gradually result in the remaining cartilage forming a shell around the mineralized tissue and bands, or plates, between the diaphysis and the two epiphyses. These cartilaginous plates become the *epiphyseal growth plates* and serve as the loci of further cartilaginous proliferation and hence elongation of the developing bone until its mature size is reached. Around the peripheral surface of the epiphyses, another population of chondrocytes continues to divide. These initially provide for growth of the epiphyses and then continue to function by secreting materials for the maintenance of the articular cartilage.

Figure 8–3. Ontogeny of the ovine skeleton. Fetal sheep collected at Days 35, 38, 41, 43, and 49 (gestational age) were fixed and stained to highlight cartilaginous and ossified tissues. Soft tissues were rendered transparent before photography. Cartilage is lightly stained while the dark staining shows calcified early bone. Note the mandible and maxilla showing ossification at Day 35, progressive ossification in the long bones of the limbs, forelimb preceding hind limb, and the distinct pattern of membranous ossification of the cranial bones. (Photograph reproduced with permission from Martina Altschul, M.S. Thesis, Cornell University, 1987.)

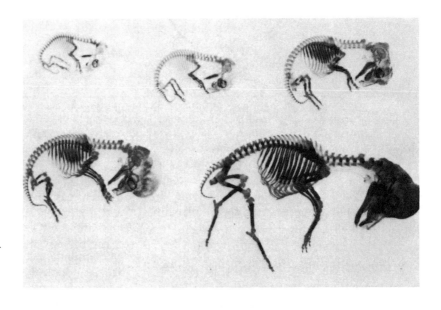

Figure 8–4. *Gross structure of a long bone.* This schematic diagram shows the relationships between the major parts of a "typical" long bone. Note the hollow nature of the diaphysis with its wall, or cortex, surrounding the marrow cavity. The external surface over the articulating epiphysis is composed of cartilage; the nonarticulating region is covered with periosteum.

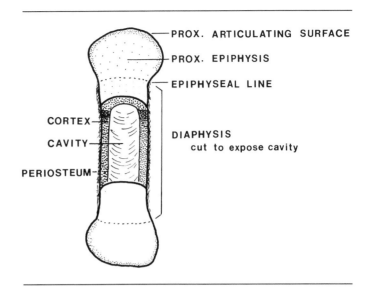

PROX. ARTICULATING SURFACE

PROX. EPIPHYSIS

EPIPHYSEAL LINE

CORTEX

CAVITY

PERIOSTEUM

DIAPHYSIS
cut to expose cavity

While elongation is taking place, bone that is already in place is undergoing remodeling by a combination of resorption and apposition. The resorption occurs centrally within the ossified shaft, while the continued apposition occurs peripherally, immediately under the periosteum where chondrocytes are still producing matrix. Continued resorption within the shaft eventually creates the cavity of the diaphysis. This will be invaded by blood vessels, reticuloendothelial

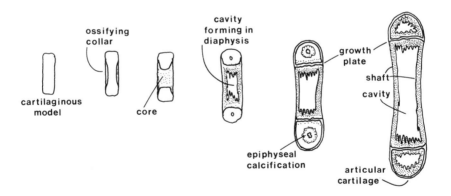

ossifying
collar

cavity
forming in
diaphysis

growth
plate

shaft

cavity

cartilaginous
model

core

epiphyseal
calcification

articular
cartilage

Figure 8–5. *Pattern of mineralization during growth of a long bone.* Initial ossification of the cartilaginous model is equatorial and takes the form of a collar. The solid core of calcified cartilage (shaded) next established is later remodeled with the formation of the shaft cavity. At later stages, ossification centers appear in the epiphyses, and the epiphyseal growth plate is discernible as a disc of proliferating cartilage, responsible for further longitudinal growth of the diaphysis. In the most mature form shown here, the bone has retained cartilage only in the growth plate and on the articulating surfaces. After closure, the growth plate cartilage disappears, although its prior location is discernible as the epiphyseal line.

cells, and connective tissue such as adipocytes to form the *bone marrow*.

Bone continues to be resorbed from the inner surface of the shaft wall and continues to form at the outer surface. This leads to an overall increase in shaft diameter and initially a thinning of the wall. Later, as there is continued accretion of mineral, the wall of the diaphysis will again thicken by accelerated apposition at the peripheral surface. This latter form of bone growth ensures increased mechanical strength without excessive weight.

The Growth Plate and Elongation of Bones

The epiphyseal growth plate is highly organized into zones with quite distinct features (Figure 8–6) and functions. Nomenclature varies somewhat, but the system adopted here uses terms that are meaningful with regard to function.

The *resting zone*, closest to the epiphysis and constituting about 20% of the total width of the plate, serves as the source of the progenitor cells, division and differentiation of which give rise to chondrocytes with distinct morphology. These differentiated cells assemble as stacks, or columns, and make up the *proliferative zone*, extending some 50% to 55% of the width of the plate. Cells in the proliferative zone are actively dividing despite their differentiated status, and they secrete chondroid matrix.

Most distal from the epiphysis is the *zone of hypertrophy*, sometimes called the degenerative zone, making up about 25% of the plate width. Cells in this region are noticeably enlarged and further distinguished by their substantial stores of glycogen and intracellular accumulation of calcium. At the distal margin, merely a couple of cells deep, calcium is actively extruded from the cells in vesicles that bud off from the plasmalemma. The calcium is used to mineralize the chondroid matrix as the first step in conversion of cartilage to bone.

The mineralized cartilage matrix is invaded by blood vessels and osteoblasts and the chondrocytes eventually disappear. Osteoblasts secrete osteoid then form bone, as described earlier. Further along in the metaphyseal region of

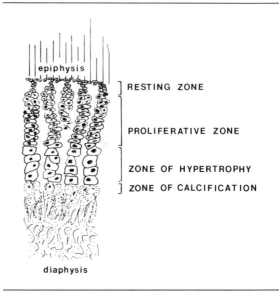

Figure 8–6. The epiphyseal growth plate. This diagram shows the various zones of an epiphyseal growth plate, labeled as described in the text. The relative widths of the zones are based on experimental data collected from the metacarpal plates of growing sheep (see Figure 8–13) by Dr. Anita Oberbauer at Cornell University.

the developing bone, residual chondroid matrix is completely removed by the action of osteocytes and the initial, nondense or "spongy" bone, called the *spongiosa*, is subsequently replaced with mature, dense bone. While it is a little difficult to grasp conceptually, the epiphyseal growth plate is progressively displaced, or grows away, from the diaphysis as additional mineralization occurs at the plate-metaphysis margin.

The process of growth at the plate continues until cells of the resting zone cease dividing and the supply of chondrocytes to the proliferative zone is arrested. The differentiated cells are finally consumed as the cells hypertrophy and then become incorporated into mineralized tissue of the spongiosa. The disappearance of the cartilaginous plate and its replacement with bone is called *closure*.

Despite intense investigation over a period of some 40 years, the nature of the hormonal control of cells of the epiphyseal growth plate is still very sketchy. Mitotic activity of cells of the resting zone seems to be growth hormone dependent and in large part under the control of the insulin-like growth factors, (IGFs) or somatomedins, noted above in relation to the cell cycle. Animals lacking growth hormone have narrow growth plates, largely devoid of mitotic activity. The first useful bioassay for growth hormone, developed in the 1930s, is based on the increase in tibial plate width in hypophysectomized rats after a few days of growth hormone replacement therapy. The somatomedins are also involved in control of the chondrocytes after they have differentiated. At least one of the peptides promotes the formation of sulfated matrix material, and this action has been the basis of one of the bioassays used to monitor concentrations of somatomedin.

Thyroid hormones are believed to be responsible for the control of differentiation of cells of the resting zone into those of the proliferative zone. Some evidence exists for the presence of a distinct chondrocyte growth factor, and insulin and glucocorticoid hormones exert nonspecific metabolic effects on the growth plate.

Androgens and estrogens are known to affect some aspects of plate function, probably by modulating the responsiveness of the cells to the other growth factors. Low-level exposure to androgens is stimulatory and thought to explain the "growth spurt" associated with early stages of puberty. High concentrations of androgens, and estrogens in some cases, may exert inhibitory actions on the growth plate, and such effects are popularly believed to be responsible for the cessation of linear growth that often occurs shortly after puberty. This analysis is not entirely satisfactory because many epiphyseal growth plates undergo closure long before puberty, even in castrate individuals. In some species, certain of the growth plates do not close until well after puberty.

Muscle

Skeletal muscle is the form of greatest interest in relation to growth. Muscle cells are very large,

highly organized, and multinucleated. Embryonic progenitor cells are called *myoblasts*. These uninucleate cells are spindle-shaped and not particularly large. The cells are capable of proliferation, and then numbers of them fuse together, producing *myotubes*, which subsequently become organized and adopt the cytologic features of mature *myocytes*. It seems that "environmental" factors determine when the myoblasts begin to aggregate into myotubes. For example, in cultured myoblasts in vitro, the density of the proliferating myoblasts is one factor. Under normal in vivo conditions, factors such as tension on the connective tissue associated with the developing muscle, perhaps as skeletal growth progressively distorts a structure such as a limb, may be equivalent to cell density changes during culture. Another possibility is that once the myoblasts have passed through some prespecified number of generations, capacity for further mitosis is lost.

Once myoblasts fuse into the syncytial form, the nuclei loose the capacity for DNA synthesis, so karyokinesis, or replication of nuclei, cannot be the reason why the mature myocytes are multinucleated. The myotube develops the densely organized myofilaments that characterize the internal structure of skeletal muscle cells and the nuclei are relocated peripherally, just under the sarcolemma. This mature form is called the myocyte, or *muscle fiber*. Muscle development requires ongoing growth of the fibers, well into postnatal life, and the cells are subjected to mechanical abuse by the very nature of their specialized function. There must be some provision for growth and replacement of myocytes that is not dependent on the myocytes themselves having to undergo mitosis; the latter is simply not possible.

Another population of cells, called *satellite* cells, is specialized for the ongoing provision of nuclei to be incorporated into existing myocytes. Mitosis therefore occurs outside of the myocyte, then further syncytial formation continues to deliver the nuclei into the highly differentiated myocyte. In addition to provision of new nuclei from outside, the muscle fiber is capable of impressive hypertrophy. Once again, physical or environmental factors are likely to be important and normal innervation by motor neurons plays a part. Muscle does hypertrophy with exercise, in the broadest possible sense of the word. The simple antigravity function of providing support for the body and the function of locomotion are stimuli for muscle development.

Numerous endocrine factors are believed to influence skeletal muscle development but surprisingly little detailed information is available. Many hormones with generalized anabolic functions, like growth hormone and insulin, and others with generalized metabolic actions, like thyroid hormones and cortisol, have effects on muscle. Many of these actions may be permissive rather than of direct regulatory importance and some may be very indirect. Growth hormone seems to act indirectly by virtue of stimulating production of IGFs. These peptides are capable of stimulating proliferation of myoblasts. Insulin is probably the major regulator of ongoing anabolism in muscle fibers and it is certainly important for general metabolic activity of the cells.

The gonadal steroids are involved in muscle development and anabolic effects of androgens are well known though poorly understood. In many other steroid-regulated systems, the steroids modulate responsiveness of tissues to other hormones by altering the receptor populations on the cells. At least part of the action of steroids on skeletal muscle is likely to be achieved in this manner. Steroids can also be expected to modulate the effectiveness of growth hormone in promoting synthesis of one of the IGFs, and they probably account for sex differences in the production of other growth factors.

Adipose Tissue

Adipose tissue, the principal depository of fat in animals, consists of morphologically distinct, or easily dissectible, depots along with diffuse populations of adipocytes in the marrow cavities and in association with the connective tissues in skeletal muscle. The major depots are located subcutaneously, on the surface of the mesentery, and around certain other viscera such as the heart and kidneys.

The adipocytes are of two types, *white* and *brown* (see Figure 1–9), and these have different cytologic features and metabolic functions. Adipose is a form of connective tissue, and the adipocytes are specialized, differentiated forms of fibrocyte-like progenitor cells. The factors responsible for triggering differentiation into adipocytes are unknown, but once differentiation has occurred, the cell is committed into its specialized function. Adipocytes in their mature form have very characteristic morphologies because of the fat locule, or multiple locules, in the case of brown fat. The ultimate appearance of the cells depends on just how much fat is being stored. A mature adipocyte with a large fat locule is not capable of further division, so changes in the extent of adipose tissue in the body reflect hypertrophic and atrophic changes. Brown fat depots, in the fetus and newborn, are capable of being replaced by white fat, and the latter form is the dominant type found in older domestic animals.

Maximal development of dissectible adipose tissue occurs relatively late in the overall life span, but fat begins to accumulate and fat depots are recognizable even in quite immature fetuses. Even before birth, the extent of adipose development reflects the metabolic status of the fetuses: newborns from undernourished mothers have less adipose and fat reserves than those from well-nourished mothers.

There are genetic factors that determine ultimate adiposity, as revealed by breed differences and the ability to select for leanness or obesity in strains of animals. It is still not clear if the genetic control is exerted on the mitotic events that contribute to proliferation of the preadipocytes—that is, control over hyperplasia—or if the final effect is obtained indirectly. For example, genetic factors influence metabolic rate and the efficiency of other anabolic and energy-consuming processes, and fat deposition could merely result from the use of the "leftovers" after nutrient requirements for the other processes have been satisfied. As in the case of other aspects of growth, genetic factors are likely to determine the potential for the growth of adipose tissue, but nongenetic factors will determine if this potential is realized.

8.3 • Patterns of Growth

The process of cell division, in which each generation of cells subsequently divides to double the number in the next generation, is the biologic basis for hyperplastic changes being potentially logarithmic. When the number of cells is plotted against time, a characteristic exponential curve (Figure 8–7) is obtained. If, on the other hand, the logarithm of number is plotted, a straight line results. It can be said that the data were *transformed* into logs before plotting, and various linearizing transformations such as this are of value in growth analyses.

For a variety of reasons, growth processes such as an increase in cell number usually do not proceed unconstrained in a purely exponential fashion as just described. Instead, the constraints cause a progressive deceleration of growth and give rise to *sigmoidal*, or **S**-shaped

Figure 8–7. Growth curves. These theoretical graphs plot growth against time. The ordinate in part *a* is cell number, and is shown to be increasing exponentially (that is, the number at each successive time interval is twice the previous number). In part *b*, the logarithm of number is plotted against time and a straight line is obtained. The taking of logs serves to "transform" the original observations into a form that is more conducive to numerical analysis.

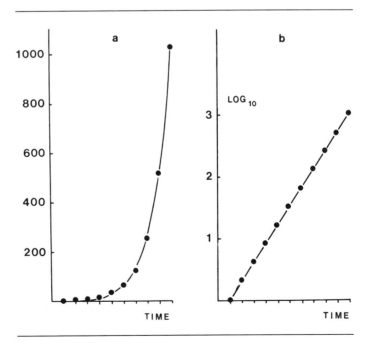

growth curves (Figure 8–8). From the general nature of this curve it can be seen that growth is initially slow, accelerates to a peak velocity, decelerates, and finally may cease altogether. When the curve shown in Figure 8–8 is differentiated to yield a new parameter, *growth velocity*, or change per unit time (the curve shown in Figure 8–9), is obtained. This form is useful in emphasizing that growth rate initially accelerates, reaches a maximum value, then decelerates.

These simple graphic representations can be applied to virtually all forms of growth, including the increase in cell number and the size and weight of tissues and organs, and finally can be used to describe changes in live weight of whole animals. The method obviously can be applied to both hyperplastic and hypertrophic events because a combination of the two is the basis for weight increase in animals. Simple sigmoidal

plots of the successive weighings of three animals, and the growth velocity curves, are shown in Figure 8–10. The curves in part show that the three animals reached the same target weight (in this case, the weight at which they were slaughtered) at different ages, so the rates of growth for each of the animals differed. Again, these differences are evident in the plots of growth velocity in Figure 8–10b.

Two descriptors of particular value in the analysis of growth of farm animals are mature body size and average growth rate. In Figure 8–10, body weights of the three animals were the same when they were slaughtered but if animal A had continued to fatten until animal C reached the arbitrarily determined slaughter weight, then, being older, it would undoubtedly have been heavier. Considered alone, weight is not a good criterion for mature body size because animals can continue to deposit fat far beyond a desirable level for efficient animal production. A more useful index for comparing mature body sizes of different animals or different breeds is obtained from mature skeletal size. This is readily determined by a simple geometric quantity such as height at the shoulder, the measurement of

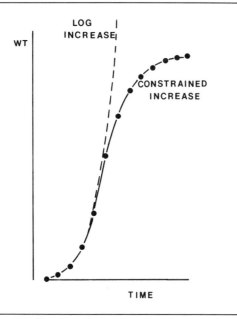

Figure 8–8. The sigmoid growth curve. After an initial exponential phase of growth, growth slows because of the influence of various constraints; the overall growth curve takes on an S-shaped, or sigmoid-shaped form. For most (but not all) species, growth will eventually cease altogether at what might be called the ultimate size.

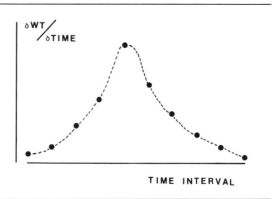

Figure 8–9. Growth velocity curve. When the sigmoid-shaped curve is differentiated with respect to time, the growth velocity or growth rate curve is obtained. Its general form shows clearly that growth rate is initially slow, increases to a maximum, then slows, and, if ultimate size is reached, will cease. The maximum rate of growth corresponds to the inflexion point of the sigmoidal curve (Figure 8–8).

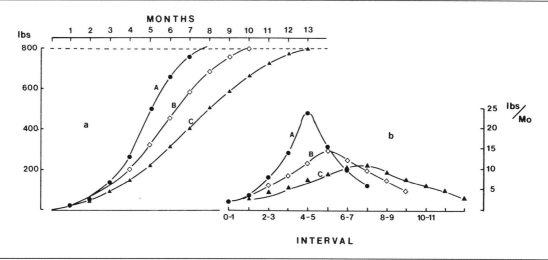

Figure 8-10. Growth velocity curves for three animals. *a:* Successive monthly weighings for three animals show striking differences in growth performance to the target weight, indicated by the dotted line at 800 lbs. Thus, the three animals reach this target at different ages. Average growth rate is greatest for A and least for C. *b:* The corresponding growth velocity curves emphasize the differences in maximal growth rate and the age at which this occurs.

which is not seriously affected by fatness. The same approach is used with bipeds such as ourselves; after adolescence, our height is far less variable than is our weight.

The reader might well ask why emphasis is placed on skeletal size when the skeletal organ system is essentially a waste product in the harvesting of meat products from animals. The most satisfactory answer stems from the relationship between muscle content and skeletal size: quite simply, animals of larger *frame* size yield more muscle in their carcass.

It was noted above that fattening can continue after mature skeletal size is obtained. Using the graphic analysis approach, one can compare the growth of component parts of animals, and one will quickly see that different organ systems grow at different times and at different rates at any given time. This phenomenon was described earlier as development. The following statements are gross generalizations about development of the major tissue types:

- The central nervous system (CNS) develops early. Indeed, mitotic activity is essentially completed by birth, and further expansion of nerves and individual neurons is mainly by hypertrophy of existing cells.

- Bone growth begins during fetal life, with the long bones developing quite extensively before birth. Many of the epiphyseal growth plates undergo closure before or about the time of birth, so further longitudinal growth of these particular bones is not possible. Some growth plates are still functional until around the time of puberty, or even later (for example, the humerus), so longitudinal growth does continue after the CNS has ceased growing.

- Muscle growth likewise begins during fetal life but the growth velocity curve is delayed slightly behind that of bone. Bone growth provides part of the stimulus for further muscle growth, and of course muscles hypertrophy with use. Finally, muscle growth may be markedly influenced by endocrine changes associated with puberty. The cessation of skeletal growth and a muscle growth spurt are both associated with puberty, so clearly the growth of these two organ systems must be asynchronic.

- The development of adipose tissue begins during fetal life, thereby accounting for the presence of brown fat in the newborn. However, major expansion of the adipose depots occurs only after the growth needs of other tissues have been satisfied. Thus, with marginally adequate nutrition, fat deposition will be unimpressive, while with nutrition greatly in excess of the anabolic needs of the other tissues, even young growing animals can be quite fat. Overall, adipose tissue deposition is most obvious after animals reach mature frame size and have acquired the bulk of their muscle tissue.

These generalizations, consistent with the growth curves shown in Figure 8–11 and the changing composition of the body resulting from development (see Figure 2–3), are important aspects to be considered in animal production. Use of this information in devising nutritional regimens, in considering ways of optimizing the economics of production, and in assessing the biologic consequences of manipulating growth represents much of the "science" of raising animals.

When the patterns of differential growth are integrated in considering whole-body development, some further generalizations are apparent. The consequences are most obvious in terms of morphologic development. For example, in Chapter 1 newborn animals were described as being "leggy." Superficially, overall growth is initially most obvious in the extremities: next, closer to the trunk; next, in the trunk itself; and finally in the loin area (Figure 8–12). In each region, bone growth precedes muscle growth, and fat deposition tends to occur last. In addition, bone growth is the dominant component in the extremities (early developing) while adi-

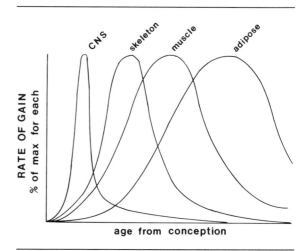

Figure 8–11. Differential growth of major tissues. This simple plot of the growth velocity curves for major tissue types shows that maximal rates of growth occur at different times (see also Figure 8–10). Notice that the curves overlap each other, indicating that, for at least part of life span, all of these tissues are undergoing growth. There is also a characteristic pattern of slowing and virtual cessation of growth of the different tissues.

pose tissue is dominant in the later developing areas, such as the loin and flanks.

As previously defined, morphology reflects underlying structure and function, so it is quite possible, though sometimes tedious, to derive the biologic basis for these patterns of development. A few examples will suffice for present description, but the reader can use this approach to consider practically any aspect of development.

The limb is concerned with support and locomotion. Distal portions are well developed at birth, and bones of the digits may have already undergone closure. Figure 8–13 shows an extensive set of data on the length of the left metacarpal obtained from intact males of two breeds of sheep at various ages. Length of the particular bone at birth was already 62% to 67% of its mature size, consistent with its rather distal location in the forelimb. Time of closure of the growth plates of major bones of the limb follows a pattern whereby the humerus and scapula, the most

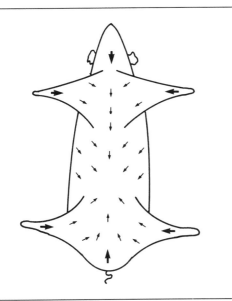

Figure 8–12. Waves of growth. This ventral view of a hog illustrates the notion of waves of growth. Growth is initially most obvious in the extremities, then closer to the trunk, and finally in the belly–loin region. A similar diagram could be constructed to indicate anterior dominance, as noted in the text. These patterns are evident in the photographs of immature sheep fetuses in Figure 8–3.

proximal of the bones, are the last to cease growing.

With consideration to function, bone weight may continue to increase after bone length ceases changing (Figure 8–13). Bone weight and density reflect mineral deposition and mechanical strength, so increases in these variables as animals increase in overall weight are quite consistent with the supportive function of the skeleton. The more distal muscles of the limb reach full size relatively early. In cloven-hooved animals, the distal portions are relatively immobile, so there is little need for continued growth of extensor-flexor and abductor-adductor pairs of muscles. More centrally, the major muscles providing extensor-flexor function for the whole limb continue to develop, as the work of locomotion increases with overall bodyweight increases. The same is true of the abductor-adductor pairs lo-

cated over the shoulder and brisket regions (see Chapter 1). In quadrupeds, the pectoral girdle and limb are more concerned in support of body weight than are the pelvis and hind limb, so the more cranial structures develop ahead of the more caudal parts.

In fattening animals, the most obvious morphologic consequences of fat deposition are apparent subcutaneously over the trunk and proximal limb regions. Deposition within the peritoneal cavity, on the mesentery, and in major pelvic depots near the kidneys leads to physical distension of the abdomen and flanks.

In addition to the foregoing general description, some aspects of growth and development are related to more specialized functional maturation. For example, growth of tissues and organs concerned with reproduction is very precisely synchronized to puberty. As noted earlier, puberty seems to be a factor involved in arresting longitudinal growth, but the mechanisms are not clearly understood. Although the skeleton of castrated animals may continue longitudinal growth beyond the time when this ceases in intact animals, certain of the growth plates are already closed by the time of puberty, and others do not close until long after puberty, even in intact animals. Nevertheless, certain bones reach enormous proportions in castrate animals compared to intact animals. For example, the mandible is usually much more massive in steers than in bulls. Bulls, however, may develop more extensive muscling over the pectoral region, and this is revealed by the depth from shoulder to brisket.

The relationship between skeletal growth and reproductive maturity might be explained teleologically if anabolic resources that could otherwise be consumed in continued growth were needed for optimal reproductive performance. This is most obvious in heifers bred as early as possible after puberty: in these animals growth is quite obviously retarded compared to that in similar animals not bred until much later. Puberty is usually delayed in animals grown under suboptimal conditions, and precocious puberty is often related to premature cessation of longitudinal growth. While the association be-

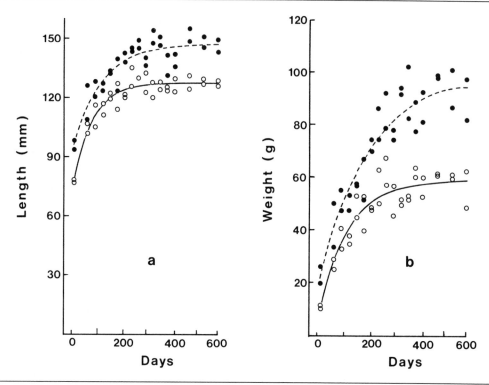

Figure 8–13. Growth patterns of the ovine cannon bone. Comparison of linear growth *(a)* and weight *(b)* of the metacarpals from birth to mature size in a large-framed breed (Suffolk, •----•) and in a medium-framed breed (Dorset, ○—○). The lines are computed from conventional exponential growth equations to best describe the overall changes with age. Note the distinct breed difference already apparent at birth and that length at birth is about 60% of mature length; ultimate length is attained by about nine months of age. In contrast, weight of the bones at birth is only about 20% of ultimate weight, the breed difference is more striking, and weight continues to increase after nine months of age. (Data replotted, with permission, from Dr. Anita Oberbauer, Ph.D. Thesis, Cornell University, 1985.)

tween the two is quite evident, precisely how growth and reproduction interact with each other is not known.

Factors Affecting Mature Size

Mature frame size is largely determined by the sequence of events occurring in the growth plates of the long bones. A cursory examination of an- imals quickly reveals very obvious differences between breeds, and the fact that selective breeding can change the gross morphologic characteristics of populations of animals indicates that mature size is genetically determined. One such difference is illustrated in Figure 8–13 with data on bone size in Suffolks, a breed of large mature frame size, and in Dorsets, a medium mature frame size breed. The metacarpal is already larger in Suffolk lambs at birth and its ultimate size, which is about 16% greater in Suffolks than in Dorsets, is reached at a later age.

It is more correct to state that genetic factors determine the potential mature frame size; whether or not this potential is realized reflects the interplay of a host of nongenetic factors. Growth biologists seek to understand how the genetic factors are expressed during development. If animals are optimally nourished and protected from parasites and environmental extremes, variability in growth performances may still be quite apparent. Selected hormones of the endocrine system are obvious candidates for mediating genetic controls over growth. A number of them, such as growth hormone, insulin, thyroid hormones, sex steroids, parathyroid hormone, and so forth, have effects on bone. With few exceptions, it has not been possible to link these endocrine factors together in any entirely satisfactory model for the control of bone growth. Even the striking exceptions such as dwarfism are seldom associated with a single endocrine deficit; hypopituitary dwarfism, due ostensibly to insufficient growth hormone, is also usually characterized by deficits in an array of other pituitary hormones.

One obvious correlate of mature frame size is age at puberty, as noted earlier. In a comparison of various breeds within a species or perhaps strains within a breed, it is generally found that animals with larger mature frame size reach puberty at later ages and at heavier body weight than do animals from smaller strains. Unfortunately this approach quickly becomes a "which comes first, the chicken or the egg?" dilemma.

Of more pragmatic concern in animal production is the minimizing of constraints that could prevent the genetic potential for growth from being realized. It is not well appreciated that growth retardation, for example because of malnutrition, has quite variable consequences, depending on the timing of the insult. For example, drastic undernutrition during the late fetal through weaning stages of development can lead to permanent stunting. In domestic herbivores, this is the period when the skeleton should be in its maximal growth velocity phase. Comparable undernutrition earlier or later, while perhaps delaying growth, may not have permanent or irreversible effects on mature body

size. Of course, the development of tissues other than bone may be compromised.

These manipulations, whether intentional or unavoidable, may involve qualitative as well as quantitative aspects of nutrition. A diet that in gross composition is totally adequate in energy, protein, vitamins, and so on but deficient in calcium available for assimilation may produce skeletal lesions that have long-lasting effects on development. Even more subtle would be the effect of a deficiency of the trace element iodine. Iodine deficiency produces hypothyroidism, which in turn delays bone development and maturation. If this occurs during fetal and early postnatal life, the effects may be long-lasting and not completely reversed by subsequent correction of the iodine status and the restoration of normal thyroid function.

Because of the relationship between frame size, rather than fatness or "finish," and muscle yield, efforts to increase the skeletal size of cattle have included the use of cross-breeding by exploiting the availability of semen from very large-framed European breeds of cattle. It has long been recognized that the genotype of the fetus is a factor determining birth size and that birth size is important in controlling mature size, in part for reasons described above.

In extreme examples of cross-breeding very large breed males with small frame size females, and vice versa, even though the fetuses have the same hybrid genotype, the offspring from small breed females (mated to large sires) are inevitably smaller than offspring from large-framed females (mated to small sires). The maternal environment provided for prenatal development obviously limits expression of the fetal genotype, and hence size at birth. In practice such extremes are avoided, but nevertheless the breeding of domestic range cattle with large European breeds of cattle, mature bulls of which may approach 1,500 kg live weight, has resulted in widespread calving difficulties, calf and dam morbidity and mortality. Based on the analysis provided earlier, the domestic cattle reach puberty relatively early and at smaller body size than heifers of the large European breeds. Their mature size, and with this their pelvic geometry, is obviously smaller, and the frequency of calving difficulties when delivering the larger crossbred fetuses is understandably increased.

Summary of Tissue and Whole-Body Growth

- Growth patterns in animals reflect the sequence of development of the major tissue types in accordance with functional development.

- Of the principal carcass components, bone reaches its maximum growth velocity before muscle, and adipose tissue develops last.

- Overall growth of the extremities precedes that of the trunk.

- Mature frame size, reflecting longitudinal skeletal development, determines in part the extent of the muscle mass and in turn is genetically determined, as is evident from gross differences between breeds.

- The frame size of an individual is constrained by various nongenetic factors. These factors have greatest effect when they operate during the period of maximal rate of bone growth; that is, prior to weaning.

- Growth is related in a complex manner to reproductive maturation, with longitudinal frame growth ceasing shortly after the time of puberty. Both intact and castrate animals continue other forms of growth after the equivalent of puberty, but the bodies assume different morphologies.

- Animals that reach puberty at relatively young ages tend to be of smaller mature frame size than those that reach puberty at later ages.

8.4 • Exercises

1. Supply the correct term for each of the following blanks:

A _____ growth curve reflects an initial exponential increase to a maximal rate of change followed by a decelerating rate, to a plateau ultimate size.

Hypertrophy is an increase in the size of individual cells without any need for cell _____ .

A _____ transformation converts cells that behave normally into rapidly dividing cells that have escaped normal control mechanisms.

_____ ossification gives rise to the formation and growth of long bones.

The term _____ is used to describe replacement of the epiphyseal growth plate by bone.

2. Identify the stage of the cell cycle at which controls determine if a cell goes on to divide further or takes on specialized features of a differentiated cell.

3. Identify one substance that satisfies the definition of being a *growth factor:* _____ .

Identify one substance known to trigger differentiation: _____ .

4. Define *bone* and *bones* in a single unambiguous statement.

5. A myocyte may be described as *syncytial*. What does this mean, and how does this condition arise?

6. Longitudinal growth of long bones is essentially complete by or shortly after puberty, but individual bones within a limb cease linear growth at different times. From the general principles of patterns of growth, indicate the likely sequence of linear growth arrest among the following bones:

      Metacarpals   Humerus   Radius

7. Using a relatively common disorder of parturient dairy cows as an example, outline a simple explanation *in terms that any intelligent layperson could understand* of the basis for considering bone as a dynamic tissue.

8. What is the basis for claiming that the potential for *adiposity* is genetically determined?

9. Identify the stage of the life cycle when severe nutritional deprivation will have most striking and lasting effects on development of the central nervous system. Consider the implications of this answer in relation to the global inequities in food availability.

10. What are the two mechanisms of growth at the cellular level? Which of these most adequately describes the ongoing process of erythropoiesis? Where does this last-mentioned process take place in adults?

11. Attempt to synthesize an explanation for the pattern of weight increase in an animal that has reached mature frame size and is gaining weight at progressively slower rates. Use the following "facts":

1. Fat deposition is energetically expensive.
2. Total body muscle is related to skeletal size.
3. Fat deposition rate is maximal after that of muscle.

Stress and Defense Mechanisms

9

Most of the material presented so far in this book has been concerned with the structural and mechanistic basis for normal animal function. The emphasis has been placed on fundamental chemical and physical principles that permit close monitoring and protection of the stability of the internal environment. Some examples of major breakdowns of the normal mechanisms have been described. In most cases the disturbances represented pathologies that stemmed not from any infectious disease vector but rather from inappropriate operation of an otherwise normal physiologic mechanism. Such pathologies reflect serious departures from homeostatic regulation.

9.1 • Stress, Adaptation, Homeorhesis, and Pathogenesis

The general concepts of homeostasis have been illustrated for a variety of physiologic variables. For example, in Chapter 5 a variety of mechanisms that regulate blood gas status were integrated as we saw how the cardiovascular, respiratory, and renal systems cooperate with each other to achieve a common objective.

The first introduction of homeostasis, in

Chapter 2, described the shortcomings of the notion of an absolutely constant steady state. The concept of a *physiologic comfort zone* was offered as an alternative. Physiologic variables can take any value within the comfort zone without invoking compensatory reactions. When a variable is perturbed to the extent that it moves out of the comfort zone, compensatory mechanisms come into play, and the variable is brought back toward a steady-state value. These adjustments are quite normal and pose no great threat or challenge to the animal's body.

When physiologic variables are greatly disturbed, however, the animal is *stressed,* and much greater effort is required to offset and correct the change. Animals then invoke more vigorous compensatory and protective mechanisms to restore stability of their internal environment because, if correction is not attempted or is unsuccessful, a *pathophysiologic* state can develop. In extreme cases, these deleterious changes in certain critical variables can be life-threatening and may actually cause death.

In stress, animals divert their resources so that the corrective mechanisms receive priority. Other activities, such as the productive functions so important in animal agriculture— growth, fiber production, reproduction, and lactation—are compromised until the stress is alleviated. For example, a heat-stressed animal will seek shade to minimize solar radiant heat gain. It is also likely to stop eating. This is partly because foraging activity is curtailed in favor of staying in the shade. Additionally, the heat production associated with the activity of foraging, digesting, and absorbing nutrients is also minimized. When intake of feed is reduced, most energy-consuming processes, particularly growth and milk production, which are energetically expensive, will be curtailed.

Animals under stress cannot be expected to perform optimally.

Stress often provokes a reasonably consistent series of reactions or responses by the animal. In the early analyses, some 50 years ago, emphasis was placed on the "fight or flight"

responses, a euphemism for profound activation of the sympathetic nervous system. The responses included emergency cardiovascular and respiratory adjustments such as increased ventilation rate, tachycardia, elevated arterial pressure, and redistribution of blood flow from cutaneous and visceral tissues to favor perfusion of skeletal muscle. Additionally, sympathetic discharge, including increased secretion of adrenal medullary hormones, provokes hyperglycemia because of mobilization of hepatic glycogen reserves.

The hypothalamo-pituitary-adrenal cortex axis (see Chapter 4) is activated and the resulting hypercortisolism prevails for the duration of the imposed stress. Elevated concentrations of cortisol favor hyperglycemia, partly because glucocorticoids play a role in gluconeogenic processes and also because they antagonize glucose utilization in many tissues. Glucose is therefore "spared" for use in critical tissues of immediate importance in life-threatening situations.

With sustained stress, animals frequently show *adaptation* and may make adjustments in a variety of physiologic systems so that homeostatic mechanisms again become effective in stabilizing the internal environment. Adaptation is a well-recognized though poorly understood phenomenon. It can relate to physiologic stressors such as inclement ambient temperatures; to social pressures such as the introduction of several new animals into a herd and the removal of young at weaning; and to environmental challenges, as are often imposed in animal management, such as confinement, isolation, and restricted mobility. Typical behavior patterns associated with acute distress and discomfort quickly change as adaptation takes place. Persistence of certain behaviors almost certainly signals a failure in adaptation.

Some adaptations can be analyzed without difficulty. One adaptation to cold ambient temperatures is the development of a coat, which increases insulation by providing a layer of still air adjacent to the skin. Other adaptations are far more complex and involve disease resistance, the immune system, and poorly understood genetic factors. For example, certain strains of pigs are virtually devoid of adaptability to nonspecific stressors and they are poorly tolerant of environmental pressures.

Even seemingly normal physiologic states such as pregnancy and lactation, which impose metabolic pressure on highly productive animals, usually trigger adaptive changes. The simplest response to the increased energy expenditure associated with pregnancy and lactation is increased appetite; this may be an adaptation to processes that otherwise would cause negative energy balance.

There is increasing interest in a different form of physiologic adjustment that, like adaptation, seems to operate on a chronic time scale. The author and his colleague, Dr. D. E. Bauman, have proposed that the term *homeorhesis* be used to describe a form of physiologic regulation that permits major alterations in how animals expend their metabolic resources, particularly when shifting between distinct physiologic states. Homeostatic mechanisms are still operative and important for acute maintenance of the internal milieu but, in addition, homeorhetic mechanisms provide for coordination and direction of metabolic activities in an "umbrella" fashion. This type of regulation can likely be achieved in many different ways, but endocrine interactions such as synergism and antagonism, introduced in Chapter 4, are likely to be most important.

Many of the marked changes in the efficiency of productive processes provoked by long-term administration of exogenous growth hormone to domestic animals can be best explained in this way. For example, the development of nonadipose tissues is favored in growth hormone–treated animals. Highly purified growth hormone, while not lipolytic in the manner of catecholamines and glucagon, nevertheless opposes the accumulation of energy reserves in adipocytes. This could be achieved by antagonizing the lipogenic action of insulin in this tissue. It could also arise from increased use of nutrients in tissues such as muscle at the expense of the alternative use for lipogenesis.

When lactating cows are treated chronically with growth hormone, milk production increases and the increased energy requirements stimulate intake of nutrients. The overhead cost of maintenance of the animal is now supporting increased productivity, hence the efficiency of production is greater.

One of the actions of glucocorticoids—antagonism of peripheral utilization of glucose to make otherwise limiting amounts of glucose available for high priority use—corresponds to a homeorhetic type of regulation. Chronic hypertension, described earlier in Box 5–8, is also a result of this type of regulation, because all usual homeostatic regulators of arterial blood pressure are functioning, but the setpoints and the comfort range for pressure are chronically adjusted upward. In some situations the comfort range for certain physiologic variables is widened, thereby reducing the requirement for rigid control.

This conceptual approach to physiologic regulation is still controversial because it is nontraditional and involves mechanisms that are not purely *compensatory*, as homeostatic mechanisms are (see Chapter 2). Experimental physiology is heavily biased toward acute mechanisms and regulation, and little effort has been devoted to elucidating the control of physiologic processes that operate over days, months, and even years. Some adaptive mechanisms have chronic time bases of a similar order but these are inevitably of a compensatory nature. The remaining chapters of this book consider a number of control systems that are *anticipatory* rather than compensatory in nature.

The Animal-Environment Interface

Animals are well protected from the environment at large by the amazing integumentary organ system, the *skin*. The skin protects animals from dehydration and protects soft underlying tissues from mechanical damage because of its toughness and flexibility. It is a very effective barrier against invasion by microorganisms that could otherwise establish themselves, to the detriment of the animal, within the soft tissues. Though less obvious than in the case of the skin, the entire epithelial covering of the exposed surfaces serves in this pivotal protective function. The linings of the airways, the digestive tract, the urinary and reproductive tracts, and so forth, are all potential loci for invasion of the internal tissues.

The protective surface tissue barriers are not, however, entirely effective, and backup defense mechanisms are necessary to protect the animal in case of failure of this first line of defense. Obvious examples of invasion are attacks by biting and stinging insects, lacerations of the skin, burns and abrasions, and colonization of the skin by fungi. Once the integrity of the skin is compromised by any of the preceding insults, sec-

ondary infections by bacteria can result, so the animal body has developed effective *isolating* strategies, physiologic versions of *biologic warfare* to deal with the invaders, and *healing* mechanisms to repair damaged structures (see Section 9.3).

The skin also serves as the major interface between the internal milieu of the animal and the strikingly variable external environment. The next section describes the mechanisms used by animals to protect the thermal stability of the internal environment in face of fluctuations in ambient, or environmental, temperature. The material is an extension of the fundamentals of metabolism and energetics introduced in Chapter 7 and provides real-world applications of the cardiovascular and respiratory mechanisms that were described in Chapter 5.

9.2 • Thermoregulatory Mechanisms

A complete analysis of interactions between animals and their environment involves consideration of metabolism, homeostasis, homeorhesis, climatology, thermodynamics, behavior, stress, and adaptation. The subdiscipline called *thermoregulatory physiology* attempts to deal with all of these aspects. Some ways in which animals satisfy their homeostatic drives in the face of thermal challenges and potential abuses from the environment will be highlighted. The discussion is intentionally selective and merely touches on factors to be considered when assessing animal functions under widely differing climatic conditions.

Heat production is an inevitable part of catabolism. The highly efficient oxidation of glucose to carbon dioxide, water, and salavageable

energy in the form of adenosine triphosphate (ATP) still results in about 50% energy loss as heat. This seemingly inefficient conversion of chemical energy from nutrients into heat production is nevertheless essential for homeotherms that are attempting to maintain deep body, or *core*, temperatures in the broad range of 35 to 40 C. Excessive heat produced is lost to the environment, so that core temperature can be closely regulated. However, some heat loss from animals is obligatory, especially in colder, less humid environments. This need for heat generation must be considered in the energy economy of animals. At a practical level, this aspect is factored into the design of animal housing and in formulating rations to meet the nutritive requirements of livestock.

Heat Exchanges

Animals lose heat to the environment through two basic mechanisms: *sensible* and *insensible*. Sensible heat loss occurs when thermal energy is directly transferred through the physical processes of *radiation, conduction,* and *convection*. Insensible or evaporative losses occur when thermal energy is used to change the physical state of water by *evaporation,* or *vaporization*. Many animals are able to *sweat,* thereby secreting aqueous solutions onto the skin surface, from which evaporation can take place. Sweating is regulated centrally by what is known as *sudomotor* control. Other animals achieve the same result by wetting their surface by *wallowing*. Additional insensible heat loss occurs because inspired air is brought to saturation by the evaporation of water off mucosal surfaces in the buccal and nasal cavities, and the trachea.

Sensible Exchanges

Radiation, which can cause both heat loss and heat gain, is the transfer of heat by electromagnetic waves without appreciable heating of the space between the emitter and absorber. This mechanism is the basis for the warming effect of the sun, either directly or with the benefit of reflection. This also occurs during the winter, even though air temperatures are quite cold. Numerous factors affect radiant heat transfer, and some generalization is needed. Radiant heat losses or gains are proportional to temperature raised to the power of 4, proportional to available surface area and therefore to surface texture, and depend on color. Radiation exchanges occur more readily to and from dark, matte surfaces than to and from shiny, light-colored surfaces. For example, a rough-coated, dull black steer will radiate more heat on a cold night than will a sleek, white-coated animal of the same size. Conversely, the latter animal will be less embarrassed by heat gain on a hot sunny day in summer.

Conduction is the physical flowing of heat energy through a *conductor* from one object at a higher temperature to another at a lower temperature. The extent of heat transfer varies with (1) *temperature differential,* (2) the area of contact, or cross-sectional area of the conductor, (3) the *conductivity* of the conductor, and (4) the distance separating the hotter and cooler objects. The reader will note the similarity to the factors governing electrical flow, described by Ohm's law (see Chapter 3), and those determining blood flow, described by Poiseuille's equation (see Chapter 5). These all describe flows through a conducting system, driven by some pressure or potential.

Biologic tissues are fairly good conductors despite the claim that "a good thick layer of fat protects one against the cold." For example, the conductivity of adipose tissue is about 16 times higher than that of air. Muscle and skin, with higher water contents, are about 30 times more conductive than air. Conductive losses may be very high when animals are confined in metal cages under barn conditions where ambient temperatures may be low and opportunity for contact with the conductor is high, especially in expanded metal cages (for instance, sanitary calf crates). There is also much opportunity for conductive losses in trucking containers and crates that are constructed of metal. Metal cages and crates are certainly more easily cleaned and sanitized than are those constructed of wood, but the welfare of the animals is better served by the poorer conducting materials.

Convective losses involve heat transfer to a flowing medium, usually air for animals, where the flow, for example wind, breeze, or even imperceptible air currents, provides a continuous heat gradient from the animal's skin to the environment at large. Convective losses are proportional to the square root of the velocity of air movement and the area of the surface over which the flow occurs. It will be noted later that convective losses from animals are somewhat reduced by a *still layer* of air, held close to the surface of the animal. Air trapped within the fibers of the coat serves to insulate the animal, especially from convective losses.

Insensible (Evaporative) Exchanges

Evaporative heat loss results from the latent heat of vaporization of water which consumes heat from the wetted surface. The main factor influencing evaporative loss is the relative humidity of the air into which the evaporation is occurring, and the ease with which the water-saturated air layer can move away from the source and out into the environment at large. The energy consumption is specified by the latent heat of vaporization, as noted in Chapter 2.

Relative Importance to Animals of These Physical Processes

It is difficult to place firm estimates on the relative importance of each of the major processes for the thermal stability of animals, but it is possible to construct quite precise heat balances for given situations. In general terms; *evaporative losses are usually more important than convective and radiant losses, which are about equal, and conductive losses are the least important.*

An exception to this, noted earlier, would be the use of expanded metal crates on trucks and in cold barns. Another situation in which conductive losses are high, accounting for about 20% of total heat loss, occurs when pigs are fed liquid dairy byproducts such as whey, obtained as a byproduct from cheesemaking. The liquid is warmed up from ambient temperature to core temperature within the digestive tract, using heat from the animal. The cost is exaggerated if the feed source has been refrigerated and is fed without prior warming.

The importance of evaporative loss varies among animals, depending on their ability to pant, sweat, or wallow. Panting increases respiratory heat loss, and some animals, such as pigs, cannot sweat because their sweat glands are essentially nonfunctional. Wallowing is a behavioral trick of coating the exterior with water or mud and allowing evaporation to remove body heat. Similar behavioral mechanisms have evolved in the kangaroo, which liberally coats its tail with saliva, and the elephant, which sprays water over its body.

Rate of Metabolism

Homeostatic mechanisms, described in detail below, enable animals to have significant short-term control over heat production and loss. Other anticipatory mechanisms operate in the long term and include the development and later shedding of a winter coat, laying down more subcutaneous fat before the winter, and so on. Although the controls that trigger these mechanisms are poorly understood, they help animals to exist in harmony with their changing thermal environment.

Heat production, or metabolic rate, bears a complex relationship to ambient temperature. At quite cold temperatures heat production is maximal and is called *summit metabolism*. At warmer, more comfortable temperatures metabolic rate decreases and is quite stable over a specified range, called the *thermoneutral zone* of ambient temperatures. Under resting conditions within the thermoneutral zone, the animal exhibits basal metabolism. Basal metabolic rate can be described in terms of joules expended, or indirectly in terms of oxygen consumption rate (see Chapter 7). Heat production then paradoxically increases at hot temperatures. At the temperature extremes, death can occur from *hypothermia*, or inadequate body temperature, or *hyperthermia*, or excessive body temperature.

There is a relatively narrow range of ambient temperatures, only about 10 C in width, where core temperature can be held constant without adjusting metabolic rate. This range of ambient temperatures is the thermoneutral zone. Note that this is ambient temperature, not the core temperature of the animal. The latter is much more strictly controlled and can vary only by a degree or two before stress conditions apply.

The upper and lower limits of the thermoneutral zone are called the *upper critical temperature* and the *lower critical temperature*. Again, it is emphasized that these limit temperatures are descriptive of the environment, or ambient temperature. They do not define the temperatures enclosing the homeostatic range of core temperatures within the animal.

Beyond these limits of ambient temperatures, metabolic energy must be expended by the animal in order to maintain core temperature within the homeostatic range. The general relationship between metabolic rate and ambient temperature is shown in Figure 9–1. In the cold, it seems reasonable that an animal increases its metabolic rate and heat production to offset obligatory losses to the environment. The adaptations above the upper critical temperatures are more complex. First, as core temperature increases, metabolic processes accelerate because of what is called the Q_{10} effect. This term, used

widely in bioenergetics, describes the doubling of the rates of chemical processes, including metabolic rate, that occurs for each increase of 10 C in temperature. More important physiologically is the energy expended in futile but often heroic attempts to lose excess body heat. For example, there is substantial energy expenditure, and therefore heat production, associated with the "heat-losing" processes of sweating and panting. This can give rise to positive feedback effects on body temperature, but only under extreme conditions. The resulting hyperthermia is an extreme, often irreversible stress

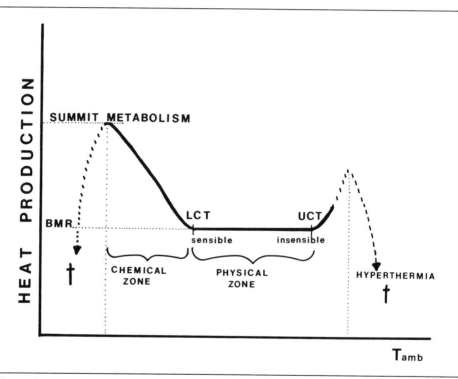

Figure 9–1. Metabolic rate and the thermal comfort zone. The thermal comfort zone is the range of ambient temperatures (T_{amb}) between a lower and upper critical temperature (LCT and UCT, respectively) over which the animal maintains core temperature without adjusting its heat production or rate of metabolism. This level of metabolism is called the Basal Metabolic Rate (BMR). Metabolism increases outside of these ambient temperature limits and, at extremes, death can occur from hypothermia or hyperthermia. Within the comfort zone, thermoregulation is achieved by sensible and insensible mechanisms, largely determining the extent by which body heat is lost to the environment. This is called the physical zone for thermoregulation. At lower environmental temperatures, thermoregulation is achieved by increased metabolic heat production within the chemical zone. The maximal rate of heat production is called summit metabolism.

that becomes terminal and causes death. Death can result from permanent damage to critical tissues, such as the brain, caused by overheating. In this case, death is secondary to an overall loss of physiologic competence.

There is widespread ignorance about the values of critical temperatures. The data in Table 9–1 may give the reader some surprises.

These values are important for several reasons. It is human nature to consider that comfortable temperatures for people should be comfortable temperatures for animals also. As a result, animals are often exposed to temperatures that exceed their upper critical temperatures, and the potential exists for them to become heat stressed. Conversely, in conditions of extreme cold, man's attempts to provide animals with an environment that is pleasing to humans are likely to have deleterious consequences: ventilation is often insufficient, humidity becomes excessive, and animals are made vulnerable to respiratory ailments. With minimal appreciation of animals' comfort ranges, these errors in management can be avoided. Temperatures that seem cold to humans often lie within the thermoneutral zone for large domestic ruminants.

Table 9–1. Lower Critical Temperatures in Selected Animals

Animal	Lower Critical Temperature
Newborn piglet	35 C
Young pig less than 20 kg	19 C
Pig less than 60 kg	15 C
Young calf	13 C
Adult cattle at maintenance	6 C
Cattle gaining at 1 kg/day	−7 C
Cow producing average milk yield	−20 C
Newborn lamb of small size with wet coat	38 C
Adult sheep with 5 cm wool at maintenance	−5 C
Adult sheep at full feeding	−18 C

In contrast, if ambient temperatures are below the lower critical temperature, animals simply expend additional energy just to maintain thermal homeostasis. Within reasonable limits of cold, the adaptations are within the flexibility of the animal's normal function and, provided the animals have adequate feed available, there is no harm done and no stress imposed. These considerations should be a normal part of the decision-making on the provision of housing, shade, shelter, ventilation, and adequate nutrition for animals.

The extremes in the critical temperature values make general recommendations about housing and maintenance feeding levels very hazardous, but the numbers give some guidelines for reasonable management relative to the physiologic flexibility of the animals. Consider the newborn piglet with a lower critical temperature of 35 C. Virtually all year 'round, the newborn pig must expend energy by increasing its metabolic rate to keep warm. It does so even on the hottest summer day!

The baby pig is disadvantaged by its small size, its relatively long, thin body, and therefore its large surface area relative to mass. The animal lacks a coat of any significance and has minimal amounts of subcutaneous fat. If the animal is not quickly dried after birth and protected from drafts, this cold stress will be increased considerably. The piglet generates the needed heat to maintain its core temperature by a combination of shivering and thermogenesis, initially using energy reserves present in its body at birth such as glycogen and its sparse supply of brown fat, and later by oxidizing nutrients obtained from its first feed after birth.

On the other hand, an adult ruminant can maintain core temperature with relative ease at quite severe sub-zero temperatures. The animal's maintenance requirements for diet do, however, increase in the cold. For example, the maintenance requirement of a 60-kg sheep with a 5-cm fleece would double if the animal were shorn to nakedness. The maintenance requirement would increase a further 50% if the shorn animal were exposed to a 10 mph wind. If additional feed is not made available, the animal will curtail energy-consuming productive processes to the extent of the deficit. If feed is still inadequate, the animal will mobilize stored reserves of adipose tissue and oxidize them for energy. It is not difficult to appreciate that the cold burden may then become worse as the insulating value of the fat is diminished. Animals can and do die from cold exposure because of the scenario just described.

On the other hand, when feed is available, shearing an animal will stimulate its appetite, largely for the reasons noted above, and there are situations, such as during late pregnancy, when the increased intake of nutrients actually improves the level of productive function. If high-quality forage is available and the animal is stimulated to increase intake of feed, its requirement for heat production may be quite adequately satisfied by oxidation of acetate. Increased production of glucose by gluconeogenesis of propionate, also absorbed during the digestion of high-quality feed, and the greater availability of amino acids from such feeds may be very efficiently used for the benefit of the fetuses.

Because management efforts are directed toward providing thermoneutral conditions for animals whenever possible, reactions to gross extremes in environmental conditions are of less immediate concern. We will now consider the thermoregulatory mechanisms that are commonly used to fine-tune deep body, or core, temperatures, under normal conditions.

It is appropriate to reiterate the principle that metabolism inevitably results in heat production because of the inherent inefficiency of catabolism. Additionally, the mere process of digestion results in heat production because of the number of active events that utilize energy (see Chapter 7).

Regulation of Core Temperature

In the thermoneutral zone, animals invoke regulatory mechanisms to balance heat production against losses without appreciably altering their metabolic rate. This is often called *physical* regulation, and it is dominated by control of sen-

sible losses at cooler temperatures, with evaporative heat loss being dominant in the warmer range. By contrast, the main function of mechanisms called into play when ambient temperature drops below the lower critical point is to increase heat production.

Most of the control over sensible loss is achieved by varying the insulative properties of tissues or the layers between the core and the environment at large. One obvious mechanism is *piloerection*. This is an elevation of the body hairs to trap a thin, insulative layer of air on the skin surface. This maneuver is not especially effective, but the long-term adaptation to cold by increasing the length and density of the coat layer is important. The major adjustment made acutely is regulation of blood flow to the surface. These *vasomotor* controls are under hypothalamic control, and they enable highly selective redistribution of blood flow, to or away from the skin. Control of cutaneous blood flow is greatest at the extremities and least effective close to the core.

When an animal is acutely exposed to cold, skin temperature over the spine might decrease to 17 to 18 C, while it may be as low as 5 to 6 C at the foot or lower legs.

Potential hazard exists on skin that is in contact with freezing surfaces, such as the paw of a dog when it is standing on ice. A process called *vasomotion* provides for cyclical changes in cutaneous blood flow to periodically warm the tissue and so prevent damage from frostbite. The mechanisms do not sustain high cutaneous flow because this would lead to excessive conductive heat loss. Instead, flow is typically minimized except for brief episodes of increased flow, which protect the tissue from freezing. These cycles vary in length for different species and different locations within an animal. The process, which could be called *cyclical cold-induced vasodilation*, is mainly under the control of local vasodilators, such as the bradykinins, that were first encountered in Chapter 5. Locally produced vasodilators have the advantage of locally adjusting blood flow according to need. Cold-exposed animals may have skin temperatures that fluctuate between 5 C and 17 C. In the ear, the cycle might have a periodicity of about 10 minutes, while the same range of temperatures may be achieved with a periodicity of 60 minutes or more in the lower leg.

Another vascular mechanism that effectively controls the thermal gradient from the core to the surface depends on the classic engineering principle of countercurrent exchange. Aquatic mammals have perfected this mechanism to minimize excessive heat loss from their fins. In terrestrial mammals there is more limited use of the countercurrent mechanism but these animals have greater ability to control blood flow through the appropriate vascular structures when thermoregulating near the lower critical temperature. The principle is very simple (Figure 9–2). Arterial blood is pumped radially outward and transfers its heat on the way to the cooler venous blood, which is flowing radially inward, in close proximity to the artery. Heat flows down the thermal gradient from artery to vein. The arterial blood is cooled by transferring heat to the venous blood flowing in the opposite direction; the venous blood is warmed. The arterial blood is therefore cooled substantially below core temperatures before it reaches the sur-

face. This simple anatomic mechanism is about 85% efficient in conserving blood heat in the major trunk vessels.

At the upper end of the thermoneutral zone, most of the control over heat loss is achieved by the regulation of evaporative mechanisms.

Sudomotor control regulates sweating rate; respiratory control regulates panting.

While sharing some features, such as the obvious consumption of heat to change the physical state of water, there are important differences between these two mechanisms. Sweat contains cations, anions, and organic compounds. Salt loss occurs with sweating, and salt appetite will therefore increase. Panting results in a loss only of water, so it causes no salt deficit. It has one potentially serious side effect, though. Hyperventilation causes respiratory alkalosis and could result in respiratory, circulatory, and neuromuscular disturbances. Panting entails very rapid and shallow breathing that causes air movement mainly in the mouth, trachea, and bronchi, without much increase in the turnover

Figure 9–2. Countercurrent heat exchange. Arterial blood passing out to the extremities is cooled by transfer of heat to the closely adjacent veins carrying cooler blood back to the core. The temperatures shown here for illustrative purposes demonstrate the gradient, always from artery to vein, along a length of a countercurrent system. This anatomical arrangement is remarkably efficient in conserving core heat.

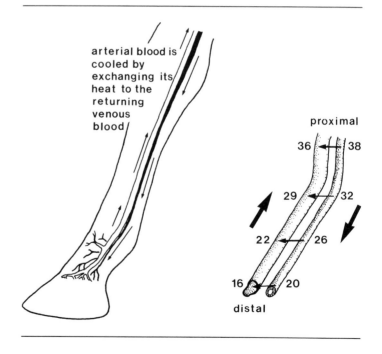

of alveolar air. Indeed, the drive to pant during heat stress completely overrides any suppressant effect on the respiratory centers that might result from mild alkalosis.

As noted earlier, animals respond to environmental temperatures outside the thermoneutral range by increasing their rates of metabolism. From the lower critical temperature down to the point where summit metabolism is achieved, body temperature can be maintained. Several mechanisms are involved, of which shivering is the most obvious.

Shivering is an involuntary muscular activity that is remarkably efficient in generating heat, despite the slight increase in convective heat loss that results from the quite obvious movement of the surface. A widely distributed series of small skeletal muscles lying immediately under the skin is twitched at high frequency, as reflected in the minor tremor-type movements of the overlying skin. About 50% of the heat generated by this contractile activity is conserved, compared to a mere 10% to 15% of the heat that is generated by vigorous exercise.

Vigorous limb and trunk movement in the cold causes tremendous convective heat loss from the skin and may chill skin temperature so much that cold-induced vasodilation is invoked to prevent skin damage. The flushed appearance that is common under these conditions reflects vasodilation and increased cutaneous blood flow. This in turn causes accelerated surface heat loss and accounts for the thermoregulatory inefficiency of such activity, compared to shivering.

An alternative heat-generating mechanism is repeated isometric tensing of muscles, which is almost as efficient as shivering. This is not simply a voluntary exercise but a quite normal reflex response to an abrupt *cold shock*. More usually, this type of effort can only be sustained by voluntary control, and fatigue usually occurs quickly.

If for some reason heat production is increased in one animal relative to another, the former will have its lower critical temperature reduced. As noted in Chapter 7, heat production in the thermoneutral zone, or basal metabolic rate (BMR), varies between species and between individuals within a species. Similarly, animals with high feed intake such as those producing high yields of milk, those in late pregnancy, or those in maximal growth phases have elevated heat production and so can tolerate colder ambient temperatures. On the other hand, they also have a reduced upper critical temperature, so they are more vulnerable to heat stress. The same general relationships hold true for humans, in whom a wide range of BMR can exist and so a similar range of comfort zones can be expected.

Physiologic Regulation of Heat Production and Loss

The control of core body temperature, or thermoregulation, has short-term and long-term, or acclimation, aspects. Acute thermoregulatory responses can be modeled quite closely on the systems used to thermoregulate a building (Figure 9–3). In the mammalian system, a wide variety of reflex mechanisms controls the heat-producing, or *thermogenic*, and heat-losing, or *thermolytic*, processes. There is an endocrine component, principally that of the hypothalamo-pituitary-thyroid axis controlling the influence of thermogenic thyroid hormones such as triiodothyronine. As noted in Chapter 4, when excessive thyroid stimulation occurs, as in *thyrotoxicosis*, there is excessive calorigenesis. In the normal situation, thermoregulation is achieved by hypothalamic mechanisms.

Body temperatures exceeding the upper physiologic limit of the comfort range activate temperature-sensitive cells in the hypothalamus. Such cells function as the body's thermostat. Cold reception is achieved by temperature-sensitive cells distributed peripherally, in skin, in the viscera, and in the mucous membranes, along with similar cells thought to be located within the spinal cord.

Afferent signals from the thermoreceptors are integrated within the hypothalamus. Groups of neurons called nuclei in the anterior hypo-

Figure 9–3. Heating and cooling control systems. The upper figure is a schematic control system for regulating room air temperature by either heat input or heat removal, under the control of a thermostat. The lower figure shows the physiological equivalent. Blood temperature, rather than air temperature, is the quantity monitored by receptors and is subject to heat producing (thermogenic) or losing (thermolytic) mechanisms.

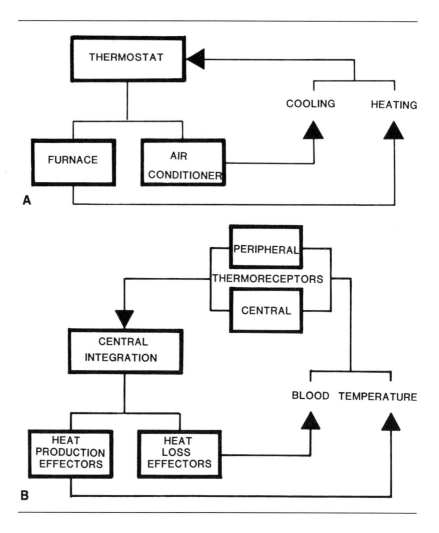

thalamus initiate and control the body's responses to excessive core temperature. A distinct set of neurons in the posterior hypothalamus controls responses to cold.

The efferent responses from the hypothalamus are mediated mainly by the thoracolumbar division of the autonomic nervous system. Responses to cold include decreased heat loss, achieved by sympathetic control over peripheral blood flow, especially that to the skin, and by a generalized piloerection. Additionally, heat-producing mechanisms are activated, and these include shivering and nonshivering thermogenesis.

Shivering and piloerection usually occur to-gether and involve cutaneous muscle structures: piloerection is achieved by contracting isolated smooth muscles that alter the orientation of hair, and shivering involves small subcutaneous skeletal muscles. Nonshivering thermogenesis describes metabolically generated heat such as that produced by brown fat, especially in the cold-stressed neonate.

The responses to heat include increased loss of body heat and decreased heat production. Increased heat loss is achieved by redistributing cardiac output to the periphery and by vasodilation of the skin vessels. Additionally, sudomotor activity under sympathetic control recruits evaporative mechanisms. Behavioral mechanisms are also initiated such as wallowing and other voluntary acts to increase evaporative losses. There is a reduction in heat production resulting from appetite depression and thereby reduced metabolic calorigenesis. It is presumably no coincidence that the hypothalamus is involved in both the regulation of body temperature and the control of appetite.

Acclimation and Long-Term Controls

The process of acclimation starts with an acute response to the environmental change, then gradual changes start to occur. These take various forms. For example, the adaptive changes alter the location of the physiologic comfort zone, meaning that the setpoints for heat-producing or heat-losing mechanisms could move to different temperatures. Changes such as these correspond to the notion of homeorhesis, introduced in the preceding section. The changes might alter the level of intake or the efficiency of use of feed by the animal. For example, during cold exposure, the acute responses would be piloerection and shivering. Gradually, heat production from nonshivering thermogenesis takes over. In some cases the oxidation of nutritive fuels is made less efficient than normal. Energy is transferred to the form of heat rather than being incorporated into bond energy in ATP.

Brown fat is also known as thermogenic fat. In contrast to normal white fat, with its large single lipid droplet dominating the interior of the cell, brown fat cells are richly endowed with mitochondria and the fat is present in numerous small droplets. Hormone-sensitive lipases, responding to epinephrine, norepinephrine, and to a lesser extent glucagon, promote lipolysis to convert the storage triglycerides into glycerol and nonesterified fatty acids. These fatty acids in brown adipocytes are then completely oxidized by beta-oxidation by the mitochondria in the cells. The fatty acids are not exported from the cells

for use elsewhere, which is what happens after lipolysis in normal fat. During the oxidative events, little ATP is generated, but enormous amounts of heat are released. The heat is picked up by the blood passing through this tissue, and then distributed to the body tissues.

Blood flow is increased in brown fat during thermogenesis so that sufficient oxygen is provided and the heat generated can be efficiently carried away. The increase in blood flow, or *hyperemia*, could easily be achieved by locally acting controls that were introduced in Chapter 5. For example, the metabolic activity of the tissue consumes enormous amounts of oxygen and produces both carbon dioxide and heat. All of these factors increase tissue blood flow.

Experimentally, nonshivering thermogenesis can be observed in animals with elevated oxygen consumption, despite being prevented from shivering by paralysis. The indirect calorimetric approach that measures oxygen consumption and/or carbon dioxide production is used to study this form of heat production.

The third stage of acclimation will usually involve increased appetite and intake, assuming that feed is available. Eventually, changes may be observed in coat thickness and possibly in the thickness of subcutaneous adipose tissue. A fully acclimated animal may have responded to chronic hormonal controls and have acquired the ability to increase its level of summit metabolism. All of these changes, considered together, mean that the animal has shifted its zone of thermoneutrality and has become more cold tolerant.

A high priority is placed on maintenance of thermal stability of the internal environment in the face of environmental abuses. This is exactly what physiologic regulation is all about.

Sometimes the environmental pressures are too great and some species have adapted by becoming more tolerant of variation in body temperature. This means that their homeostatic comfort zone is wider in range than is normally the case. The camel has this perfected and hence is superbly adapted to its desert environment, where night temperatures can be very cold and days exceedingly hot.

Specialized mechanisms may exist to protect the most "heat-sensitive" tissues at the expense of other less fastidious organs. For example, a countercurrent-type vascular cooling system protects the brain from excessive blood temperatures in some species (Box 9–1). The spermatogenic function of the testes (see Chapter 10) is protected in most species by the testes being suspended outside of the body cavity, where they are maintained at a cooler temperature than the body core temperature.

Summary of Thermoregulation

The foregoing material is not simply an exposition of the incredible versatility that physiologic systems confer on complex animals; it also has very obvious practical significance. Several aspects of thermoregulatory physiology have relevance in animal husbandry:

- The calf in a metal "sanitary" crate;

- The newborn piglet, potentially cold stressed at 35 C;

- A black steer radiating more heat than a white animal;

- The high-producing cow being very cold tolerant yet readily heat stressed;

- An explanation for the affinity of pigs to a mud-bath;

- A case for warming a liquid diet before offering it as feed;

- A rationale for the increased appetite in sheep after being shorn;

- The reason why a panting dog does not need extra salt.

Most importantly, an analysis of thermoregulation in its various forms requires consideration of a wide array of physiologic support systems that together act harmoniously in maintaining homeostasis. The discussion has provided examples of mechanisms of central integration of sensory inputs, control of numerous autonomic systems, hormonal control mechanism, the cardiovascular, respiratory, and digestive systems, metabolism, salt balance, and aspects of animal behavior.

Box 9–1   The Carotid Rete

In some species, especially the herbivores that evolved in ecosystems in which they were the prey of carnivores, the brain is protected from hyperthermia by a specialized countercurrent cooling system. At the arterial input at the base of the brain, the artery branches into a complex meshlike set of vessels enclosed in a venous sinus called the *carotid rete*. This structure is located close to the roof of the nasal sinuses and pharynx. Thermal exchange to venous blood, or to the airways, takes place so the arterial blood is precooled before it passes on to the brain. Heat-stressed sheep can maintain brain temperature within 0.5 C of normal even though the temperature of their aortic blood may be as much as 6 C above normal core temperature during extreme exercise. This form of exchange is, of course, aided by the fact that during such exercise, the rate of respiration is greater, so there is more air flow across the exchange surface and venous blood in the sinus is cooler.

9.3 • Reactions to Injury

Inflammation

Many forms of injury provoke a relatively uniform series of reactions by the animal's body. The most important response is *inflammation*. This serves to isolate and destroy noxious agents, to clean up damaged tissue, and to prepare the tissue for healing. Central to inflammatory reactions is the part played by vasoactive substances such as histamine, serotonin, and bradykinin, all of which have been described in previous chapters. By way of introduction, the following description applies to the reactions following a cutaneous injury.

After an immediate vasoconstriction, to guard against hemorrhage at the site of injury, a phase of vasodilation follows. This causes the redness and warmth that are frequently noted at injury sites. Thereafter capillary permeability increases, so plasma and often cells are exuded from the vessels to cause local swelling, or edema. Usually, the swelling caused by accumulation of interstitial fluid stimulates sensory nerve endings and gives rise to the sensation of dull, persistent pain. Bradykinins and prostaglandins are also responsible for sensitizing the pain-receptive nerve endings.

In very severe cutaneous injuries, as in third-degree burns, the sensory nerves themselves are destroyed, so, paradoxically, there may be very little pain sensation despite the massive trauma to the skin.

Cellular Responses

The leukocytes, or white blood cells, emigrate from the capillaries by squeezing through between the endothelial cells to accumulate in the interstitial space at the site of injury. The leukocytes are a complex family of blood cells, some further details of which are provided in Table 9–2. The data are provided for the purposes of illustration and the reader is not expected to learn specific details from the table. It now appears that the motility of some of the leukocytes and control of the direction of their migration is brought about by chemical "attractants" and the process of activating the leukocytes is called *chemotaxis*. Some chemotactic molecules are derived from invading microorganisms, some are endocrine in nature, and one class of paracrines includes *inflammatory proteins,* derived from the blood at the site of the injury.

The leukocyte invasion of damaged tissue leads quickly to *phagocytosis*, particularly by the monocytes and the polymorphonuclear leukocytes (PMNs), or neutrophils. These cells engulf foreign particles, such as bacteria, after extending pseudopodia out to surround the object. The particle is then incorporated into a vesicle that is enclosed within plasmalemma from the leukocyte and the invaginated vesicle attracts, then adheres to, lysosomes present within the leukocyte. The lysosome's complement of hydrolytic enzymes then proceeds to digest the engulfed particle, thereby neutralizing any threat it may have posed. In addition, hydrogen peroxide (H_2O_2) is generated and this is an extremely potent microbiocide. When the leukocyte has completed its task, it dies and the fluid residues accumulate at the site of conflict as *pus.*

With time, the pus is reabsorbed by the nearby tissues, or if a capsule forms around the damaged tissue, the pus may be extruded to the surface, as in an abscess. Gradually the exudate, either from the initial edematous reaction or from pus, dries and contributes to the formation of a scab. Epidermal cells begin to migrate into the scab from the periphery and from under the dry scab to reestablish a complete cell barrier. Subepidermal tissues are replaced or repaired, connective tissue and collagen fibrils are laid down

Table 9–2. Distribution of White Blood Cells

Species	Total (×10⁶/mL)	Neutrophils[a] (%)	Lymphocytes[b] (%)	Monocytes[b] (%)	Eosinophils (%)	Basophils (%)
Pigs	15–22	30–35	55–60	5–6	2–5	<1
Horses	8–11	50–60	30–40	5–6	2–5	<1
Cattle	7–10	25–30	60–65	5	2–5	<1
Sheep	7–10	25–30	60–65	5	2–5	<1
Goats	8–12	35–40	50–55	5	2–5	<1
Dogs	9–13	65–70	20–25	5	2–5	<1
Cats	10–15	55–60	30–35	5	2–5	<1
Chickens	20–30	25–30	55–60	10	3–8	1–4
Humans	7	50–70	20–40	2–8	1–4	<1

Compiled from Swenson M.J.: *Duke's Physiology of Domestic Animals*, 9th ed. Ithaca, N.Y.: Cornell University Press, 1977; and Vander A.J., Sherman J.H., Luciano D.S.: *Human Physiology: The Mechanisms of Body Function*. New York: McGraw-Hill Book Co., Inc., 1980.
[a]Polymorphonuclear leukocytes (PMNs).
[b]Agranulocytes.

to support the new skin, and new blood vessels invade the tissue. These specific cellular events are controlled by a multitude of growth factors, similar to the somatomedins (see Chapter 4). There is solid evidence supporting the existence of *endothelial growth factor* and *epidermal growth factor*. The former stimulates proliferation of endothelial cells and their organization into new capillary networks. The latter is a powerful stimulant of epithelial cell proliferation and so is a likely candidate for controlling the healing process and perhaps the formation of scar tissue.

The reactions to tissue damage as just described are obviously *cell mediated*, they are rapid in onset, and are relatively short-lived. The great advantage of these mechanisms arises from their nonspecificity. Essentially the same process of inflammation, cell migration, and tissue replacement occurs irrespective of the form of the initial insult.

The most frequently encountered and economically most important inflammatory condition in animal agriculture is *mastitis*, or inflammation of the mammary gland. The anatomy of the gland and the nature of the secretion it produces predispose this organ to infection. Bac-

teria gaining access to the lumen via the streak canal (see Chapter 11) multiply rapidly in the milk present in the gland. For example, if an organism has a doubling time of 20 minutes (that is, 1 becomes 2 in 20 minutes, 4 by 40 minutes, and 8 by 60 minutes), then a single organism, if allowed to multiply without constraint, can give rise to more than 1 billion (<2³⁰) organisms in about 10 hours. Of course, some of the organisms die during this period and the chemotactic substances released from them provoke a massive influx of leukocytes from the cow's blood into the gland.

The leukocytes engage in phagocytosis and may eliminate the infection completely. With wholesale phagocytosis taking place, the gland becomes palpably turgid, or "hard," warmer than usual, and is described as *inflamed*. Cell wall components released from certain types of bacteria may have systematic actions in the cow. These may include fever, tachycardia, shallowing of respiration, and concurrent sweating and shivering. These reactions constitute *toxemia*. Local tissue damage, some tissue sloughing, and bleeding into the gland lumen can occur.

Neutrophils are normal constituents of milk,

reflecting their continuous low-level emigration from the circulation into the lumen of the gland. An extremely high number of these cells in milk is indicative of inflammation and therefore infection. However, the efficacy of the neutrophils in protecting the gland from infection indicates that a certain population of the cells, even in the complete absence of infection, must be regarded as beneficial.

The Immune Response

Animals have yet another line of defense that has unique properties and incredible power to protect the integrity of the internal environment. Study of the immune system, or immunology, has progressed rapidly to the extent that it has budded off as a distinct discipline area. It is of great importance in animal health, and knowledgeable use of immune biology certainly has a major place in modern animal management.

Substances that are foreign to an animal are often capable of initiating an immune response when they are introduced to that animal. The substance is first recognized as foreign, or *non-self*, by cells of the lymphoid system, and a complex series of reactions is set in motion, often leading to the production of *antibodies* by the immunized animal. Substances that are capable of evoking an immune response are called *immunogens*. These can be isolated molecules, or molecular components of foreign cells. There is a tendency for larger molecules to be more effective immunogens than smaller molecules. For example, large proteins, especially the glycoproteins, initiate antibody production more readily than do very small peptides. Complex carbohydrates and lipids are also potent immunogens, so it is no surprise that the plasmalemma of foreign cells, or the cell wall substances of microorganisms, may be quite immunogenic.

Small molecules that are not intrinsically immunogenic can be chemically coupled to larger molecules to make artificial immunogens. This has enabled the raising of antibodies to an infinitely large array of substances and has permitted the development of powerful research and diagnostic reagents that exploit the unique properties of antibodies (see Box 9–2).

When the inflammatory response was described earlier, it was indicated that leukocytes invaded the site of damage or infection. These cells then proceed to engulf damaged cells and foreign particles. After performing their task, these cells die and in turn may be phagocytosed by macrophages, cells derived from the monocytes of the white blood cell population. A portion of the cells and partially processed foreign substance is picked up by the lymphatic drainage from the injury site and transported to lymph nodes. The nodes are aggregations of lymphoid tissues, consisting of reticuloendothelial cells located at strategic sites in the paths taken by lymphatics on their way back to the great veins. Some of these lymphatic trunks were described in Chapter 6.

There are additional specialized lymphoid tissues such as the *thymus* in the neck, the *spleen* adjacent to the stomach, the *tonsils* in the pharynx, and a major form in the *marrow* of the long bones. As lymph flows toward the major veins, it passes through the lymph nodes where opportunity exists for the leukocytes containing foreign immunogens to be filtered off and retained in the node.

One class of leukocytes, the *lymphocytes*, are especially important in mounting the immune reaction. In the simplest possible terms, lymphocytes after appropriate stimulation become programmed to produce a class of proteins that are collectively called *antibodies*. These are globulin molecules that can be further classified into forms that react with soluble antigens, with cells, and so on. Antibodies are capable of incredible selectivity in their binding so that one or just a few very similar molecules are recognized by the antibody, while others are ignored. For example, by means of hapten immunization, as described in Box 9–2, antibodies prepared to react with estradiol-17β may be 50,000-fold selective for this steroid versus the closely related estra-

Box 9–2   Hapten Immunization and Immunoassays

Small molecules, while usually not immunogenic in their native form, can be engineered to elicit antibody production by chemically coupling the small molecule to a large protein so that antibodies are raised against the whole complex. In this strategy, some of the antibodies will be capable of recognizing the small molecule, or *hapten*. This technique has been a powerful tool in the experimental preparation of antibodies against molecules such as steroids, drug compounds, and so forth, for use in the powerful analytical methods known as *immunoassays*. The great specificity of an antibody for the immunogen against which it was raised, and the very high affinity of binding between the two, is the basis for such assays. They take various forms.

In immunohistochemistry, thin sections of tissue are exposed to the antibody under conditions where the antibody molecules can bind to the corresponding immunogens present within the tissue. The bound antibody is then visualized by any of several methods at the light or electron microscopic level. Another form of immunoassay is called *radioimmunoassay* because radioisotopically labeled immunogens are used to quantify the amount of the immunogen of interest, usually in biologic fluids. These laboratory methods have provided most of what is known about normal and pathologic changes in the concentrations of hormones in man and domestic animals. For example, with these immunologic methods it is quite feasible to quantify picogram (10^{-12} gm) amounts of steroid hormones in plasma and solid tissues.

diol-17α. The only difference between the two steroids is that the 17-hydroxyl group stands up above the plane of the molecule in one case and is held down below the plane of the molecule in the other.

The binding between antibody and antigen can be extremely tight so that once bound there is virtually no chance that the antigen will ever dissociate and be freed. In some cases, after antibodies have attached to the surface of cells to which they have been raised, other serum proteins are attracted to the complex and can lead to a complex of events finally resulting in lysis of the foreign cell.

Immune reactions often involve the participation of a phenomenon that is a little like memory. After primary immunization and an initial transient phase of antibody production, the capacity exists to rapidly mount a more vigorous antibody response should the animal be subsequently challenged with more antigen. In some cases the subsequent exposure to the antigen can be delayed for years without compromising this ability, so some form of memory exists and is passed on to daughter cells of the original lymphoid cells. Presumably, specific portions of the DNA of the lymphoid cell have been switched on, or programmed, to code the RNAs controlling synthesis of particular globulin antibody molecules.

A given lymphocyte, once activated into synthesizing antibody, produces a single form of the globulin molecule and no others. This great specificity and memory has been exploited during the last decade in the technology of producing monoclonal antibodies (Box 9–3).

Immunization may, in some cases, make use of very small and therefore noninfectious doses of a live organism, or the infectious agent, be it a bacterium or a virus, may be killed before it is used. The surface characteristics are still present in the dead microbe and these are the compo-

Box 9–3   Monoclonal Antibodies

The recently developed technique of *monoclonal antibody* production depends on the specificity of immune reactions, coupled with virtually unlimited cell division potential of certain cancerous lymph cells. Antibody-producing lymphocytes are harvested from the spleens of immunized but otherwise normal mice and are fused in vitro to tumorous lymphocytes to make hybrid cells, called *hybridomas.* Lines of cells called *clones* are then developed from single

hybridomas. Clones that generate desirable types of antibodies are selected and proliferated. The specificity of antibody type is passed on from the parent lymphocyte, while the capacity for rapid cell proliferation is obtained from the cancer cell. These artificially constructed hybridomas can be multiplied, virtually infinitely, either in vitro in cell culture or in vivo in other mice, and large quantities of a single molecular type of antibody can be prepared.

nents in a vaccine that elicit the antibody response.

Passive Immunization

Very young animals of many species lack the ability to make antibodies. In some cases, antibodies of maternal origin cross the placenta into the fetal blood, so the fetus becomes *passively immunized* and uses these maternally derived antibodies until its own immune system is functional. Such transfer across the placenta is not always possible, so other species use *neonatal passive immunization.* Antibody molecules produced in the dam accumulate in the first mammary secretions, the *colostrum,* as will be described in Chapter 11. The intake of colostrum by the newborn animal is particularly important because, for a brief period after birth, antibody globulins escape peptic hydrolysis in the stomach and the intact proteins can be absorbed by pinocytosis from the small intestine (see Chapter 6). This ability is quickly lost, within at most a day or two after birth, as a new population of intestinal epithelial cells becomes established. Additionally, peptic digestion is established within a day or so after birth and from that time the globulins in milk are digested. The antibodies acquired passively from placental or colostral

transfer remain effective in the recipient animal for several weeks, until full immune competence in the young has become established.

Miscellaneous Immune Phenomena

Similar processes to those described above underlie the phenomena of transfusion reactions, transplantation rejection, and immune reactions to tumors. Occasionally the ability to distinguish between non-self and self breaks down, and antibodies may be raised against endogenous body constituents. This is called autoimmunity, and it accounts for the pathogenesis of a number of diseases and is likely to be part of the mechanism of physiologic deterioration that accompanies aging. In Chapter 4, a couple of endocrine diseases were described as having an autoimmune basis. In the case of *autoimmune thyrotoxicosis,* antibodies raised against thyroid tissue include globulins that are capable of binding to and activating the thyroid-stimulating hormone receptor. In this condition, the thyroid is excessively stimulated and normal feedback control mechanisms cannot function. In some forms of *diabetes,* antibodies bind to and block the insulin receptor and prevent activation of the target tissue by insulin, thereby causing *insulin-resistant diabetes.*

9.4 • Exercises

1.   Select an item from the left column that logically relates to one from the right. In the space provided, note the basis for your choice.

Epinephrine	Immunogen
Heat conservation	Fatty acid oxidation
Hapten	Countercurrent flow
Ketogenesis	Heat production
Thermogenic fat	Hormone-sensitive lipase

Choice 1. _____

_____

Choice 2. _____

_____

Choice 3. _____

_____

Choice 4. _____

_____

Choice 5. _____

_____

2.   a. What generic term is used to describe a substance that is capable of eliciting antibody production?

   b. True or false: Monoclonal antibodies are made by hybridomas which are unusual cells because they occur exclusively in leukemic animals.

   c. True of false: Passive immunization describes antibody production by animals without use of a vaccine.

   d. True or false: Autoimmunity describes the condition where antibodies are raised against self rather than just against non-self.

3.   Label the following heat exchange processes as being examples of either *sensible* or *insensible* mechanisms:

A dark-colored beast radiating heat to a clear, cold, night sky.

An animal standing in a fine spray of warm water on a hot, still, sunny day.

A newborn, but dried, foal standing in a draft.

A calf lying on an expanded metal grating in a cold, but not drafty, barn.

A dog leaning over the side of a speeding pickup truck on a hot day.

A chilled newborn lamb being immersed in warm to hot water in an attempt at resuscitation.

A dog standing quietly (and miserably) on a frozen pond.

A chilled newborn piglet under an infrared lamp.

An animal completely immersed in a cold lake on a very hot day.

A dog that has been exercising on a hot day and is breathing rapidly with its tongue lolling and dripping saliva.

4. Provide simple definitions for the following phenomena using everyday language and examples:

Stress: _____

Vasomotion: _____

Nonshivering thermogenesis: _____

Inflammation: _____

Homeorhesis: _____

Pathogenesis: _____

Reproductive Mechanisms

10

10.1 • Functional Anatomy of the Reproductive Tracts

The reproductive organs have a primary function in producing gametes and the hormones that support reproductive function. In males, the tract is specialized for the delivery of *gametes* to enable fertilization. In females, the major role is in providing an environment for fertilization and then the development of the *conceptus* to a suitable degree of maturity before its birth. The female mammal subsequently provides for most of the early postnatal needs of the young through the function of the mammary glands. Lactational biology will be dealt with in Chapter 11.

Anatomy of the Female Tract

The female reproductive organs consist of a pair of *ovaries*, two *oviducts*, a *uterus* and *cervix*, *va-*

gina, and the *vulva*. There is considerable variation among species in the anatomic organization of the oviducts and uterus. For example, the uterus may be extensively divided into two horns, or *cornua*, with a relatively small body, or *fundus*. The cornua may be greatly elongated in the case of litter-bearing animals, such as the pig. In the rabbit, the two cornua communicate with the vagina via two cervices, but most species have a single cervix.

The general organization of the female tract is depicted in Figure 10–1. The following description applies to mammals in general, but because of the between-species differences already noted, the details may not be correct for any given species. The tract is suspended from the dorsal wall of the caudopelvic region of the abdominal cavity on connective tissue ligaments. The cranial portions are covered by peritoneum, as are the other viscera, but the more distal parts

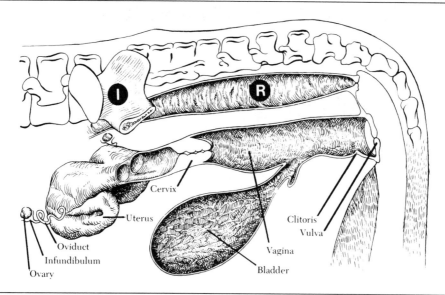

Figure 10–1. Female reproductive tract. A lateral view from the left side of the bovine reproductive tract, shown in relation to the ilium (I) of the pelvis and the rectum (R). Part of the tract is sectioned medially and shows the partial separation of the uterine fundus, giving rise to the two cornua. (Reprinted with permission of the publisher. From Anderson, G.B.: "Reproduction, Artificial Insemination, and Embryo Transfer," in Cole, H.H. and Garrett, W.N. (editors): *Animal Agriculture,* 2nd edition, San Francisco: W.H. Freeman and Company, 1980.)

lie outside the peritoneal cavity. With the exception of the ovaries, the reproductive organs are specialized structures derived from a hollow, smooth-muscle walled tube. This takes the typical form noted earlier in Chapter 1 (see Figure 1–17). The outer portion is smooth muscle that merges gradually into the superficial ligament. The ligament provides general support, provides the route of access for blood vessels and nerves, and maintains an appropriate spatial orientation between the component parts of the tract. For example, in most species the oviduct defines the outer border of the broad ligament, the ovaries are located dorsolaterally on the ligament, and the body of the uterus is medial. This arrangement permits the vascular supply and drainage of the ovaries and uterus to be partially in common, an important requirement for some functional specializations of ruminant animals, to be described later. Part of the tract lies within the pelvic opening, and

the more caudal portions lie dorsal to the ischium. Thus the birth canal passes through the bony pelvic cage, an important obstetric consideration.

The smooth muscle wall usually consists of the outer, longitudinal layer and an inner, circular layer of muscle. In some cases there is an additional oblique layer or at least numerous bundles of smooth muscle arranged obliquely to the longitudinal and circular portions. The inner lining of epithelium, the *endometrium,* is present in various forms along the tract. In parts of the oviduct the internal lining is ciliated and participates in movement of gametes and the embryo within the lumen of the tubes. Elsewhere the endometrium is secretory and produces fluids having a nutritive function for the embryo, or the secretion may be mucous in nature and likely to have a protective function. The secretions are under hormonal control. Both volume and composition vary in a predictable fashion.

The cervix is a specialized fibroelastic portion of the tract that contains some smooth muscle, continuous with the lower segment of the uterine fundus. It contains a central canal which may be relatively uncomplicated or may be thrown into a series of convolutions. The cervical canal is usually occupied by a thick, viscous plug of mucus which provides an effective barrier between the uterine lumen and the external portions of the tract. The vagina is also somewhat fibroelastic, may contain smooth muscle in its wall, and is lined with epithelium, the function of which changes with physiologic state. Changes in the properties of the secretions and in the nature of the epithelial cells themselves can be monitored and used to assess the endocrine status of the female. The reproductive and urinary tracts come together either within the vagina itself or they open separately, within the vulva. The epithelium undergoes a transition to the more protective, keratinized form at the vulva.

Functionally, the ovaries are the source of the female gamete. The oviducts are the conduits between the ovaries and the uterus and provide the site for *fertilization* and very early *embryo* development. The embryo passes to the uterus, the endometrium of which serves as the site of implantation. The uterus serves to accommodate the developing embryo and, later, after organogenesis, the *fetus* with its elaborate set of extraembryonic membranes including the *placenta*. The cervix has a protective function throughout pregnancy by mechanically closing the birth canal and by virtue of the mucus which serves as a barrier against the entry of microorganisms into the uterine cavity. When the fetus achieves a suitable degree of maturation in preparation for birth, the uterus and cervix undergo changes that lead to the birth process. The fetus is born and separates from its placenta to begin postnatal life. The placenta is also delivered and the maternal tissues begin an involutionary process that reverts them to the nonpregnant condition, in preparation for a subsequent pregnancy. These events are described in the remaining sections of this chapter.

The Ovaries

The ovaries are paired, mixed-function organs lying caudad to the kidneys on either side. Embryologically, the gonads, which are ovaries in females and testes in males, arise from primitive structures that are common to the reproductive and urinary systems. The gonads are initally *indifferent*, meaning that there is no obvious difference in form between the structures that develop into ovaries and those that become testes. Sexual differentiation begins in mammals with endocrine, paracrine, or autocrine signals, controlled by the Y chromosome, triggering development of the indifferent gonad into a testis. In the absence of this signal, as in females lacking a Y chromosome, the indifferent gonad begins development into an ovary. This developmental sequence can be deranged in some species, for example in cattle, when they are carrying twin fetuses of mixed sex. If there is any co-circulation of blood between the two fetuses, the presence of the Y chromosome–derived signal from the male fetus will interfere with normal development of the female co-twin. Such females will subsequently be infertile, and they are called *freemartins*. If, however, there was total independence of the fetal circulations and no opportunity for blood-borne signals to pass from the male to the female fetus, the female is likely to be quite normal.

The adult ovary has two major functions. Its primary reproductive role is in the production of *ova* (singular, ovum), the female gametes; additionally, it serves as an endocrine organ. The inital events in oogenesis occur during the fetal life of the female, then a prolonged arrest phase sets in and there are no further events of significance until the female reaches puberty. The ovary in the newborn and prepuberal female contains thousands of *primordial follicles*. Indeed, the total number of potential gametes is determined before birth. Only a minute fraction of these primordial follicles will ever develop and be ovulated during the reproductive life of the female. The remainder will degenerate.

Maturation of the ova and their release by the process of ovulation occur periodically throughout the reproductive phase of the life cycle. This will be described in some detail in Section 10.2. The reproductive capacity of females is finite. When the initial investment of primordial follicles present at birth is consumed, functional reproductive activity ceases.

The follicular structures are located in a stroma of interstitial cells. The outermost layer of connective tissue cells forms a capsule known as the *tunica albuginea*. In the fetal ovary, the germinal epithelium lies directly under this capsule. Cells from this layer divide and migrate into the medullary portion of the ovary where the cells become organized into the primary follicles.

Within each follicle there is a single oocyte, or ovum, an enlarged cell with only half of the normal complement of chromosomes. Gametes, both sperm and ova, are *haploid*, which distinguishes them from the remaining *diploid* cells of the body. Surrounding the oocyte is a layer of follicular cells. The presence of the primary follicles in the mass of the ovary gives the organ a somewhat textured superficial appearance.

The active ovary of the postpuberal animal contains additional structures (Figure 10–2). Follicles at varying degrees of maturation are present and can be visualized superficially. There may be a *corpus luteum*, or several corpora lutea in species that ovulate several follicles at any one ovulation. The follicles mature cyclically, as will be described in the next section, and at a given time several representative stages may be present. Maturation of the follicle involves further divisions of the original single follicular layer. The oocyte is surrounded by a thickened acellular membrane called the *zona pellucida* and then by a clump of granulosa cells that form the *cumulus*. The granulosa cells divide to form a shell of cells enclosing a fluid-filled cavity, the *antrum*. The size of this cavity is an approximate index of the degree of follicular maturation. The outer border of the follicle is made up of cells derived from the stroma; this layer is called the *theca interna*. The endocrine function of the ovary resides in the granulosa and thecal cells.

A very distended, thin-walled follicle, immediately adjacent to the capsule, is probably

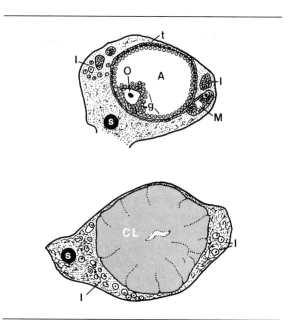

Figure 10–2. The ovary. The upper figure represents a section of the ovary that might be obtained at estrus. The structure is dominated by a large pre-ovulatory follicle distended with its fluid-filled antrum (A). The ovum (O) is surrounded by granulosa cells (g) that continue around the inner surface of the follicular wall. Thecal cells (t) are found in a shell immediately external to the granulosa layer. Additional follicles are usually evident within the stroma (s); they can be classified on the basis of size as being immature (I) or maturing (M). The lower figure is a section of the ovary obtained during the mid- to late-luteal phase of the estrous cycle. The dominant structure is the corpus luteum (CL), shown here with a small cavity. Numerous immature follicles (I) are evident within the stroma of the ovary.

preovulatory. The mature follicle has a characteristic size in each species, and in the large domestic animals, follicles that are maturing in prepartation for ovulation can be palpated through the wall of the rectum. Cystic ovarian disease, a not infrequent pathologic condition causing temporary infertility, can be diagnosed by palpation. The ovary is grossly enlarged because of the presence of numerous very large follicles. For some reason ovulation has not occurred and the normal cyclicity of reproductive behavior is disturbed.

The follicle normally ruptures after pituitary gonadotropins have brought about its maturation. The external follicular wall ruptures and the fluid contents and the oocyte, along with cumulus cells, are shed into the peritoneal cavity. The ovarian end of the oviduct is expanded into a wide funnel-like structure called the *infundibulum*, located in close proximity to the ovary, or in some species even completely surrounding it. The oocyte is usually picked up by the infundibulum and carried down the oviduct to the fertilization site. The now empty follicle is gradually occupied by residual follicular cells that are functionally transformed by the same hormone, luteinizing hormone (LH), that was responsible for ovulation. The cells continue to divide and become extensively vascularized, eventually forming a firm, almost spherical structure that partly extends out from the ovary at the ovulation point. This temporary endocrine organ is the corpus luteum. The name means yellow body, but the appearance is more usually reddish orange, a result of the abundant blood supply it receives and a high cellular content of carotene, a yellowish orange pigment.

The corpus luteum may have a central cavity but the overall firmness of the organ allows it to be readily distinguished, by palpation, from follicles of comparable size. The corpus luteum also has endocrine function, as it is the major source of progesterone during what is called the *luteal phase* of reproductive cycles, and during early pregnancy. In some species this function persists throughout pregnancy, but in others the placenta takes over the major role of producing this key hormone of pregnancy.

After the corpus luteum becomes nonfunctional, it regresses and eventually becomes a small piece of connective or scar tissue within the stroma of the ovary. In the early stages the regressing tissue is called a *corpus albicans* and it is readily discerned visually as a pale, essentially avascular structure.

The Oviduct

The oviducts, also known as the uterine tubes or fallopian tubes, provide a means of communication between the infundibulum and the cornua, or horns, of the uterus. The free margin at the end of the infundibulum is called the *fimbria*. Cells lining the highly convoluted oviduct are either secretory or ciliated. The cilia contribute to the passage of ova from the fimbria toward the uterus and may assist in the transport of sperm in the opposite direction. Fertilization occurs within the lumen of the oviduct, as does the very early stages of embryo development. Passage of the embryo to the uterus requires a few days. When the lumen of the utuerus is reached, the endometrium is normally ready to provide for the needs of the embryo by its secretions, or it provides an optimal environment for implantation. The oviduct therefore provides for communication, transport of gametes, fertilization, embryonal development, and delayed transport of the embryo into the uterus.

The Uterus

The uterus is the most highly specialized segment of the female reproductive tract by virtue of its enormous plasticity in morphology and function. Prior to puberty, and in castrated animals, the organ is infantile and consists of rudimentary endometrium surrounded by a sparse smooth muscle and connective tissue coat. The organ undergoes steroid-dependent growth at puberty with the endometrium thickening and the muscle layers expanding by the combination of cell division and hypertrophy. The contractile apparatus within the smooth muscle cells develops in response to steroids, particularly estrogens, and motile function is established.

The function of the uterus changes cyclically in the absence of pregnancy, reflecting the interplay of estrogens and progesterone at various stages of each ovulatory cycle (see Section 10.2 for more detail). The most important cyclical changes occur in the endometrial lining. In women, the endometrium undergoes a major proliferative phase, then hypertrophic and secretory phases, that are synchronized to the time when a fertilized egg can be expected to reach the uterus. In the absence of conception in humans, the corpus luteum regresses and the production of progesterone is abruptly terminated. Lack of progesterone leads to disruption of the endometrium; large portions slough off, along with blood lost from ruptured blood vessels. This process is called *menstruation*. The endometrium is then repaired and replaced prior to the next ovulation.

Most species exhibit less dramatic changes in the endometrium than do humans. The cells are cyclically programmed to provide an optimal environment for the developing embryo at the appropriate time, relative to ovulation and fertilization. If conception fails, the corpus luteum regresses by one of several mechanisms described below, and progesterone support of the endometrium is withdrawn. The endometrium regresses without menstruation and is then prepared afresh in anticipation of another conception.

The most specialized organization of the endometrium is observed in ruminant animals. The tissue is thrown up into focal thickened areas, called *caruncles*, that dominate the internal surface of the uterus. The endometrium in the caruncles is aglandular, in contrast to the secretory or glandular nature of the remainder of the inner lining of the organ. The caruncles are specialized implantation sites, and during pregnancy they become considerably enlarged as the maternal portions of the placenta.

Vascular Supply and Drainage

The reproductive tract is supplied with arterial blood through three major pairs of arteries. In animals with long cornua, the arteries form an anastomosing network to supply the uterus, while in others, the three pairs supply distinct portions of the tract. The cranial uterine arteries supply the ovaries and oviducts, the middle uterine arteries supply most of the uterus, and the caudal uterine arteries, branching off the vaginal artery, perfuse the lower uterine region and the cervix. The arteries have characteristic form and take a very convoluted path across the broad ligament, especially in the ruminant animals. The blood supply to the ovary arises from a common artery located closely adherent on the major veins draining the uterus and ovary. It winds back and forth over the surface of the ovarian vein (Figure 10–3), finally branching as it enters the ovary. The major vessel, the middle uterine artery, fans out as a series of branching arteries in the broad ligament, close to the uterus.

Figure 10–3. Vascular system of the uterus and ovary in ruminants. The ovarian artery (OA) and uterine artery (UA) closely adhere to the corresponding veins—the uterine vein (UV) and the ovarian vein (OV)—which come together as a common vessel—the utero-ovarian vein (UOV). The arteries (solid) and veins (shaded), along with the ovaries (O) and oviducts (ov) are supported by the broad ligament (bl). Other identified structures are the vagina (V), cervix (C), uterus (Ut), infundibulum (inf), and corpus luteum (cl) on the right ovary.

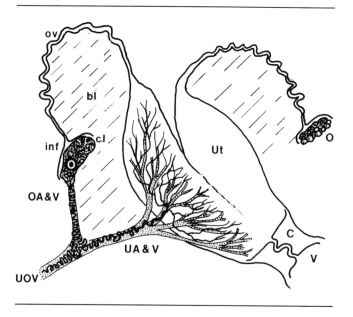

Blood flow through this vessel increases substantially during pregnancy to satisfy the perfusion needs of the placenta and the enlarged uterine mass. The size of this artery and the volume of blood flow are partly dependent on estrogen, and there is reason to believe that the artery is indeed a target organ for estrogen action.

The venous drainage of the ovaries and uterus combines into common vessels, popularly called the utero-ovarian veins, located on either side. These vessels curve dorsally and drain into the abdominal vena cava. As noted above, in many species, and in the ruminants in particular, the arterial supply courses tortuously over the surface of these major veins. This anatomic vascular arrangement is of significance because it provides a means of communication, specific details of which are still elusive, between the uterus and the ovaries. In some way, the uterus is able to signal to the ovaries that no pregnancy has been initiated and, as a result, the corpora lutea undergo regression and a new ovulatory cycle is initiated. This will be described in more detail in the following sections. The mechanism can only operate if the normal intimate arrangement of the ovarian arteries with the utero-ovarian veins is intact.

The Male Reproductive Organs

The reproductive organs of the male (Figure 10–4) include the gonads, (*testes,* in this case), the *spermatic ducts, accessory glands,* and the *penis.* The testes, like the ovaries, are mixed-function cytogenic and endocrine organs responsible for producing male gametes, or *spermatozoa,* and sex steroids. Sperm are produced from germinal epithelium within the testes, they are shed into tubules and pass from the body of the testis into the *epididymis,* the beginning of the spermatic duct. After appropriate phases of maturation, the sperm are mixed with secretions obtained from the accessory glands and delivered through the urethra within the penis. The distal portion of the spermatic duct is therefore common with that of the urinary system. The penis serves as the organ of copulation and provides for delivery of the ejaculate, a suspension of sperm in a vehicle of seminal fluid, into the vagina. There is much in common between the reproductive tracts of the male and female, not surprisingly, considering the embryonic origins, but there are distinctions of significance. As will be described further in Section 10.2, the production of gametes in the male is generally not episodic but is continuous from puberty. The rate of sperm production may, however, vary seasonally and there may be obvious behavioral signs of seasonal changes in *libido,* or sex drive.

Spermatogenesis is adversely affected by elevated temperatures so the testes are suspended outside of the peritoneal cavity in a sac of skin called the *scrotum.* As noted earlier, the testes have a common embryologic origin with the ovaries, but in contrast to the female gonad, the testes migrate out of the abdominal cavity, a process that is usually completed by or shortly after birth.

The Testes

The testes are masses of *seminiferous tubules* enclosed within the *tunica albuginea,* a heavy connective tissue capsule which provides support to and defines the shape of the gonad. Peripheral to the testes and underlying the skin of the scrotum are additional layers of connective tissue that are derived from the peritoneum. The testis is attached ventrally to the scrotum by a ligament, the *gubernaculum.* Interspersed between the seminiferous tubules, the location of the germinal epithelium, are found interstitial or *Leydig* cells. These function to produce testosterone, the major male sex steroid.

The Epididymis and Spermatic Duct

The tubules are connected, by means of *efferent ductules* that pass through a rich vascular network, to the *head of the epididymis,* usually found on the dorsal pole of the testes (Figure 10–5). The epididymis contains a convoluted series of

Figure 10–4. Anatomy of the male reproductive tract (sheep). The left testis (lt) is shown with the tunica albuginea (ta) intact and connected to the distal portion of the cremaster muscle (cm). The tunic and cremaster are removed from the right testis (rt) to show the epididymal (E) structures: the head (h), body (b), and tail (t). The right spermatic cord (sc) is shown with its proximal cut end exposing spermatic artery and vein (sa&v). The vasa deferentia (vd) fuse at the ampulla (a), just dorsal to the bladder (bl). Seminal vesicles (sv) are cranial to the pelvic urethra (pu), while the bulbourethral gland (bu) is located between the os ischii of the pelvis (the tuber ischium on the left side is sectioned sagittally in this preparation). The penis (pe) is shown from the region of the ischiocavernosus muscle (icm) and bulbocavernosus muscle (bcm), through its sigmoid flexure (sf), along its body or corpus, to the distal extremity, the final urethral process (up). The penis is shown retracted within the prepuce (pr) because the retractopenis muscle (rpm) is contracted. (Author's drawing is based on a mounted anatomical preparation at the University of Zurich.)

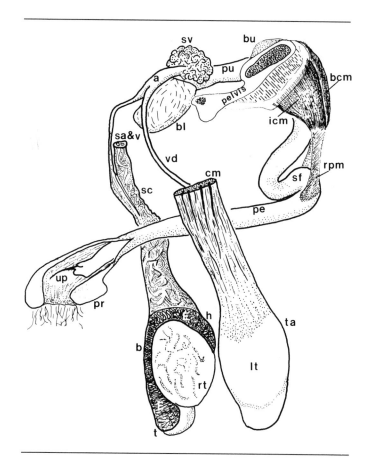

ducts which eventually come together at about midtestis level in the *body*. Most ventrally, the epididymal *tail* turns back on itself and connects to the *vas deferens*, which leaves the scrotum along with blood vessels and nerves as the *spermatic cord*. The spermatic cord passes back into the inguinal region of the body, then the vasa deferentia, one from each side, leave the cord and come to the midline where they join the urethra. A common urogenital duct passes caudally through the pelvis, curves ventrally and then cranially, finally forming the canal of the penis.

Accessory Sex Glands

A series of secretory glands, often paired and sometimes absent from certain species, add the fluid vehicle that makes up the bulk of the seminal plasma. The glands are under the control of male sex steroids and so their growth and function is established about the time of puberty. The secretions are important for part of the maturation of sperm, their nutritive support, and they give the ejaculate a slightly alkaline reaction. During mating, this serves to buffer the sperm from the acidic environment of the vagina.

The *ampullae* are glandular portions of the final segment of the vas deferens. The *seminal vesicles* empty into the pelvic portion of the urethra in close vicinity to the vasa. The *prostate*, an unpaired gland, is located beside the pelvic urethra and has multiple openings into the urogenital duct. Finally, in most species a pair of *bul-*

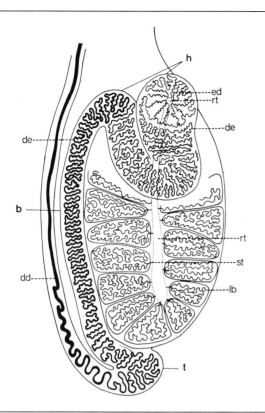

Figure 10–5. The testis and epididymis. A schematic drawing of the tubular system of the testis and epididymis in the bull. The testis is enclosed within the tunica albuginea (see Figure 10–4) and a few of the seminiferous tubules are shown within lobules (lb) of the gland. The seminiferous tubules collect via straight tubules (st) into the rete testis (rt), which communicates with the head (h) of the epididymis. Efferent ductules (ed) come together forming the duct of the epididymis (de) which passes in convoluted fashion through the body (b) and tail (t) of the epididymis. The ductus deferens (dd) leaves the testis via the spermatic cord as the vas deferens, as shown in Figure 10–4. (Reprinted, with slight modification to labeling, by permission of the publisher. From Ashdown, R.R. and Hancock, J.L.: "Functional Anatomy of Male Reproduction," in Hafez, E.S.E. (editor): *Reproduction in Farm Animals,* 4th edition, Philadelphia: Lea & Febiger, 1980.)

bourethral glands is found at the caudal extremity, just before the urogenital duct swings ventrally into the base of the penis.

The accessory glands vary greatly in size, and presumably in importance, among species. Animals with voluminous ejaculates, such as the stallion and boar, tend to have large seminal vesicles. The bulbourethral glands of boars are notably large. The glands contain smooth muscle which contracts under sympathetic control, causing delivery of the secretions into the spermatic duct.

The Penis

The penis consists of erectile tissue, the *cavernosum,* a fairly open series of blood sinuses, a urethral canal, and tough fibrous connective tissue. Distally, the free extremity of the penis may be specialized, forming a *glans,* and there may be a delicate urethral process extending beyond the glans, as in the ram. The external opening usually lies within a sheath, or *prepuce.* In the boar, a prepucial pouch exists within the prepuce and is the source of the unmistakable odor of sexually active boars.

More proximally, the body of the penis is also known as the shaft, and most proximally, the penis arises from two roots attached to the pelvis. In some species, for example in cattle, sheep, goats and pigs, there is relatively little erectile tissue but the body of the penis is twisted into an **S**-shaped *sigmoid flexure.* In the nonerect state the penis is withdrawn back into the sheath because the *retractor penis* muscle is tonically contracted (see Figure 10–4). During erection this muscle is relaxed, the sigmoid flexure straightens, and the penis extends from the prepuce. In species lacking the sigmoid flexure, erection is achieved by engorgement of the cavernous sinuses with blood. The organ increases in diameter and straightens.

The complete erection of the penis usually accompanies mounting of a receptive female, or surrogate, as in the case of collecting semen for artificial insemination. Partial erection usually precedes mounting and is the result of psychic stimulation, mediated via parasympathetic nerves controlling the vessels supplying the cavernous sinuses. The arterioles supplying the sinuses are usually constricted, thereby largely excluding the entry of blood into these spaces. Parasympathetic nerves effect dilation of the arterioles, the sinuses engorge with blood, and the distension then passively compresses the veins that drain the sinuses. In addition, there is minor control over sympathetic vasoconstrictor innervation of the arterioles.

The erectile response is, in part, a spinal reflex, afferents for which respond to mechanoreceptor stimulation of the penis. There is opportunity for higher, or cranial, influences to facilitate or inhibit the reflex. A variety of stressors negatively influences the erection reflex. The development of the penis, morphologically and functionally, is dependent on testosterone. Sexual drive, or *libido*, is also testosterone dependent but is influenced by psychic factors.

Sexual competence is achieved at puberty but, in contrast to the female, is then continuous because gonadal steroidogenesis is maintained thereafter. Loss of sexual drive with aging is therefore due to psychic or behavioral deficits rather than to inadequate testosterone levels. In domestic animals, dominance factors arising from competition with younger, more vigorous males can account for the loss of libido. In species where the male exhibits seasonal changes in gonadal function—obvious in deer, less so in sheep and goats—there are corresponding behavioral changes. These will be noted in a broader context in the next section.

Development of the Male Tract

The testes develop, distinct from the indifferent gonad, at a stage during fetal life that varies between species. During fetal growth, the testes are drawn out of the peritoneal cavity, taking with them folds of peritoneum that leave the abdominal cavity through the inguinal canal. The vascular supply, nerves, lymphatics, and the vas deferens, making up the spermatic cord, are also drawn toward the scrotum. Descent of the testes is usually complete at or shortly after birth. *Cryptorchidism* describes the condition in which one or both testes remain within the body. Puberty is unaffected because the steroidogenic capacity of the cryptorchid testis is intact. However, gametogenesis is severely compromised by the elevated temperatures to which the testis is exposed, unless it is located in the scrotum.

The process of spermatogenesis and other functional aspects of reproduction in the male will be described below.

10.2 • Control of Gonadal Function

The Ovarian Cycle

The maturation of ova in the female is discontinuous, or periodic, and the complex of secondary reproductive and behavioral changes may be referred to as *cycles*. In species in which the female exhibits enhanced receptivity to the male (*estrous behavior*) at or close to the time of ovulation, the cycles are called estrous cycles, and it is convenient to time the length of the cycle from one estrus (day o) to the next (day x, or the next day o). Some animals are not cyclic but are effectively in constant estrus unless they are pregnant or pseudopregnant.

Many primates are only cyclically receptive, near the time of ovulation, while others will copulate at any opportunity. Because many primates menstruate at regular intervals, the term *menstrual cycle* is commonly used. Some confusion exists because the cycles can be timed from the onset of menstruation or, with somewhat less variation, from the day of the preovulatory peak in plasma concentrations of LH or follicle-stimulating hormone (FSH).

In all species of interest, the cycles are most obviously controlled by interactions between LH, FSH, estrogen, and progesterone. In some of the domestic species, prolactin and/or prostaglandins, described earlier in Chapter 4, contribute to the control of the ovarian cycle. Another hormone, not previously encountered, is the protein of follicular origin called *inhibin*. This hormone serves as the feedback arm of part of the control of FSH secretion from the pituitary. Salient aspects of the central control of gonadotropin secretion are described in Box 10–1.

Because much of the following description involves frequent mention of the gonadal steroids, a summary description of the actions and roles of the major classes—estrogens, progestins, and androgens—is provided in Box 10–2.

The cycle can be subdivided into a preovulatory or *follicular* phase and a postovulatory or *luteal* phase. In animals with estrous cycles, the follicular phase is relatively brief and is characterized by a series of events:

1. Cessation of secretory function of the corpus luteum of the previous cycle *(luteal regression)*, resulting in a decline in circulating concentrations of progesterone.

2. Increased frequency of secretory pulses of LH, reflecting a change in the pattern of secretion of GnRH from the hypothalamus (see Box 10–1). This is provoked by the removing of a feedback influence of progesterone directed toward the hypothalamus.

3. Follicular development occurs and results in

a mature preovulatory follicle that produces large quantities of estrogen and inhibin, a protein that inhibits FSH secretion from the pituitary and thereby prevents an inappropriately large number of follicles from maturing.

4. The substantial increase in circulating concentrations of estrogen, acting on CNS tissue that has been relieved of a prior influence of progesterone, causes behavioral estrus. There are characteristic events that vary somewhat in form and pattern of development between the species (see Section 10.4).

5. The estrogen feeds back both positively and negatively on the hypothalamo-pituitary tissues, sustaining LH secretory pulses and then a more massive release called the ovulatory surge of LH.

6. LH serves as the ovulatory hormone and, within hours of achieving peak concentrations, causes a weakening of the wall of the follicle, rupture and release of the ovum, and the beginning of the events termed *luteinization* that affect the cells remaining in the ruptured follicle. These changes result in formation of a new corpus luteum.

The events described here follow characteristic time courses so that the onset of estrus, the peak in LH, and ovulation occur at reasonably predictable intervals.

The luteal phase of the estrous cycle corresponds to the interval between ovulation and the beginning of the next follicular phase. In domestic animals, the life span of the corpus luteum seems dominant in controlling the interestrus interval, while in primates the length of the follicular phase seems to vary more between individuals than does the luteal phase.

The corpus luteum evolves from the ruptured follicle by a thickening of the follicular wall and a rich investment of blood vessels. This transient endocrine gland secretes progesterone in

Box 10-1 Hypothalamo-Pituitary Regulation of Gonadal Function

The location of the hypothalamo-pituitary endocrine unit favors opportunities for regulation of endocrine targets by the neural integration of diverse types of input information. Factors influencing gonadotropin secretion include environmental cues, with the ratio of hours of light to dark being especially important; steroid feedbacks; stress; drugs; and biogenic amines, both the catecholamines and the specialized amines of the pineal gland, such as melatonin and serotonin. *For the present purposes, it can be assumed that these various inputs are integrated within the brain to result in control over gonadotropin-releasing hormone (GnRH) production, gonadotropin secretion, and the function of the target tissues, or gonads.*

It is now apparent that the hypothalamus has a built-in oscillator, with a basic frequency of about 40 to 60 minutes, that controls brief phases, or pulses, of GnRH secretion. The frequency of these GnRH pulses is slowed by feedback effects of progesterone on the hypothalamus. The single hypothalamic factor, GnRH, provides the positive drive for secretion of both LH and FSH by the anterior pituitary. Feedback effects of estrogens modulate the LH secretory response to the GnRH, and inhibin, derived from the maturing follicles, influences the magnitude of FSH secretion in response to the GnRH (Figure 10–6).

Figure 10–6. Control of gonadotropin secretion. The hypothalamus exerts primary control over gonadotropin secretion by the anterior pituitary through the pulsatile secretion of GnRH. The frequency of these pulses is dictated by an intrinsic rhythm of activity in the neurons of the hypothalamus. The frequency of GnRH pulses is slowed by feedback effects of progesterone. At the pituitary level, additional feedback mechanisms, mediated by estradiol and inhibin, moderate responsiveness to GnRH. As shown, pituitary secretion of LH and FSH are affected differently.

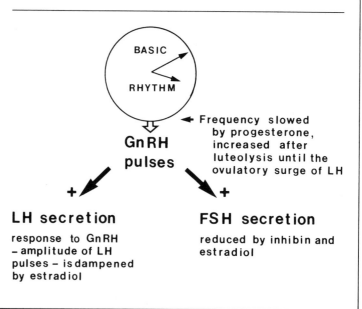

response to an array of stimulating hormones, collectively known as the *luteotropic complex,* that is characteristic for each species.

The complex may include any of the following: LH, prolactin, estradiol, prostacyclin (one of the prostanoids, first noted in Chapter 4). The life span of the corpus luteum is controlled by one of two general mechanisms:

1. Failure of the luteotropic complex caused, for example, by insufficient concentrations of LH; or

Box 10–2   The Gonadal Steroids

Steroids are synthesized from cholesterol by a well-defined series of enzymic changes that fit a general sequence of cholesterol being converted into progestins, then androgens, and finally estrogens. The adrenal cortex has the potential to secrete some or all of the members of these classes of steroids. As a result, some adrenal pathologies have severe reproductive consequences. For example, overactivity of the adrenals may cause precocious puberty.

The functions of *estrogens* (Figure 10–7) include well-known effects on the central nervous system that underlie sex-specific behavioral characteristics. Less well appreciated are the effects on metabolism, body composition, water, and electrolyte balance. The major reproductive effects are those affecting the oviduct, myometrium, endometrium, cervix, and vagina. Important actions, to be described in Chapter 11, are also exerted on mammary tissue. It is now apparent that some rather minor effects of estrogens on nonreproductive smooth muscles, including vascular and gastrointestinal muscle, can be exaggerated during pregnancy, and when pharmacologic amounts of synthetic steroids are taken for contraceptive purposes.

Progesterone is synthesized and secreted by the corpus luteum, the placenta in some but not all species, the adrenal cortex, and in small amounts by nonluteal ovarian tissue. Progesterone influences many of the tissues that are also subject to estrogen action (Figure 10–8). Actions of estrogens and progestins are often cooperative yet may be antagonistic. Additionally, progesterone, which has weak mineralocorticoid activity, may overlap with aldosterone in action, and so may cause sodium retention and therefore influence water balance. Progesterone has important actions on excitable tisues, possibly by direct action on cell membranes, rendering them less excitable. An extreme example of this underlies the anesthetic effects of massive amounts of the steroid. Effects of progesterone on the myometrium will be noted in Section 10.6.

The *androgens,* and testosterone in particular, have equally diverse actions on the body (Figure 10–9). Actions in the central nervous system (CNS) influence the *aggressiveness* that is supposed to be typical of males, and sex drive, or libido. Generalized metabolic effects are known, and the specific case of actions by androgens on protein metabolism and anabolism is well recognized, though poorly understood. Androgens influence the activity of sebaceous glands and body hair distribution in some species, and underlie the deepening of the voice coincident with puberty. Many of these effects are also noted during excessive androgen production in females with disorders of the adrenogenital system. They are also encountered quite frequently in postmenopausal women.

Testicular-derived testosterone acts locally to influence the whole process of spermatogenesis; and in nearby accessory sex glands such as the seminal vesicles, prostate, and so forth this steroid controls growth and secretory function. By such actions, testosterone regulates the production of both the gamete and non-gamete components of an ejaculate. Finally, the growth and copulatory function of the penis have a requirement for elevated circulating concentrations of testosterone.

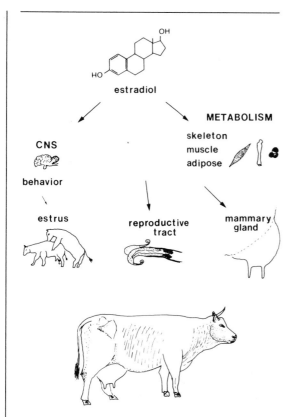

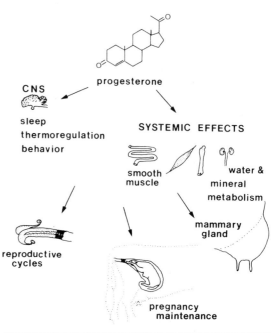

Figure 10–7. Summary of estrogen actions. Estradiol-17β, the most potent of the steroidal estrogens, exerts widespread influence on behavior, metabolism, development, and (most obvious) the organs of reproduction. In animals, the behavioral actions are best exemplified by estrus, with overt mating-like activity and acceptance of the male. Within the reproductive tract, estrogens influence motility and secretory function, and modify the connective tissue of the cervix. They may increase blood flow to the tract. Estrogens, along with progestins, influence mammary development by direct action on the parenchyma (see Chapter 11) and by actions that are mediated by other hormones. Systemic effects on metabolism and nonreproductive smooth muscle are complex, but underlie the morphological and functional changes apparent in females passing through their life cycles.

Figure 10–8. Summary of progestin actions. Progestins, best represented by progesterone, influence the tissues and processes subject to control by estrogens. Actions of the two classes of steroids are partly cooperative and partly antagonistic. Progesterone is known to reduce excitability of some neural and smooth muscle tissues. Reduced excitability of neural tissue influences sleep state, affects body temperature, and contributes to some behaviors. Reduced excitability of uterine smooth muscle accounts for the major role of progesterone—that of helping maintain pregnancy. Similar effects on the smooth muscle of cardiovascular and gastrointestinal systems are recognized, but not characterized as well. The steroid controls secretory activity of the endometrium, especially during the luteal phase and in early pregnancy. Progesterone contributes to mammary development while preventing the initiation of its secretory function. Targets for metabolic regulation include the skeleton, muscle, and adipose tissue; additionally, progesterone exerts some mineralocorticoid activity, thereby influencing mineral and water balance.

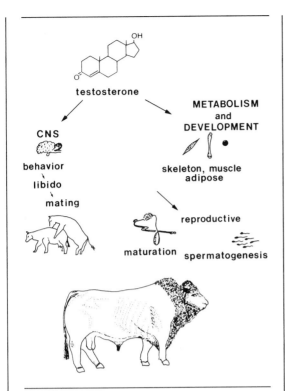

Figure 10–9. Summary of androgen actions. Androgens, represented here by testosterone, exert behavioral actions related to libido, including typical male behaviors, aggressiveness, and mating responses. Their effects on the development of the reproductive apparatus are most obvious and are accompanied by changes of functional consequence such as spermatogenesis, secretory activity of the accessory glands, and the competence to deliver an ejaculate. Additional actions influencing whole body metabolism, growth, and development are best known for skeletal, adipose, and muscle tissues. These underlie the characteristic morphology of mature males.

2. An overriding luteolytic influence that initiates degenerative changes in the luteal cells despite the continued presence of the luteotropic stimuli.

The former process seems to be the most important in primates. The *luteolytic mechanism* is more important in domestic animals.

Luteal function is generally prolonged when

pregnancies occur, but there are exceptions. In animals capable of developing a pseudopregnant state in response to nonfertile copulation, or cervical stimulation during estrus, luteal life span is again greater than normal. This lengthening of luteal life span may occur because the luteotropic complex is reinforced reflexly by copulation. This serves as another example of a neuroendocrine reflex, where afferents, or sensory nerves, pass to the thalamus and hypothalamus to control prolactin secretion. Prolactin is luteotropic in both the rat and the bitch. Both species are known for the ease with which pseudopregnancy can be established.

In some species the products of conception, and specifically the extraembryonic membranes (described in Section 10.4), may secrete gonadotropin. Humans produce an LH-like *human chorionic gonadotropin (hCG)* that is said to "rescue" the corpus luteum. In the absence of pregnancy, and therefore in the absence of hCG, the corpus luteum fails by mechanism 1, above.

In most of the domestic animals, it is believed that the life span of the corpus luteum is not normally compromised because of any shortage in gonadotropic support. Rather, the nonpregnant uterus normally triggers luteal regression, also called *luteolysis*, unless a pregnancy has become established, in which case this uterine luteolytic mechanism is blocked in some way. In the previous section, in the description of the vascular arrangement of the ovaries and uterus, it was noted that the intimacy of the ovarian artery on the utero-ovarian vein was important. With reference to Figure 10–10, an endocrine signal that most likely includes prostaglandin $F_{2\alpha}$ is released from the endometrium of the nonpregnant uterus toward the end of the luteal phase. This signal influences the function of the corpus luteum in the adjacent ovary by means of some local pathway.

If the close contact between the ovarian artery and the utero-ovarian vein is disrupted, this signal is ineffective. Similarly, if a pregnancy has been initiated, this luteolytic mechanism does not operate and the corpus luteum continues to function, producing progesterone to support the pregnancy (Figure 10-11).

The availability of pharmaceutical quantities

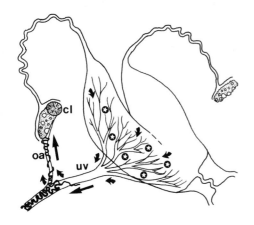

Figure 10–10. The luteolytic pathway in ruminants. In ruminant animals several days after ovulation, the endometrium produces a luteolysin (stars)—most likely prostaglandin F$_{2\alpha}$—if pregnancy has not been initiated. This passes into the uterine venous drainage (uv) and in some way influences the function of the corpus luteum (cl) on the ipsilateral ovary. The mechanism is not well understood, but the integrity of the vascular pathway—including the very intimate contact between the ovarian artery (oa) and the uterine veins—is required. Thus, the nonpregnant uterus is able to trigger regression of the corpus luteum, and the decrease in progesterone secretion in turn initiates changes in gonadotropin secretion to start a new follicular phase.

of prostaglandin, approved for use in domestic animals since the early 1980s, has enabled relatively simple control of the occurrence of estrus in farm animals. Except for the very early and very late stages of the normal estrous cycle, injected prostaglandin will cause reliable luteolysis, a reduction in the plasma levels of progesterone, and the triggering of the events leading to estrus and ovulation. Thus all steps from 1 to 7 (above) can be initiated at will. Estrus can be synchronized in large groups of animals, and this may aid certain managerial operations and facilitate the use of artificial insemination, particularly in range cattle. The corpus luteum in a pregnant animal can also be regressed with injection of prostaglandins, and this strategy could be used to abort unwanted pregnancies, for example in young, incompletely grown females that had been mated unintentionally.

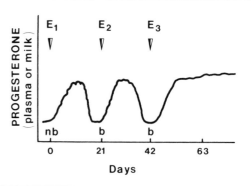

Figure 10–11. Progesterone changes in early pregnancy. Plasma or milk concentrations of progesterone reflect the secretory activity of the corpus luteum. This cow displayed estrus (E) at normal 21-day intervals when progesterone levels were lowest. She was not bred (nb) at the first estrus (E$_1$). She was bred (b), though unsuccessfully, at the second estrus (E$_2$). Note the decrease in progesterone levels preceding the estrus at day 42 (E$_3$). A second breeding at day 42 resulted in conception, sustained levels of progesterone, and a failure to show estrus around day 63.

In the menstrual cycle of primates, the preovulatory or follicular phase is of greatest importance in determining the length of the cycle. Estrogen production continues during the luteal phase and estrogen is likely to act locally on luteal cells to stimulate progesterone synthesis. As noted earlier, in the absence of pregnancy in primates, luteal regression occurs because of inadequate luteotropic support. Progesterone and estrogen secretion then wane, the endometrium degenerates, and menstruation follows. These latter events are, of course, blocked if pregnancy and hCG production maintain luteal secretion of progesterone.

Some species that do not display cyclicity are described as being *induced ovulators*, in contrast to the foregoing species in which the events described correspond to *spontaneous ovulation*. In induced ovulation, the stimulus of coitus activates afferent nerves leading from the cervix and anterior vagina to the CNS. This is yet another example of a neuroendocrine reflex mechanism. Suitable inputs trigger the release of LH, which causes ovulation and then the formation of corpora lutea. Some representatives of this group, such as the rabbit, will then either become pregnant or pseudopregnant, and for a period of a couple of weeks, luteal function is indistinguishable in the two states. If the rabbit is pseudopregnant, the activity of the corpora lutea wanes between days 14 and 20, and thereafter an estrous state is resumed. If the rabbit is pregnant, luteal function persists until about day 30, then progesterone secretion is arrested and parturition follows. This indicates that either the absence of pregnancy is recognized and causes luteal failure between day 14 and 20, or that the pregnant uterus provides something that adds to the luteotropic support of the corpora lutea.

Spermatogenesis

In most species, comparable cyclicity of gonadal function, both in steroidogenesis and gametogenesis, is not observed in the male. Indeed, the males of many species are continuously fertile, secreting testosterone and producing spermatozoa, from puberty until death.

The male gametes, spermatozoa, arise from the germinal epithelium within the seminiferous tubules by a series of cell divisions. As the cells divide and undergo morphologic changes, they migrate toward the lumen of the tubule and are eventually released as free cells. It is convenient to separate the several stages from the original *spermatogonium* within the germinal epithelium through to the final form, a motile *spermatozoon*, complete with a tail.

The primary spermatogonia, which are still diploid cells with the same complement of chromosomes as all other cells, replicate by mitotic divisions. The diploid status is retained and the daughter cells, called *primary spermatocytes*, begin to relocate toward the lumen of the tubule. The next division is by *meiosis*, in which the chromosomal number is halved to produce two *haploid* cells, called *secondary spermatocytes*. These in turn divide by mitosis, each giving rise to two *spermatids*. Thus, the original primary spermatocyte divides by meiotic and then mitotic mechanisms to give rise to four spermatids. This completes the cell divisions of spermatogenesis.

The spermatid is transformed from an attached, nonmotile cell into a detached, motile cell with a tail. The process is called *spermiogenesis*, and the resulting cell is a *spermatozoon* (Figure 10–12). The important changes occurring during this morphogenesis include the isolation of the nucleus from most of the cytoplasm, forming the bulk of the *head*. The nucleus is surrounded by a nuclear membrane, then by an *acrosome*, a saclike organelle that contains enzymes required for fertilization. Externally, as in any other cell, the head is covered with a cell membrane.

Behind the head there is a sparce but highly organized cytoplasm. The cell extends for the equivalent of several head diameters as a flagellum, or *tail*. Contractile fibers, exactly 20 in number, run the length of the tail and are arranged in two concentric rings surrounding two central fibers. The contractile apparatus originates from centrioles, located just behind the head. This apparatus confers motility on the cell. Behind the centriole, the *neck* region is dominated by tightly packed mitochondria arranged helically between the contractile fibers and the outer cell membrane. These mitochondria provide the energy to power contractions of the filaments.

During the development of the spermatid, closely adjacent *Sertoli* cells in the seminiferous tubule function to nourish the germ cells. The mature spermatozoon is released into the lumen of the tubule and then begins a further phase of maturation within the epididymis. The initial basis of movement within the ductules of the testis, the epididymis, and even within the vas deferens is passive and due to secretion of fluid into the lumen along with contraction of the smooth muscle cells of the wall of the duct system. Sperm take anywhere from 1 to 3 weeks to pass along the epididymis, then they are stored in the tail of this structure. Two possible fates await them: they may be ejaculated (see Section 10.4), or they may die and be phagocytosed. Within the epididymis, the sperm are morphologically mature; and although they are fully equipped for motility, this function is not expressed until the cells are mixed with secretions of the accessory glands during ejaculation.

Figure 10–12. Structure of sperma-tozoa. The head consists of the nucleus, partly covered by the acrosome, and the cell membrane, or plasmalemma. The mid-region is dominated by a helical array of mitochondria surrounding the contractile filaments (dotted) that continue down the length of the tail. In cross-section, the tail consists of a pair of central filaments (cf) and two sets of filaments (9 outer and 9 inner, f) in concentric arrays. The outer surface is a continuation of the plasmalemma (p), or sperm cell membrane.

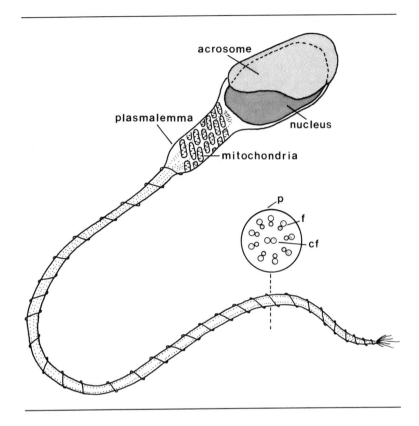

Spermatogenesis involves truly astronomical numbers of cells. Daily production rates, based on numbers recovered by ejaculation, are of the order of billions of sperm per day. This figure contrasts strikingly with the very few ova that are actually ovulated during the entire reproductive life of females.

10.3 • Reproductive Phases and Seasonal Effects

Seasonal Effects on Reproduction

Great variation exists between species in the incidence of annual fluctuations in reproductive activity. For domesticated animals, considerable variation may also exist between breeds within a species. For example, there are striking differences among breeds of sheep. This indicates that there is a genetic basis for animals being reproductively active only during the fall months, compared to others that are active during most of the year. There are enormous economic possibilities for selecting animals that lack seasonality of breeding. The seasonal changes are most obvious in females, because estrous cycles and estrus occur only within the so-called *breeding season*. In contrast, the males may attempt to mate at any opportunity. As noted in Section 10.1, deer and goats are well-known examples of species in which males exhibit dramatic seasonality in reproductive activity. Such annual cycles, while present, are much less obvious in the males of highly domesticated sheep, cattle, and pigs. In the male goat, peak reproductive function is signalled by the powerful odor that is characteristic of sexual prowess. In deer, there is a marked seasonality in gonadotropin secretion, testicular growth and involution, and marked changes in testosterone secretion. These provoke striking consequences: the antler growth cycle, changes in spermatogenesis, morphogenic changes in the neck and shoulder regions, aggressiveness, vocalization, and mating behavior.

Females subject to seasonal changes in reproductive capacity may be classed as *seasonally polyestrous* or *seasonally monestrous*. Polyestrous implies that recurring estrous cycles will occur in the absence of pregnancy. Monestrous describes the situation in which a single estrus is exhibited in a given season. In the former group, sheep and goats, with pregnancies of about 150 days, tend to be polyestrous during the fall in temperate to cold climates. Their young are therefore born in the early to mid-spring, about 5 months later. The basis for this form of seasonality is decreasing daylight hours, characteristic of the fall months. Not unexpectedly, breeds of sheep from the Mediterranean and tropics, where there is little circannual change in day length, are often continuously reproductively active. Breeds that evolved much farther from the equator are highly seasonal and their breeding season is shorter in duration.

Artificial manipulation of the light-to-dark ratio can be used to control the breeding season. Horses, with pregnancy lengths approximating 11 months, move out of the breeding season, or become *seasonally anestrous*, during the fall. Artificial control of lighting, for example by use of continuous light, or at least 16 hours of light each day, can prolong the breeding season. It is tempting to suggest that the species have evolved mechanisms maximizing the chances of their young being born at an optimal time of the year, presumably in the spring to early summer.

An important aspect of seasonality that has economic consequences stemming from reproductive efficiency is the change in ovulation rate commonly observed within the breeding season. Ovulation rate in sheep, for example, is usually low early in the breeding season, and if animals are bred at this stage, the number of lambs produced will be constrained.

Reproductive Phases of the Life Cycle

Reproductive competence is present only during part of the whole life cycle, yet distinct events associated with reproduction may occur at all possible times. It is convenient to consider the life cycle in four stages:

1. Fetal, neonatal, and prepuberal,

2. Puberal,

3. Adult, and

4. Senescent.

The embryology of the reproductive tissues is relatively complex. Prenatal development, as briefly outlined in Section 10.1, is closely linked to that of the renal-urinary system. Partial maturation of germ cells occurs prenatally, especially in the female, where primary, or primordial, follicles form, but subsequent development is arrested until puberty. In the fetal horse, the gonad is very active endocrinologically for part of gestation. Despite the small size of the fetus, its gonads may be larger than those of the dam and certainly more active in steroidogenesis. It is now known that androgen production by the fetal equine gonad is partly responsible for the enormous production rate of estrogens during equine pregnancy.

In some species, development of the CNS and the establishment of the basis for adult sexual behavior is programmed during fetal or neonatal life. A neonatal male rat injected with estrogen will exhibit female reproductive behavior as an adult, and vice versa in the case of females that are neonatally treated with androgens. Some female fetuses may be masculinized as a result of exposure to androgens or even excessive amounts of progestins. The consequences are primarily morphologic and may include an enlargement of the clitoris and partial fusion of the labia. Similarly, *freemartinism*, a developmental defect of female cattle that were co-twins with, and shared part of the circulation with, a male fetus, was described earlier.

The onset of puberty is accompanied by some well-characterized endocrine changes, although the precise cause of puberty in most species is not known. Sexual or reproductive competence is acquired gradually and involves a multitude of physiologic, morphologic and behavioral aspects. In a formal sense, puberty is reached when viable and potent gametes are produced and released from the respective gonad. It seems that puberty is influenced by age and/or body weight in most species. In some but not all species, puberty is delayed if the young animal has been subjected to serious undernutrition or has suffered retarded growth. Likely triggers of puberty include an altered pattern of GnRH secretion from the hypothalamus, altered pituitary sensitivity to GnRH, and therefore altered secretion of gonadotropins. In addition, an increased gonadal sensitivity to the pituitary hormones is apparent. This sensitivity aspect likely reflects the development, or ontogeny, of hormone receptors in the gonad, and the acquisition of steroidogenic capacity.

During adult life, reproductive competence is subject to the seasonal constraints noted earlier for some species, but in general terms the capacity to produce and release gametes is exhibited by both sexes for an extended period of time. In females, the overall duration of the reproductive phase is determined by the availability of follicles. Many, many more follicles degenerate by a process described as *atresia* than ever mature and ovulate. This process of follicular depletion underlies the phenomenon of menopause in women, but it is of little concern in the case of domestic animals. Most female animals are removed from breeding herds long before their ovaries are depleted of follicles. This form of loss of reproductive competence may be encountered in companion animals that have reached advanced age.

In most domestic species, fertility improves over the first few years, is maintained relatively constant for some years, and then finally declines. In part this pattern is explained by changes in ovulation rate, by changes in the ability of the animal to support the burden of reproduction, and in many cases, by progressive or accumulative deterioration of the reproductive tract.

There is no similar constraint on spermatogenesis, although the frequency of sperm defects increases with age, and the male may lose the ability to effectively deliver them. With age, there may be functional impediments to copulatory activity, or psychic and dominance problems may prevent effective reproductive behavior.

The whole process of aging is a fascinating and largely unexplored sub-discipline of biology. In reproductive terms, efficiency of the mechanisms described earlier dwindles or ceases. For humans of both sexes, these changes are psychologically far more important than they are physiologically. In domestic animals, loss of reproductive potency due to aging is seldom encountered because of the turnover of animals, and the indirect effects of animal deterioration on reproductive capacity usually precede any specific problem in the reproductive system. For example, tooth wear in older grazing animals may severely compromise their nutritional wellbeing; ovulation rate may be affected secondarily.

10.4 • Mating and the Initiation of Pregnancy

The females of most species permit copulation only during estrus. They may exhibit intense interest in the male, even to the point of mimicking male mating behavior by mounting other females in their company. Different species exhibit their characteristic estrous behaviors, presumably providing visual cues to the male, such as tail elevation and wagging. Most species also provide olfactory cues by producing *pheromones*, or volatile chemical products, capable of triggering the mating response in receptive males. Additionally, characteristic vocalization patterns may aid in attracting and communication with the opposite sex. Some of these behaviors are recognizable by experienced human observers, and others, such as the pheromones, can be detected by trained dogs. However, in many species estrus can only be detected reliably by the male of that species. Estrus detection, which is necessary for any program of artificial breeding, is frequently less than optimal and is a significant cause of reproductive inefficiency in intensive dairy operations.

The reverse of the preceding behavior—that is, the male communicates his status to the female—may also occur. A related phenomenon is known in small ruminants, where the presence of an active male may initiate the onset of the breeding season or even synchronize the cycles of a group of females.

In some species the female will actively seek the male, then exhibit estrous behavior as a prelude to mating. In others, such as sheep, the male routinely examines each female at regular intervals in an attempt to determine their acceptance of efforts at mating.

Standing estrus is defined as the stage when the female will not engage in avoidance activity when mounted. Before and after this stage, the female may exhibit many of the signs of estrus but nevertheless will not permit the male to mount her. An ovariectomized female can be induced into estrus by injecting steroids. Estradiol is responsible for triggering estrus, but prior exposure of the CNS to progesterone will enhance the behavioral response. Physiologically, the secretion of estrogen by the maturing, preovulatory follicle is responsible for estrus. The ovarian cycle of follicular and luteal phases, separated by ovulation, can be monitored by repeated occurrences of estrus. The interval between these occurrences is reasonably constant and is called the *interestrus interval*, or the length of the *estrous cycle*. Typical values for this interval are provided in Table 10.1. Failure of estrus to occur may indicate the initiation of a pregnancy, with sustained function of the corpus luteum serving to block any new follicular phase. Alternatively, in seasonally polyestrous animals, the cessation of repeated estrus may indicate that the breeding season has ended.

Because the ovary has been inactive prior to the first ovulation at puberty, or at the beginning of a new breeding season, the CNS will not have had a recent exposure to progesterone and so these first ovulations may not be accompanied by estrus. These are called *silent ovulations*. In some species, and the goat is a good example, the first interestrus interval is frequently abnormally short. In cattle resuming cyclic activity some weeks after calving, the first estrus is preceded by a phase of low-level production of progesterone. This presumably primes the CNS so that estrogen can elicit a full estrous response.

Copulation is achieved with the penis serving as the organ of intromission and its full erection usually accompanies mounting a female that is in standing estrus. In some of the domestic animals, full extension of the penis occurs by contracting abdominal or pelvic muscles; and in some species the sigmoid flexure of the penis is straightened immediately before ejaculation.

Ejaculation is the forcible emission of semen, comprising spermatozoa suspended in a spe-

Table 10–1. Estrus and Ovulation*

Species	Interestrus Interval	Estrus Duration	Ovulation Time
Cattle	21 d	18 hr	10–18 hr after end of estrus
Sheep	17 d	24–36 hr	18–24 hr after onset of estrus
Pig	21 d	48–54 hr	30–36 hr after onset of estrus
Horse	21 d	5 d	Last couple of days of estrous period

*These values are subject to considerable variation. For example, cattle may have quite normal cycles of anywhere from 17 to 25 days, estrus may last up to 5 days in sows, etc.

cialized nutrient-containing vehicle produced by the accessory sex glands. Ejaculation is largely a spinal reflex employing sympathetic motor nerves to the smooth muscles of the glands and genital duct and some innervation of skeletal muscles at the pelvic base of the penis. The process involves a series of fairly rapid contractions, with the ejaculate being expelled in portions.

In contrast to the ovum, spermatozoa are not fully potent for fertilization on their release from the gonad. As noted earlier, further maturational events take place in the epididymis and elsewhere within the vas deferens, or male reproductive duct. The maturation changes include the acquisition of motility and alteration of the properties of the surface membrane of the sperm.

A second phase of maturation is needed before fertilizability is maximized. This occurs within the female tract by a process termed *capacitation*. The properties of the acrosome seem to be affected in a way that facilitates penetration of the cumulus and zona pellucida of the egg. The acrosome is the lysosome-like structure lying superficial to the sperm nucleus (see Figure 10-12). When activated, its enzymes aid in hydrolytically creating a fertilization path through the egg envelope.

Spermatozoa pass from the anterior vagina into the uterine lumen largely because of their inherent motility. The nature of the cervical canal and the secretions it contains do influence the ease of access. The canal is usually closed by a plug of mucus that isolates the uterine lumen from the outside. The consistency of the mucus changes noticeably when the animal is under the influence of estrogen, as at the time of estrus. The change in mucus properties makes it more penetrable by sperm.

Once within the uterus, a combination of sperm motility and contractile activity of the myometrium enables the sperm to move to the oviducts, then progress along the oviduct to the fertilization site. Capacitation occurs during this transit, and once contact is made with the cumulus cells, the sperm penetrates between the cumulus to gain access to the *zona pellucida* and egg envelope. The acrosome breaks down and hydrolytic enzymes digest a path through the vitellus until the sperm head contacts the plasmalemma of the ovum (Figure 10–13). The membranes fuse and nuclear material from the sperm admixes with the egg nuclear material. Fertilization has now occurred and the diploid state is obtained.

Polyspermy, or fertilization by more than one sperm, is normally blocked, presumably because of changes in the remaining zona pellucida triggered by entry of the first sperm. This means that a second sperm cannot gain access to the *zygote*, or newly fertilized egg, and contribute additional nuclear material. The initial cell divisions are also triggered, enabling the zygote to begin development into an embryo.

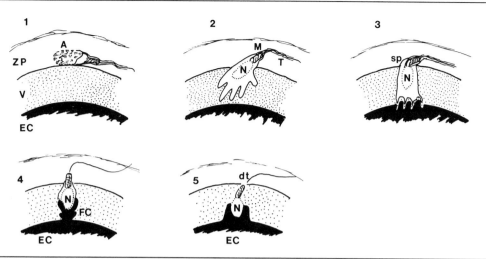

Figure 10–13. *Fertilization.* The fertilizing spermatozoan is shown in 1, lying within the zona pellucida (ZP), adjacent to the egg envelope or vitellus (V). The acrosome (A) is fragmenting which releases hydrolytic enzymes capable of digesting a fertilization path (2) through the vitellus. The sperm nucleus (N), mid-piece (M), and tail (T) are identified. Interaction between the sperm and egg is most obvious in 3, with the sperm plasmalemma (sp) forming intimate contact with the egg plasmalemma, lying between the egg cytoplasm (EC) and the vitellus. In 4, the cytoplasm of the egg is thrown up around the sperm nucleus in what is called the fertilization cone (FC), and the sperm and egg plasmalemmas fuse so that the sperm nucleus becomes part of the egg. The remainder of the sperm disintegrates at this time; for example, the tail is shown to be detached (dt) in 5.

Embryonic Development and the Formation of the Placenta

The inital cell divisions of the zygote, called the first, second, third cleavage divisions, and so on, result in a progressive reduction in the size of each crop of cells (Figure 10–14), the number of which increases exponentially. These initial divisions occur within the confines of the zona pellucida and give rise to a ball of cells termed a *morula.* Each cell is a *blastomere.* In the very early stages, any one blastomere is identical with all others at the corresponding stage of development. If the cells in the two-cell stage or the four-cell stage are separated by micromanipulative techniques, each cell can be made to give rise to a normal embryo, fetus, and then off-spring. The cells capable of developing into complete individuals are said to be *totipotent.* At the four-cell stage, this type of manipulation could give rise to four genetically identical individuals, or *clones.*

After the four-cell stage, a single blastomere loses this capacity, but multicellular portions of more advanced morulae may retain the capacity to develop into an individual. For example, later stage morulae can be sectioned simply by being cut into two or four portions, and these portions can go on to develop into clones. For unknown reasons, a small proportion of morulae spontaneously divide, and if the two part-morulae survive development, they are born as identical twins. More correctly, these are *monozygous* twins because, while they have identical genetic makeup, they may exhibit differences that are nongenetic in origin. For example, birth weight

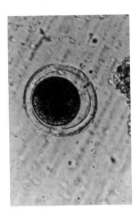
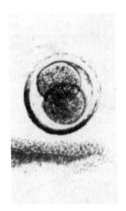
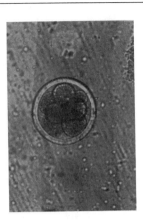

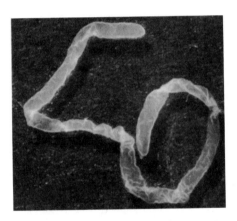
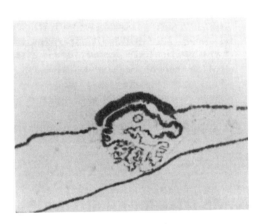

Figure 10–14. Early embryogenesis in cattle. The earliest events in embryogenesis show the progressive reduction in the size of cells during the exponential phase of cell multiplication. *Top, left to right:* Unfertilized ovum, 2-cell, and 8-cell stages obtained from the oviduct 2 to 3 days after estrus. The first, second, and third cleavage divisions result in reasonably synchronous doubling of the number of cells, but note that the 6-cell stage shows blastomeres of different sizes because 2 of the 4-cell stage blastomeres have not yet undergone the third cleavage division. *Bottom, left:* Fourteen-day stage, called the chorionic vesicle, 70 mm in length showing marked expansion of the fluid-filled trophoblast. *Bottom, right:* Section through the embryonic disk at day 14 with the beginning of embryogenesis and formation of the secondary embryonic membranes (shown schematically in Figure 10–15). (Original photographs, courtesy of Dr. Wm Hansel, New York State College Of Veterinary Medicine, Cornell University. Reproduced by permission of the publisher. From Hansel, W. and McEntee, K.: "Female Reproductive Processes," in Swenson, M.J. (editor): *Duke's Physiology of Domestic Animals,* 9th edition, Ithaca, NY: Comstock Publishing Company, Inc., 1977.)

is not solely determined by the genetic makeup of the fetus, so monozygous twins can differ in size.

During passage down the oviduct, the cells of the morula divide further and begin early differentiation (see Figure 10–14). As the number of cells increases, they become wedge-shaped and contact is made between the plasmalemmas of adjacent cells. Intercellular junctions form and seal the spaces between the innermost cells and the exterior of the morula, still within the zona pellucida. Fluid accumulates within the morula, creating a cavity between the cells that is called a *blastocoele*. At this stage in most species, the embryo is within the cavity of the uterus and when the blastocoele has formed it is called a *blastocyst*.

Differentiation, probably controlled by variations in the microenvironment existing within the embryo, has given rise to two populations of cells. The two types of cells are the peripheral *trophectoderm* cells and the rest make up *the inner cell mass*. The trophectoderm will grow to form the *trophoblast*, eventually a portion of the embryonic membranes, and finally part of the placenta. The inner cell mass is the portion that develops into the embryo and eventually the fetus.

The embryo *hatches* from the zona pellucida at about this size and survives for a while as a free-living blastocyst, deriving nutrients by absorption across the trophoblast membrane and through the fluid-filled blastocoele, or blastocyst cavity.

The blastocyst enlarges rapidly and may press against the endometrial lining of the uterus, thereby initiating an implantation reaction. In some species such as cattle, horses, and pigs, the blastocysts expand and may remain with very tenuous contact with the endometrium for 4 to 5 weeks before a definitive placenta is formed.

The mechanism of implantation and placentogenesis varies enormously across the species, and the details are beyond the scope of this description. In essence, all of the events are aimed at establishing an adequate exchange surface, without mixing, between the maternal circula-

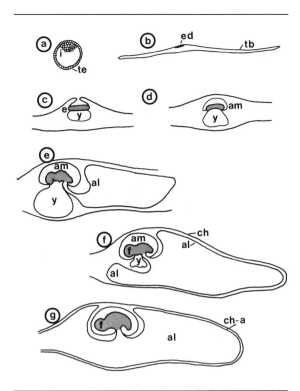

Figure 10–15. Development of the embryonic membranes. a: The blastocyst consists of an inner cell mass (i), differentiated from the single shell of trophectoderm cells (te) that delimits the blastocoele, or cavity. *b:* The trophoblast (tb) is undergoing marked elongation as the chorionic vesicle; the inner cell mass is organized into the embryonic disk (ed, see photograph in Figure 10–14). *c:* The trophoblast is forming dorsal folds and the yolk sac (y) is forming from the embryo (e, shaded). *d:* The folds have come together to create an extraembryonic space, the amniotic cavity (am) adjacent to the embryo. *e:* The yolk sac (y) is maximally developed, and presses against the trophoblast to provide for the early diffusion function between the developing embryo and the maternal tissues. The embryo is acquiring distinct form and has sent out another membrane vesicle called the allantois (al). *f:* The yolk sac is undergoing involution as the vascularized allantois expands to make close contact with the outer membrane. The embryo now has a distinct fetal shape; the trophoblast is known as the chorion (ch) from this stage on. *g:* The allantois has expanded to occupy much of the space delimited by the chorion and forms the compound structure, the chorioallantois (ch-a). This is vascularized from the fetus and forms the fetal part of the placenta.

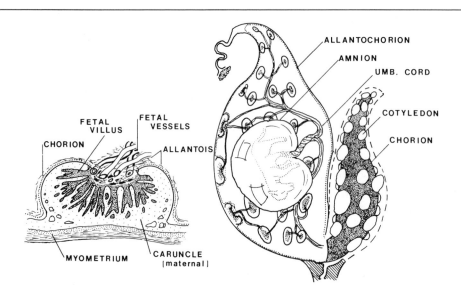

Figure 10–16. Placentation in small ruminants. The figure to the right is a construct that shows the inner aspect (left) and outer surface (right) of the extraembryonic membranes found in ruminants. The inner view shows the fetus within an intact amnion connected by the umbilical cord to a series of placentomes. The placentomes collectively make up the placenta. Each fetal portion is also called a cotyledon and is highly organized chorionic tissue supported and vascularized by the closely adjacent allantois. The outer view, shown on the right, is obtained if the maternal tissues are dissected and peeled away from the intact allantochorion. The cotyledons are morphologically distinct on the surface of the chorion (heavily shaded). The left figure is a section though a placentome to show the fetal portions in intimate contact with the maternal caruncle, the specialized, thickened areas of endometrium found in all ruminants. The morphology of the whole structure shown here is approximately concave and is the form found in sheep and goats. The placentomes are more flattened to convex in cattle, but otherwise the arrangement is similar. The chorion forms villous extensions (shaded) into crypts formed in the maternal tissue. Adjacent to the placentome, the chorion continues in the membranous form shown at far right. Vessels of the umbilical circulation pass across the allantois to reach the villous chorion. The maternal side of the placenta is vascularized by arteries and veins that develop from those originally present in the caruncular endometrium of the non-pregnant state.

tion and the rapidly developing fetal and membrane vasculature.

In the earliest stages, illustrated for simple mammalian embryos in Figure 10–15, the inner cell mass expands into an *embryonic disk,* located superficially on a rapidly expanding blastocyst. The blastocyst folds around the embryonic disk and finally encloses it with what will become the *amnion,* delimiting the fluid-filled *amniotic cavity.*

The embryo develops a *yolk sac* that extends across the cavity of the blastocyst, and this temporary structure serves as the initial organ of exchange. A second outgrowth from the embryo, the *allantois,* expands to occupy much of the space delimited by the trophoblast. As the allantois develops it carries with it fetal blood vessels that will take over the exchange function from the yolk sac, which is concurrently involuting. In many species close apposition between the allantois and the most peripheral membrane, the trophoblast, produces the compound structure known as the placenta.

In the ruminant animals, the *chorion,* as the trophoblast is known after the earliest stages, is pressed against the endometrial caruncles. The chorion then begins to invade the maternal tissue by sending out villous extensions that erode and reorganize the endometrium. Fetal blood vessels are carried within each villus so an intimate exchange surface is created (Figure 10–16). There are somewhat different arrangements in other species but the function is essentially the same. The placenta is primarily an organ of materials exchange between the fetal and maternal circulations. There are additional functions, such as the production of hormones, but these are definitely secondary.

In some species the placenta has the capacity to variously synthesize steroids, prostanoids, peptides, proteins, and glycoprotein hormones.

It is emphasized that there is great variation among species in placental endocrine competence. For example, the chorionic gonadotropin mentioned in connection with luteal function is found in primates, although a somewhat similar molecule, called pregnant mare's serum gonadotropin (PMSG), or, more recently, equine chorionic gonadotrophin (eCG), is also found in the equids. Placental lactogens, though more widely distributed than chorionic gonadotropins, are nevertheless absent from many species.

The further development of the embryo into the fetus involves a strictly programmed sequence of cell divisions, differentiations, foldings, and fusion of bands of cells to create the beginnings of organs. The specific details of embryology, beyond that provided in relation to the formation of the placenta, are outside the scope of this text.

10.5 • Fetal Development and Maternal Adaptations

Fetal Development

Most fetal organs develop from primitive structures laid down in the process of *organogenesis,* which begins at or shortly after the time of implantation. This accounts for the greater sensitivity of the early embryo or fetus to *teratogens.* Teratogens are substances that are able to cause developmental anomalies resulting in birth defects of nongenetic origin. The sequence of development of organs, then the beginning of function, occurs at physiologically appropriate stages: for example, essential vital organs such as the heart and liver develop early.

The heart and vasculature develop at about the time of implantation so that nutrients absorbed at the placental membrane can be distributed throughout the fetus. The liver is the dominant visceral organ throughout fetal life, and it serves a similar critical function in the fetus as that described for the animal after birth. In addition, during early fetal life, the liver is the main site of erythropoiesis.

In the case of the pulmonary system, the respiratory muscles are in place and exercised during late gestation in preparation for their continuous use from the moment of birth. This is a fascinating example of developmental anticipation, because the lungs serve no obvious function to the fetus before birth. Maturation of type

II pneumocytes, noted earlier in Chapter 5 for their ability to secrete surfactant, occurs shortly before birth in anticipation of postnatal lung aeration.

The kidneys function during fetal life to produce urine, which is initially bypassed from the bladder through the urachus into the allantoic cavity. The urachus is a duct running from the bladder to the umbilicus in the midabdominal region. It eventually becomes nonfunctional, involutes, and is found as a ligament between the bladder and the ventral abdominal wall in older individuals. Later in fetal life, micturition occurs and urine is regularly passed through the urethra, to accumulate in the amniotic cavity.

The earliest changes in the embryos and fetuses of domestic animals, which have been discribed in much detail, are morphologic. The morphologic changes follow underlying anatomic and functional developments, but they are more easily detected. Tabulations of the appearance of external features by stage of gestation are readily available. One such tabulation is provided in Table 10–2.

The control of fetal growth and development has been intensely studied during recent years as techniques have become available for prolonged monitoring of the fetus in utero. A major development was the ability to maintain and monitor surgically modified, or instrumented, fetuses; another important development has been the use of noninvasive visualization methods such as ultrasonography. It is a relatively simple task to obtain repeated linear measurements of the whole fetus, or parts of the fetus such as a limb or head, so that its development can be followed. Movements of the chest wall can be visualized, as can gross movements of the limbs.

One area of particular interest to the author is the programmed acquisition by the fetus of endocrine competence. In most cases, fetal and maternal hormones are not exchanged between the two circulations. Instead, the fetal endocrine system is considered to be autonomous. Endocrine tissues may develop before complete control systems are in place. The pituitary is present, and contains the array of hormones described in Chapter 4, long before the neural pathways

Table 10–2. Prenatal Development in Cattle*

Gestation Day	External Features of the Embryo or Fetus
24	Three primary brain vesicles and forelimb bud present.
25	Embryo assumes characteristic C shape.
26	Mammary ridge present, hind limb bud forming.
30	Optic cup formed, eyes pigmented, olfactory pits forming.
34	Acoustic meatus present, grooves evident between forelimb digits.
38	Eyelids and external ear forming, hind limb digits separating.
40	Late embryo stage (Figure 10–17).
45	Hair on muzzle and above eye; tongue visible.
50	Eyelids cover eye—distinct fetal appearance.
56	Palate fused, abdomen closed.
60	External genitalia differentiated, hooves forming.
75	Hair follicles widely distributed over skin.
80	Teats present, hooves keratinized.
83	Scrotum present.
100	Hooves firm and opaque.
110	Tooth eruption beginning.
150	Coloration evident, eyelashes present, descent of testes.
182	Hair on tail tip, prepuce or vulva, and near umbilicus.
196	Eyelids separated; hair-covered except on belly and medial aspect of limbs.
230	Body fully covered with hair.
250	Eyes open.
276–292	Birth—distinct breed differences in gestation length.

*Adapted from data compiled by Evans H.E., Sack W.O. "Prenatal Development of Domestic and Laboratory Mammals: Growth Curves, External Features and Selected References," *Anat. Histol. Embryol.* 1973;2:11–45.

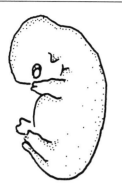

Figure 10–17. *The late embryo–early fetus in cattle.* The definitive fetal stage of development in cattle is reached at about 40 to 50 days after conception. Note the anterior dominance and immature morphology of the limbs, although digits are evident on the hind limbs by about day 40.

influencing the hypothalamus and its ability to secrete hypophysiotropic factors are mature.

The total extent of development that occurs prenatally, or the degree of maturity of the fetus at birth, varies enormously among species and remarkably little within species. In similar fashion, maturation of certain physiologic systems may occur before or after birth, depending on the species. Newborn rats are unable to thermoregulate and acquire this ability only some 2 weeks after birth. In sheep, this particullar homeostatic mechanism is in place about a week before normal term.

Major changes in cardiovascular and pulmonary function take place at the moment of birth and shortly thereafter. A somewhat detailed description of the fetal circulation and changes at birth is provided in Box 10–3.

Box 10–3   The Fetal Circulation and Neonatal Adaptations

The fetus communicates with the mother via the placental exchange system. The structural nature of the placenta was described earlier and illustrated in Figure 10–16. The placenta provides for intimate exchange, but never mixing, between the blood systems of the fetus and mother.

The vascular supply from the fetal side is by means of the umbilical arteries that leave the abdominal aorta, pass across the abdominal cavity, then exit from the fetus at the umbilicus. The vessels pass along the umbilical cord, then ramify within the allantois to supply the exchange tissues within the chorion (see Figure 10–16). In ruminants with their cotyledonary placenta, each placentome receives an arterial supply and drains via veins that collect together to become the umbilical vein. The umbilical vein therefore transports freshly exchanged blood back to the fetus.

Within the fetus itself, the umbilical vein runs cranially and ventrally from the umbilicus to the liver. Some of this blood joins the portal vein and some bypasses the liver through the *ductus venosus* (Figure 10–18) to enter the posterior vena cava. About 50% of fetal cardiac output is used to perfuse the placental circulation.

The fetus has a number of vascular specializations that operate to favor perfusion of the most critical fetal tissues. Many of these must be shut down promptly at birth; if they are not, the well-being of the newborn is compromised. During fetal life, blood returning to the heart from the head and foreparts of the fetus passes through the right atrium and right ventricle, just as in postnatal life (Figure 10–19). However, in contrast to the adult animal, little blood perfuses the lung via the pulmonary arteries, partly because there is no opportunity for oxygenation at this time, but most importantly because the lungs are collapsed (nonaerated), and there is a very high vascular resistance in the pulmonary bed.

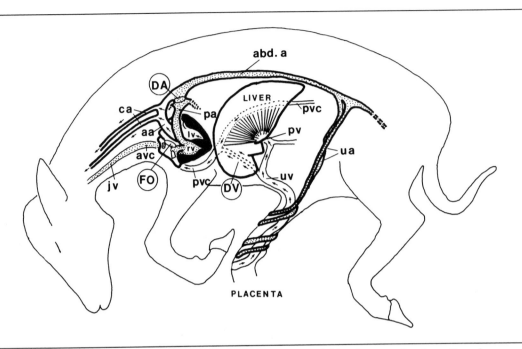

Figure 10–18. The fetal vasculature. Umbilical venous (uv) blood, returning from the placenta, in part joints the portal vein (pv) to pass through the liver and into the posterior vena cava (pvc). It in part by-passes the liver through the ductus venosus (DV). This freshly oxygenated blood, upon reaching the right auricle, passes through the foramen ovale (FO) to the left auricle and is then pumped by the left ventricle (lv) into the proximal portion of the aortic arch (aa). It is selectively delivered via the carotids (ca) to the head. Venous blood, returning from the head via the jugular veins (jv) and anterior vena cava (avc), passes through the right auricle and ventricle (rv) and leaves via the pulmonary artery (pa), only to be diverted through the ductus arteriosus (DA) to reach the abdominal aorta (abd.a). This blood perfuses the lower trunk and, most importantly, it is delivered back to the umbilical arteries (ua) for exchange at the placenta.

During fetal life, a bypass called the *ductus arteriosus* exists between the pulmonary artery and the aorta, just beyond the exits of the major trunk arteries that run cephalad to give rise to the carotids. This arrangement enables blood that is returned from the head to pass through the right-hand side of the heart and then to be directed caudally into the abdominal aorta, to the umbilical arteries, and to the placenta (see Figures 10–18 and 10–19).

The newly oxygenated blood that returns from the placenta also reaches the right auricle, but it is handled differently from that just described. This blood passes through an opening between the right and left ventricles, called the *foramen ovale,* and enters the left side of the heart. After passing on to the left ventricle it is ejected during systole into the proximal portion of the aortic arch and is directed cephalad. In this way the freshly exchanged blood returning from the placenta is preferentially sent to the brain.

In fetal life, pressure within the pulmonary artery is greater than that in the

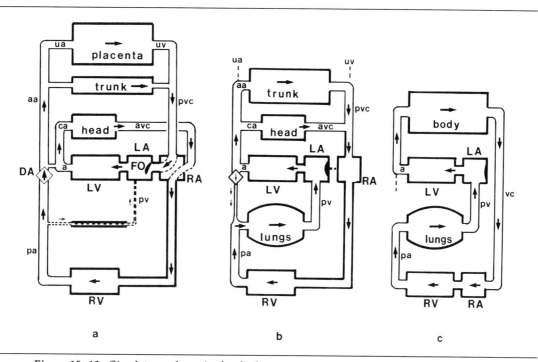

Figure 10–19. *Circulatory schematics for the fetus, neonate, and adult. a:* The fetal circulation through the left and right heart (LA and LV, RA and RV, respectively) is shown to be parallel. Refer to Figure 10–18 for a detailed explanation. Perfusion of the lungs via the pulmonary artery (pa) to the pulmonary vein (pv) is minimal (dotted) because of high vascular resistance in non-expanded lungs and because the ductus arteriosus (DA) is open, shunting blood from the pulmonary artery to the abdominal aorta (aa), and then to the trunk and placenta. Notice that the right auricle has been located in proximity to the left auricle—and connected to it via the foramen ovale (FO)—rather than in association with the right ventricle. Oxygenated blood leaving the aorta (a) flows preferentially cephalad and supplies the carotid arteries (ca). Venous return from the head, in the anterior vena cava (avc), is handled differently than that from the placenta and trunk, via the posterior vena cava (pvc). *b:* In the neonate, the two sides of the heart operate in series (follow arrows from the right ventricle, through the lungs, to the left heart), because the umbilical vessels (ua and uv) have shut down, thereby raising total peripheral resistance in the remaining vasculature supplied by the aorta (a). Aortic pressure increases and vascular resistance in the lungs decreases because of their expansion. Increased flow through the pulmonary veins to the left auricle shuts the foramen ovale. There is now greater pressure in the general circulation than in the pulmonary circulation. Until the ductus arteriosus closes, some aortic blood from the left ventricle is shunted back into the right side, simply because of the pressure gradient. *c:* When the ductus is completely closed, the adult condition is reached.

aorta, and blood freely passes through the ductus arteriosus. This allows the right side of the heart to develop and exercise before the time that pulmonary perfusion must begin. The arrangement for selectively handling venous return to the heart, depending on which vena cava delivers it, sends the most oxygenated blood to the brain and the blood with highest P_{CO_2} and lowest P_{O_2} to the placenta for exchange.

These properties of blood in the umbilical artery maximize the efficiency of exchange processes that take place in the placenta. It should be noted that the shunts present during fetal life cause blood to be pumped by the two sides *in parallel,* in contrast to *in series,* as in postnatal life (compare parts a and c in Figure 10–19). Obviously, striking changes must take place at birth.

At delivery, constriction of the vessels in the cord causes an increase in total peripheral vascular resistance, so intraaortic pressure increases. This pressure will now exceed that in the pulmonary artery. Asphyxia develops in the fetus once its placental supply of oxygen is cut off, and the hypoxemia provokes a gasp to generate negative intrapleural pressure (see Chapter 5). This is responsible for the first postnatal inflation of the lung and, if there is any residual placental circulation, the negativity serves to draw part of the placental blood back to the fetus (see discussion of the thoracic pump in Chapter 5). The inflation of the neonatal lung suddenly reduces pulmonary vascular resistance, and blood from the right ventricle in the pulmonary artery now tends to flow into the lung, rather than be shunted through the ductus arteriosus. Indeed, because intraaortic pressure is now much higher than during fetal life, flow through the ductus actually reverses (see Figure 10–19).

The wall of the ductus is sensitive to PO_2 and as soon as neonatal oxygenation improves, the ductus constricts, or closes down. This closure is normally completed within the first day of postnatal life. The foramen ovale closes because pressure within the left auricle increases from the increased flow in the pulmonary vein. The foramen is covered by a flaplike valve that is pressed back against the opening and eventually seals it closed.

Maternal Adaptations

While these events are occurring in the fetus, gradual changes are evident in the dam. Again, interspecies variation exists, and this variation helps in assessing whether a given mechanism, event, or change is likely to be of critical importance. For example, it has already been noted that many species produce a hormone called placental lactogen that may resemble prolactin or growth hormone. The pattern of secretion of placental lactogen during pregnancy in goats is shown in Figure 10–20. However, many species, including horses, pigs, cats, and dogs, do not produce any such hormone. These interspecies differences make it difficult to claim that a hormone such as this one plays any indispensable role in pregnancy. Another example is provided by vascular adaptations, including striking increases in maternal cardiac output and blood volume in some but not all species. Expansion in blood volume may or may not be accompanied by adequate changes in erythropoiesis, so that packed cell volume, or hematocrit, may actually decrease during pregnancy. This seems to be the reason for *pregnancy anemia* in the bitch.

Maternal adaptations to pregnancy include a redistribution of the cardiac output to favor increased perfusion of the pregnant uterus. At least part of this adaptation is due to increased production of estrogens during pregnancy, causing an increase in uterine blood flow. Sometimes the setpoints for systolic and diastolic arterial pressures are changed so that a transient *physiologic hypertension* prevails. Dietary preferences may also change. These may serve to sup-

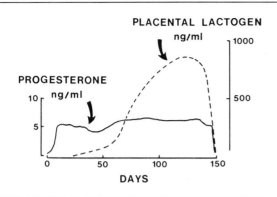

Figure 10–20. Progesterone and placental lactogen in goats. This graph illustrates changes in the plasma concentrations of progesterone (solid line) and of placental lactogen (dotted) during pregnancy in a goat with twin fetuses. Progesterone levels remain fairly constant throughout pregnancy, reflecting the continued secretory activity of the corpora lutea. Placental lactogen is first detected by about day 45 to 50 and then increases to high concentrations during the last third of pregnancy. The concentration of placental lactogen is generally higher in animals carrying twins than in those with a single fetus. Concentrations of both hormones decrease before parturition at day 150.

during pregnancy. The fate of the major nutrients such as glucose may be slightly different during pregnancy, because glucose is a key nutrient for the developing conceptus. In ruminants especially, glucose-sparing mechanisms become of greater importance, so the conceptus gets priority for use of this nutrient. In an earlier description (see Chapter 7) of metabolic adaptations in animals, pregnancy toxemia was provided as an example of a metabolic disorder in pregnant sheep. It dramatically exemplifies the extent to which the pregnant animal is affected by the demands made by the fetus on the dam.

Because pregnancy is normally a prelude to lactation, part of the maternal adaptation involves preparation of the mammary glands for the anticipated secretory function that will follow parturition.

There is reason to believe that many of these maternal changes are under ultimate control that originates in the fetus. Thus the fetus may control production of placental hormones influencing maternal physiologic events to ensure adequate flow of nutrients to the conceptus. Even more intriguing is the possibility that the fetus influences maternal mammary development that will eventually contribute to the postnatal welfare of the fetus. In sheep and goats, for example, the development of secretory tissue in the mammary glands is greater in animals carrying twins than in those with single fetuses.

plement the intake of energy and selected minerals that may be required in greater amounts by the fetus. There is some evidence that the intestinal absorption of calcium is more efficient

10.6 • Maintenance of Pregnancy and Initiation of Labor

The uterus is an organ that is superbly suited to its role as an incubator of the conceptus. Because it is subject to a variety of hormonal controls, it can undergo substantial growth and retain distensibility, so that little or no pressure is exerted on the contents, despite the continuing growth and development of the conceptus. Uterine growth is controlled in part by estrogen and in part by the very slight but sustained stretch that the contents impose on the uterine wall. The typical smooth-muscle attributes of spontaneous or myogenic activity, contraction in response to stretching, and sensitivity to various agonists, are all suppressed during pregnancy. In large part this adaptation to the pregnant state results from the tonic influence of progesterone on the myometrium.

At the end of pregnancy all of these properties are suddenly switched around. The uterus is converted into a powerful expulsive organ that brings about parturition and then begins the process of uterine involution that reduces the organ back to near its nonpregnant size. In some species, such as the rabbit or goat, the *evolution of labor* seems to result from cessation of, or at least a marked reduction in, progesterone secretion. In other species, such as the sheep, a comparable change in progesterone is less obvious and increased prepartum estrogen secretion seems to be more important. *In either case, the relative influences of progesterone and estrogen switch from progesterone being dominant to estrogen being dominant, in the same time period that uterine changes take place.*

Where progesterone withdrawal is most obvious, this requires regression of the corpora lutea in species dependent on their presence for pregnancy maintenance, such as rats, rabbits, goats, and cattle. Others, such as sheep, that have established the capacity for placental progesterone secretion, require some mechanism capable of supressing this endocrine function of the placenta. The mechanisms employed by the small ruminants are the best understood and are described in Box 10-4.

Labor is the term used to describe the phase in which uterine contractions evolve into their most powerful expulsive form, the cervix changes to permit distension by the fetus, and, finally, delivery is achieved. Uterine activity can be monitored by measuring intrauterine pressure or by direct electromyography of the myometrium, using implanted macroelectrodes. The tracings shown in Figure 10-21 are electromyograms and pressure recordings obtained from two sites on the uterus of a pregnant cow. During much of

pregnancy, electrical bursts lasting for several minutes occur about once every hour (Figure 10-21). During labor and immediately after parturition, the contractions occur with highly synchronic electrical bursts lasting about 30 to 45 seconds and occurring at a frequency of about one per minute. The evolution of these expulsive contractions (Figure 10-21) that characterize labor is a gradual process that takes several hours in most domestic species. During this time, dramatic changes occur in the relative concentrations of estrogen and progesterone (Figure 10-22). The fetus assumes its typical presentation attitude (Figure 10-23) during this phase of labor. Under the influence of increasing amounts of estrogens, just at the end of pregnancy, the tough connective tissues of the cervix become markedly softened and there is copious secretion of mucus.

The uterine contractions gradually push the presenting parts of the fetus, usually the extended feet of the forelimbs, into the internal opening of the cervix. The cervix, now suitably prepared, is forcibly distended by the fetus, and stretch receptors in the cervical wall are activated. These communicate via sensory nerves to the spinal cord and then up to the thalamus and hypothalamus, where they trigger a massive release of oxytocin. The oxytocin feeds back positively on the myometrial contractile effort to aid in the final stages of delivery. This neuroendocrine reflex is known as the genital reflex, or *Ferguson's reflex*. The myometrium is maximally sensitized to oxytocin at this time because the shift in estrogen relative to progesterone has prompted the appearance of oxytocin receptors in the sarcolemma of the muscle cells. The same afferent nerves synapse at integrating centers in the spinal cord controlling efferent nerves to abdominal muscles. They are also contracted at this time, in strenuous efforts that are closely synchronized with forced expiration against a closed glottis. The result is the generation of substantial intraabdominal pressure. These combined efforts usually culminate in rapid expulsion of the fetus.

Parturition is a critical event in the life span of an individual. The fetus is at real risk of hy-

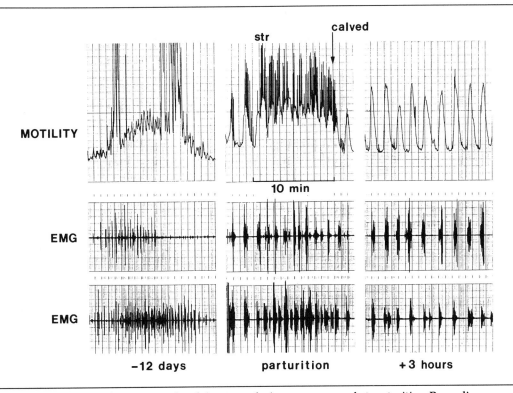

MOTILITY

EMG

EMG

str   calved

10 min

−12 days   parturition   +3 hours

Figure 10–21. *Electromyography of the uterus during pregnancy and at parturition.* Recordings of uterine contractions (motility) and voltages (EMG) detected at two locations on the uterus of a cow during late pregnancy and at parturition. Recordings made 12 days before spontaneous parturition show characteristic long bursts of electrical activity occurring with some synchrony at each site and associated with a sustained mechanical response of the uterine wall. These events are of about 6–12 minutes duration and they occur about once each hour during most of pregnancy. During parturition, the electrical bursts and mechanical responses are quite different; they correspond to what is called labor. Bursts of potentials last for 20–35 seconds; they are usually quite discrete from each other, but they are highly synchronic at the two recording sites. The uterine contractions are also discrete events—except during the final delivery stages when partial fusion of contractions is evident. Part of the motility signal is due to imposed pressures from abdominal straining efforts (str) at this time. Note the sudden change in the character of the signals immediately after the calf is delivered. Following parturition, uterine activity is highly synchronic, and the mechanical events are perfectly synchronized with discrete electromyographic episodes. This activity, recorded here within a few hours after calving, wanes gradually over a few days. To make these recordings, stainless steel electrode wires were sewn into the myometrium, and a strain-sensitive transducer was placed in the uterine wall during surgery under regional anesthesia. Leads from these sensors were exteriorized and protected from the animal. During recording, the wires were connected to a multichannel physiological recorder. The raw signal was amplified, electronically filtered to remove artifactual signals, and then written onto moving chart paper. (Tracings were kindly provided by Dr. H. Kuendig, Institut für Zuchthygiene, Universität Zürich.)

Box 10–4   Control of the Initiation of Labor

In small ruminant animals, there is good evidence that the fetus plays a critical role in triggering the initiation of labor. The duration of pregnancy is remarkably constant within a breed: a day or so variation around a mean value of about 146 days for sheep and 150 days for goats seems to be normal. There are quite consistent breed differences, so pregnancy length in some sheep may be about 142 days, while for others 150 days is typical.

The initiation of labor is closely synchronized to the final stages of maturation of the fetus in its preparation for postnatal life. Central to all of the mechanisms activated at this time is a major change in the function of the fetal adrenal cortex. This gland has grown at much the same rate as the remainder of the fetus, but it has little obvious function until approximately the last 15 days before parturition. In sheep and goats, the adrenal cortex begins to secrete significant amounts of cortisol, starting around day 135 after conception. There is a further increase in cortisol secretion rate during the last 3 to 5 days before birth. These events in the fetal cortex are dependent on adrenocorticotropin (ACTH) from the fetal pituitary, but little is known about why adrenal function picks up at this time.

The initial clues to the control of parturition came from an analysis of several syndromes in which pregnancies are abnormally prolonged. A genetic condition in cattle can cause prolongation of pregnancy, and this condition is associated with striking hypofunction of the adrenal cortex. If afflicted calves are delivered surgically at the expected time of parturition, they show signs of adrenal insufficiency, such as immature lungs, and are not viable. In sheep exposed to certain plants at specific stages of pregnancy, pregnancies are grossly prolonged. One plant contains substances that act as teratogens and derange the normal development of the fetal hypothalamus and pituitary. Such lambs are not born spontaneously. They grow to a size that is greatly in excess of normal birth weight and eventually die in utero. If they are delivered surgically, they are nonviable; at necropsy immature lungs and tiny nonfunctional adrenals are found.

These conditions can be simulated in otherwise normal fetuses by experimental in utero ablation of the pituitary gland, or sectioning of the fetal pituitary stalk. These fetuses are carried beyond term, have hypoplastic adrenals, and immature lungs, and cannot survive a surgical delivery. The lung and viability traits, typical of immaturity, are observed in normal lambs that are delivered surgically prior to about a week before normal expected term. Some such neonates survive with difficulty, but they may suffer functional deficits as a result of the difficulty in breathing, and perhaps hypoxic damage to the brain resulting from insufficient pulmonary surfactant and inadequate lung inflation.

In contrast to the foregoing, if an immature fetus is treated in utero with ACTH, or with glucocorticoid hormones such as dexamethasone (see Figure 4–24), maturation of a whole host of fetal systems is brought about. Most importantly, fetuses treated in this way initiate premature labor and are born. Thus, the fetal hypothalamo-pituitary-adrenal axis is implicated in triggering the initiation of labor.

In fetal sheep, hypercortisolism causes a change in the placental synthesis of steroids. Progesterone production wanes and estrogen synthesis increases. This change promotes prostaglandin synthesis and activation of the uterus into labor. In goats, progesterone is produced by the corpora lutea during pregnancy, and the elevated concentrations of cortisol in the fetus cause prostaglandin release, luteolysis (see Sec-

Figure 10–22. Estrogen and progesterone at parturition in goats. Plasma concentrations of progesterone decrease quite sharply, starting almost exactly 24 hours before fetal delivery. In goats, virtually all of the progesterone is produced by the corpora lutea, so this change reflects pre-partum luteolysis. Throughout the last two days, estrogen is produced by the placenta as part of the maturational events occurring in this tissue along with those in the fetus. The decrease in progesterone and increase in estrogen cause a very marked change in the steroid regulatory environment imposed on the uterus.

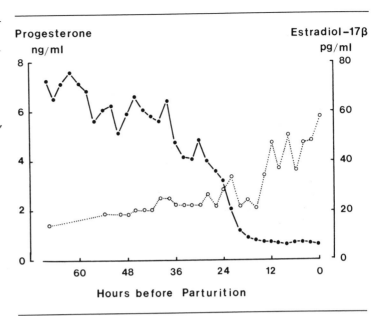

tion 10.2), and an abrupt decline in maternal plasma progesterone concentrations about 24 hours before parturition (see Figure 10–22). In this species the decline in progesterone and the relief of the inhibition it has conferred on the myometrium are responsible for the initiation of labor. These events are summarized in Figure 10–24.

Species have evolved with slight variations of this best-known mechanism. For example, cattle seem to be somewhat intermediate between the sheep and goat in terms of the importance of the corpora lutea and placental production of progesterone for pregnancy maintenance. The role of fetal adrenal activation, however, is equally effective irrespective of the source of the progesterone, and the overall mechanism described seems to account for the initiation of labor in cattle. It is much less certain that other domestic animals use more than just a few component parts of this control scheme. For example, the pig with a litter of maturing fetuses somehow manages to arrest the production of progesterone by the corpora lutea so that labor can evolve. It is still not known with certainty how this is achieved. However, from a practical standpoint, it is known that an injection of prostaglandin is able to cause luteolysis and then to initiate labor.

poxic damage as soon as any pressure or traction is applied to the umbilical cord. The sooner delivery is completed the better, as far as the fetus is concerned. The cascade of events just described results from a change in the regulatory milieu imposed on the myometrium by progesterone and estrogen (Figure 10–24). The events include a mixture of endocrine, neuroendocrine, and purely neural mechanisms. All these mechanisms reinforce one another so that parturition is completed expeditiously.

The interval between fetal and placental de-

Figure 10–23. Normal fetal positioning for delivery. The fetal ruminant is shown with its forelimbs extended towards the cervix (c). The general orientation is indicated for interest. The bones of the pelvis shown are the ilium (il) and ischium (is). The femur (f), vagina (v), uterine wall (uw), and the regressing corpus luteum (cl) on one ovary are also indicated. The fetus normally assumes this position during labor; uterine contractions push the foreparts into the softened cervix. The limbs and head form a wedge-like shape to offer maximum mechanical advantage on the cervix. If the fetus is positioned differently than that shown, for example with even one forelimb flexed rather than extended, the delivery will be far more difficult (dystocia) and may be impossible without obstetrical repositioning.

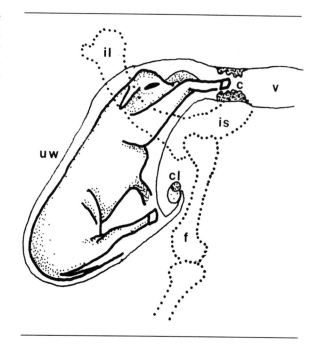

Figure 10–24. Control of the initiation of labor. This diagram illustrates the control of the initiation of labor and the completion of fetal delivery in goats and cattle. Arrows indicate the direction of change in concentration of hormones in blood. The ratio E/P is given a central place in the control of myometrial activity; it is also shown (+) to facilitate the reflex secretion of oxytocin in response to distension of the birth canal and the responsiveness of the uterus to oxytocin. For goats and cattle, the initiation of labor is always preceded by the regression of the corpus luteum, which is due to the release of prostaglandins as luteolysins (described in Box 10–4).

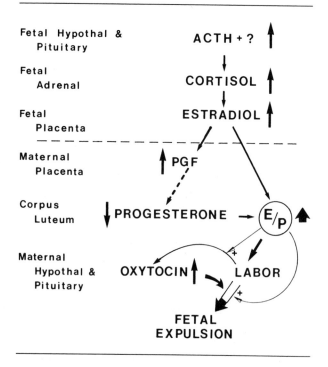

livery varies among species. In litter-bearing animals such as the pig, the placenta detaches readily and is delivered with each fetus. In the mare, the placenta separates easily and is delivered several minutes after the foal. In ruminants, separation of the numerous cotyledonary attachments (see Figure 10–16) takes much longer, and placental delivery might not occur for several hours. If placental delivery is delayed or is not completed by 24 hours, a condition called *retained placenta* exists. This has serious consequences because the cervix cannot close down properly, tissue is left to autolyse within the uterine lumen, and inflammation and infection can occur. These factors all lead to a delay in the normal uterine regressive events that follow parturition.

Maternal Postpartum Adjustments

Uterine involution begins at about the time of fetal and placental delivery and proceeds for some weeks in the larger animals until the organ is almost as small as in nulliparous animals, those that have never completed a pregnancy. Substantial quantities of protein are mobilized from the involuting tissue, but substrates are also required for repair of the endometrium in preparation for a subsequent pregnancy. Some species, for example the horse, are capable of initiating another pregnancy almost immediately after parturition, so it is difficult to generalize on the consequences of the involutionary process.

Many animals, best exemplified by cattle, enter a phase of *postpartum anestrus* and are reproductively inactive for a time. Others, such as goats, may be seasonally anestrous at the time they normally bear their young, so they too will be inactive for some time. In sheep that have been selected for insensitivity to season, such as ewes of the Dorset breed, cyclic ovarian activity will often resume shortly after the lambs are weaned. Although the mechanism is not completely understood, the pituitary-ovarian axis is often inhibited during heavy lactation.

The normality of uterine involution may be assessed by palpation through the rectal wall in cattle and horses. In humans and small domestic animals, noninvasive methods such as ultrasonography can be used to determine the size of the uterus. The rate at which involution takes place is a factor determining the time before cyclical ovarian activity is resumed, and the opportunity to initiate another pregnancy. This is of economic importance in cattle. It is not unreasonable to assume that while uterine involution is proceeding, there is continued release of prostaglandins from the endometrial tissues, and these can be expected to negatively influence ovarian function.

The most striking maternal adjustment occurring in the periparturient period is the initiation of lactation. The mechanisms underlying the development of the mammary glands and the switch to active lactation will be discussed in the next chapter. The female completes her pregnancy, having sustained the metabolic burden of the conceptus as it develops, and then reorganizes her function to provide for the needs of the offspring. At the same time her reproductive tract is repaired and readied for a subsequent pregnancy.

10.7 • Reproduction in the Chicken

Anatomy

The testes in the chicken are abdominal and located ventrad to the anterior portion of the kidneys. Vasa deferentia lead back to the middle segment of the cloaca where they enter dorsally, just lateral to the ureters. In females, only the left ovary persists and is found dorsally to the left of the midline, proximally to the kidney and suspended on the mesovarium. The functionally active ovary contains follicles at all stages of development (Figure 10–25). The reproductive tract is often called the oviduct, but, for consistency with description of the mammalian tract in Section 10.1, it will be considered here to consist of

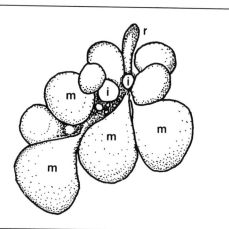

Figure 10–25. Chicken ovary. The single functional ovary of the chicken has follicles at all stages of maturation. The body of the ovary contains primary follicles and there will usually be a number of immature (i)—but nevertheless growing—follicles. The most obvious structures are the maturing follicles (m) that form a hierarchy of sizes enabling prediction of the order by which they will ovulate. The mature follicles have accumulated substantial quantities of yolk. A ruptured follicular structure (r) is shown. Note that there are no structures equivalent to the mammalian corpora lutea.

ovary, infundibulum, magnum, isthmus, uterus, and vagina (Figure 10–26). The tract develops functionally on the left side. It shares some features with the mammalian tract; namely, transport of gametes and provision of the fertilization site. The differences are more important than the similarities, however. Portions of the tract are specialized for massive secretory activity so the yolk, released from the follicle at ovulation, becomes surrounded with albumin (the egg white), then is enclosed in membranes and, finally, inside a shell. The uterus (shell gland), somewhat homologous to the mammalian uterus, is specialized to accommodate the egg as it completes its development and is capable of powerful expulsive activity to enable ovipositioning (the laying of the egg—its movement from the uterus, through the vagina to the cloaca, and its leaving the vent).

Ovary

The ovary, while dominated by relatively enormous follicles being prepared for ovulation, is histologically similar to the mammalian organ described in Section 10.1. Externally, a capsule of germinal epithelium encloses stromal tissue. Blood vessels and nerves are concentrated in the inner, medullary portion. Each follicle contains an oocyte (ovum), a variable amount of yolk, a layer of granulosa cells, and follicular thecal cells. The size of an individual follicle reflects the amount of accumulated yolk; two broad classes of follicles include those undergoing rapid growth (about a dozen) and hundreds of small follicles from primary stages to those of a few millimeters in diameter. Yolk expansion is one of the functions of the follicular cells because, controlled by estrogens, the cells selectively transport lipids of plasma origin and synthesize proteins to be deposited as lipoprotein complexes in the yolk. In laying chickens, the ovary contains a hierarchy of follicles of different sizes,

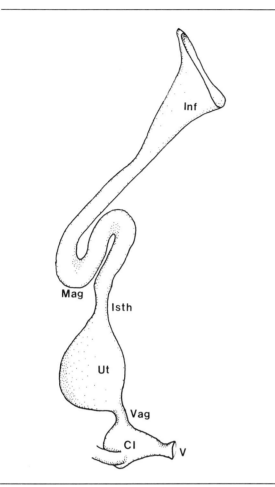

Figure 10–26. The reproductive tract of the chicken. The unilaterally developing oviduct is shown here dissected from its in situ orientation. The infundibulum (Inf) is closely adjacent to the ovary. The oviduct comprises segments named the magnum (Mag), isthmus (Isth), the uterus or shell gland (Ut), and vagina (Vag). The vagina communicates with the exterior via the cloaca (Cl) and vent (V).

each of which will be ovulated at approximately 25- to 28-hour intervals: the largest follicle will be the next to be ovulated, the second largest will be ovulated a day later, and so on.

The Oviduct

The general form of the oviduct is as described for mammals. Suspended on connective tissue ligaments formed from folds of peritoneum, the tube-like structure consists of a serosal, connective tissue ligament; an outer longitudinal smooth muscle layer; an inner circular muscle layer; a supportive submucosa of connective tissue; and an innermost mucosal epithelium.

The infundibulum is funnel shaped, located near the ovary, and captures the ovum at ovulation. Fertilization occurs toward the magnum but is not a prerequisite for egg formation and ovipositioning. Sperm may be held in the vicinity of the fertilization site awaiting arrival of the ovum. The infundibulum contributes to egg formation by secreting a mucoid substance that coats the membrane of the ovum (vitelline membrane). During transit of the magnum, the mucoid material is twisted into a characteristic form at each pole of the yolk, and the whitish twisted material, readily discerned in a broken egg, is called the *chalazae*.

The magnum is the longest portion of the tract and is especially important because it secretes the albumin layers that surround the yolk. The first portion immediately covers the chalazal layer and is *thin albumin*. Next is the *thick albumin* (about 50 to 60% of the total), and the outermost layer is a viscous liquid enclosed within the *inner shell membrane*.

The isthmus provides the inner and outer shell membranes to the developing egg. The inner membrane totally encloses the outermost liquid portion of albumin. The outer membrane, highly keratinized and rough surfaced, is the substratum upon which the shell is deposited (Figure 10–27).

The uterus contains epithelium capable of secreting all components of the shell. The dominant component is a crystalline form of calcium carbonate, which is deposited on a proteinaceous matrix. If the shell is to be pigmented, this process also occurs in the uterus. Finally, a superficial cuticle of protein is deposited shortly before ovipositioning. The uterus responds to the neurohypophyseal peptide (*arginine vasotocin*), which is closely related to oxytocin and vasopressin (ADH), and will also contract in response to prostanoids (see Section 4.4).

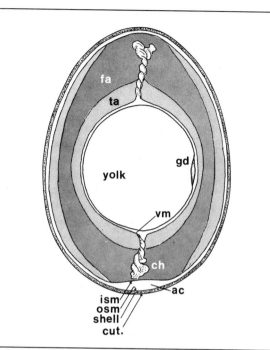

Figure 10–27. The chicken's egg. The chicken's egg is a multi-layered structure, formation of which is detailed in the text. The yolk is somewhat organized, although this is not depicted here beyond showing the germinal disk (gd) lying under the vitelline membrane (vm). The chalazae (ch) are the twisted structures of mucoid material that coat the yolk. The egg white consists of concentric layers of thin albumin (ta), firm albumin (fa), and a final viscous layer (unlabeled) underlying the inner shell membrane (ism). At one pole of the egg, a distinct air cavity (ac) separates the inner and outer shell membrane (osm), though to distinguish these membranes, the cavity is shown here to extend all around the periphery. The shell is deposited on the outer shell membrane and in turn is covered by cuticle (cut.).

The Ovulatory Cycle

The timing of ovulation and of ovipositioning is interrelated and because ovipositioning can be monitored very easily (and even recorded automatically for caged birds using very simple sensors), it is convenient to describe laying patterns and then to consider the ovulatory events.

Chickens typically lay a number of eggs on successive days, skip a day, and then start another series of daily layings. The eggs produced on successive days constitute a *sequence* consisting of a variable number of eggs *(sequence length)*. In the highly selected strains of chickens used in commercial egg production, a large proportion of birds have long sequences without skip-days; such birds are the most productive. Each successive oviposition within a sequence occurs at a slightly later time of the day.

Ovarian function is subject to regulation by gonadotropins of pituitary origin. Removal of the pituitary (hypophysectomy) arrests follicular development and initiates regressive changes (atresia) in partially developed follicles. The follicle wall matures through a process whereby its endocrine secretory function changes in a predictable fashion according to the number of days until that particular follicle is ready for ovulation. The follicle is capable of producing progesterone, androgens, and estrogens along with prostanoids and peptides similar to the hormones involved in ovipositioning. There is no corpus luteum produced from the ruptured follicle.

While ovarian steroidogenesis depends on stimulation by gonadotropins, the steroids provide part of the control over the massive release of LH (the ovulatory surge). An important component of control over this increased secretion of LH is the stage of the light:dark cycle. For the first ovulation of a sequence, this photoperiodic factor is probably the dominant control. Ovulation occurs some hours after the surge in LH secretion and that ovum completes development to be laid about 26 hours after ovulation. The timing of the LH surge, ovulation, and ovipositioning of the second egg in the sequence are similarly related but are delayed by 0.5 to 2.5 hours from the events for the first ovulation. This pattern of time offset continues with subsequent ovulations within the sequence until the next expected surge of LH would occur at an inappropriate time of the light:dark cycle. The LH surge fails to occur, the preovulatory follicle is not ovulated on the day of the last ovipositioning of the sequence, and so the laying sequence is broken on the next day. During the night after the last ovipositioning of the sequence, the LH surge that is triggered primarily by time into the dark phase of the light:dark cycle enables the arrested follicle to be ovulated; this is laid about a day later as the first egg of the new sequence.

Mating, Fertilization, and Development

Copulation in the chicken is part of an elaborate pattern of mating behavior involving advances by the male and initial escape and avoidance maneuvers on the part of the hen. Finally the female assumes a position called the mating crouch and is mounted by the male. In chickens intromission is not used for insemination; rather, the cloacas of both sexes are everted and make superficial contact. Sperm are held in folds of the lining of the uterovaginal region from which they are released periodically, usually temporally related to ovipositioning, to travel through the oviduct to the fertilization site. Fertilizability is retained for about 10 days after insemination.

Sex determination in birds differs from that in mammals. All sperm carry the same sex chromosome so the female gamete determines sex of the progeny. The ovum either has the sex chromosome (the same as in the sperm) or it

does not. If the embryo is homozygous for the sex chromosome (i.e., one from the sperm along with one from an ovum) it will develop as a male. If the union involved an ovum lacking the sex chromosome, the embryo contains only the one chromosome derived from the sperm and so it must develop as a female.

Initial stages of chick embryo development are very rapid, and a cell mass is present by the time of ovipositioning about 24 hours following fertilization. It should be obvious that all of the nutritive needs of the prehatched chicken must be provided within the egg. Additional needs include warmth, humidity, and rotation and are provided by the hen or by mechanical incubators. The normal period of incubation is 20 days and is followed by hatching, a process that is initiated by the chick, though still incompletely understood. The maturing embryo undergoes a predictable programmed ontogeny. More is known about the embryology of the domestic chick than any other species.

Hatching may be logically viewed as an escape phenomenon and is likely initiated by a combination of deprivation of nutrients within the egg; inappropriate balance of respiratory gases; maturation of the chick's nervous, endocrine, and metabolic systems; and so on. The role of the uterus in expelling the egg and the role of the embryo in initiating the hatch shows surprising similarity to the events described in Section 10.5 for mammals.

10.8 • Exercises

1. What is the name of the inner epithelial lining of the uterus?

List two functions of the active ovary.

What is the term used to describe the process of regression and involution of the corpus luteum?

The corpus luteum is transformed into/arises from a mature follicle by the process of luteinization (strike out one).

Efferent ducts from the testes collect into the head/the body/the tail of the epididymis (strike out incorrect choices).

Provide an alternative word for cornua.

What is the name of the duct connecting the epididymis to the urethra?

The testicular cells responsible for testosterone production are Sertoli cells/Leydig cells (strike out one).

What is the technical term for sex drive?

2. Outline the events that take place at the end of one luteal phase, encompassing a follicular phase, ovulation, and the beginning of a new luteal phase, in a ruminant animal.

What is different in an animal that conceived on mating at the previous estrus, and in which no subsequent estrus is observed?

What could be used as a simple means of detecting pregnancy, given your analysis of the foregoing?

3. Identify, from the list lettered a–f, where the events in the second list take place:

a. seminiferous tubules   b. oviduct
c. uterine lumen   d. epididymis
e. vagina   f. endometrium

_____ early cleavage divisions

_____ normal fertilization

_____ sperm capacitation

_____ coitus

_____ placentation

_____ blastocyst hatching

_____ implantation

_____ sperm maturation

_____ tubal pregnancy

_____ spermatogenesis

4. Outline the sequence of events leading up to the completion of fetal delivery in a ruminant animal in which maintenance of pregnancy depends on continued secretory function of the corpus luteum.

5. Either (1) describe the control of maturation of the fetal lung and the events leading to the initiation of breathing immediately after delivery, or (2) outline the cardiovascular adjustments that distinguish the pattern of circulation in fetal versus postnatal life.

Lactational Biology

11

Lactational biology is a specialty area of mammalian physiology that has much in common with reproductive physiology, nutrition, metabolism, growth, and development. It is of particular importance in the biology of domestic animals, both in regard to the needs of the young mammal in its early postnatal life and because the secretory product, milk, is a valuable agricultural commodity, the harvesting of which is the basis for the dairy industry.

A comprehensive treatment of lactational biology begins with embryologic differentiation of ectodermal cells into the primitive mammary streak, a process that occurs about the time that the embyro assumes a C-shaped form, early in gestation. As there will be much reference to the histological elements of the mammary gland, a description of the various tissues making up the mature gland will be provided first.

11.1 • Functional Anatomy

The functional glandular, or secretory, unit of mammary tissue is the *alveolus*. As introduced in Chapter 1 (see Figure 1–7) when epithelia were first described, the alveolus can be considered as a flasklike structure, the inner lining of which is made up of cuboidal secretory epithelium. The lumen of the alveolus contains secretory products awaiting ejection into and through the duct system during milking or suckling. The ducts connect the lumina of variable numbers of alveoli in a progressively expanding series of collecting ducts. In some species, such as the ruminants, these larger ducts drain into a *cistern,* which then communicates to the exterior.

Other species lack cisterns so the largest of the ducts serve as reservoirs for secreted product. They communicate directly to the exterior through multiple openings in the *nipple.* Where a single channel leaves the cistern to the exterior, it is enclosed within a *teat.*

Immediately exterior to the layer of secretory epithelium, the alveolus includes specialized *myoepithelial* cells. These are spindle- or stellate-shaped, muscle-like cells that wrap around the alveolus and are capable of contracting, thereby exerting pressure on the alveolar contents to cause milk ejection (Figure 11–1). The cells are physiologically stimulated by oxytocin as part of the milk ejection reflex. This was described in Chapter 4 as an example of a neurohumoral reflex, and further description will follow in this chapter.

Surrounding the epithelium and the myoepithelium is a basement membrane that provides structural support for the alveolar cells. The basement membrane separates the alveolus from nearby capillaries and lymphatics and attaches to the connective tissues of the gland.

The next level of organization is the *lobule.* Lobules are aggregations of many alveoli, along with the finest of the ductal units, making discrete macroscopic structures. They are invested with fine supporting connective tissue elements that constitute the stroma of the gland. In turn these connective elements are attached to the more rugged connective tissue components of the gland, forming the system of mammary ligaments.

The ligaments are the basis for the gross morphology of the mammary gland. They provide support, particularly for the pendulous glands of quadrupeds, and they separate the individual glands. For example, the cow has four

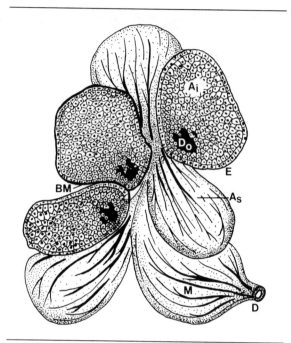

Figure 11–1. The mammary alveolus. This construct shows a group of alveoli, some viewed in section to show the internal appearance (A_i) and some from their serosal surface (A_s). The walls, made up of secretory epithelium (E) are shown for two adjacent alveoli, separated by the basement membrane (BM). Each alveolus drains (D_o) into a system of ducts (D). Myoepithelial cells (M) are shown, with their typical stellate geometries, on the serosal surface of the alveoli.

glands, called *quarters,* arranged as two halves, each with a forequarter and a hindquarter. A medial ligament separates the left and right halves, and there is a bilateral pair of suspensory ligaments. The latter are located external to the mass of secretory tissue, or *parenchyma,* and lie under spongy, subcutaneous connective tissue and the skin. Ligamentous tissue also separates the forequarters and hindquarters but is less obvious than the median and lateral structures (Figure 11–2).

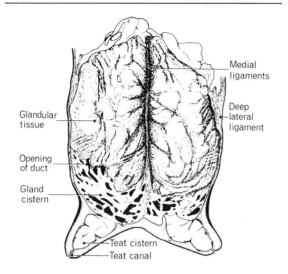

Figure 11–2. Gross structure of the bovine mammary gland. Section cut in the transverse plane shows the relative organization of the mass of secretory parenchyma, or glandular tissue, with the duct and cistern system. The form of the glands is defined by the supporting ligaments, medial and lateral. The gland cisterns communicate with teat cisterns and with the exterior via teat, or streak, canals. (Reproduced by permission of the publisher. From Cowie, A.T. and Buttle, H.L.: "Lactation," in Hafez, E.S.E.: *Reproduction in Farm Animals*, 4th edition, Philadelphia: Lea & Febiger, 1980.)

Vascular Supply and Drainage

The vascular supply to mammary tissue is extensive, particularly during lactation. It is organized into a branching system that is duplicated bilaterally. The major vessels run in the heavy connective tissues and arteries branch off to penetrate the parenchyma by arborizing throughout the interlobular connective tissues. Grossly, the mammary glands of cattle are supplied with arterial blood from four *mammary arteries* that are branches of the *pudic arteries*, each of which arises from the external iliac arteries on either side (Figure 11–3). There may be some additional arterial input from the perineal vessels and sometimes from the abdominal arteries. At the finest level, arterioles and capillary beds are found in intimate association with the fine connective elements surrounding each alveolus.

There is a similar venous organization and a well-developed lymphatic drainage system, complete with lymph nodes within the mammary mass. The major veins draining the bovine gland are the *subcutaneous abdominal veins*, readily discerned running forward near the midline on the ventral surface, and the paired *pudic veins*, which pass internally into the iliac veins. The

Figure 11–3. The circulatory system of the bovine udder. The major vessels of the mammary gland are shown, with veins unshaded. The bulk of the arterial supply is via the pudic arteries (PA), shown here arising via the external iliacs (IA) from the abdominal aorta (AA). The remainder is obtained from perineal vessels (VP). Notice the complex of major vessels, mammary artery and vein (MA&V), just dorsal to the bulk of the udder. This anastomosing ring of veins supplies the subcutaneous abdominal mammary veins (MV_{ab}) as well as pudic veins (PV).

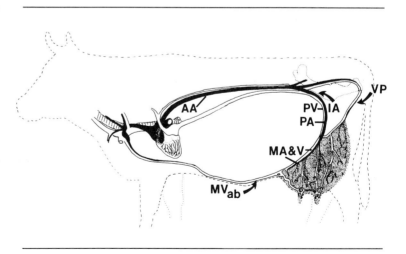

major veins collect venous blood from an anastomosing "ring" of vessels located at the dorsal base of the udder (Figure 11–4).

Mammary tissue is a specialized derivative of cutaneous tissue, which originates in the ectodermal tissues of the embryo. For this reason, blood supply to the gland is controlled by many of the same mechanisms that control perfusion of other cutaneous structures. The shared system of control is important in understanding the dynamics of mammary blood flow and the effects of stress on mammary function.

Development of the Bovine Mammary Gland

The process of development of mammary tissue is described by the term *mammogenesis*. Mammogenesis can be conveniently considered in five phases: fetal, prepuberal, postpuberal, pregnancy, and early lactation.

Prenatal Development

Prenatal development begins very early, with organogenesis of what will become mammary tissue taking place just a few weeks after conception. The ectodermal tissues that will eventually give rise to all skin and skin-derivative organs flatten out on the ventral surface as a band of cells known as the *mammary streak*. During these very early stages, when the embryo is merely 1 cm or so in length, there is no discernible difference between fetuses destined to develop as males and those destined to develop as females. The gonad is indifferent at this time, but the embryo will either have XX or XY sex chromosomes, so its genetic sex is unquestionably determined.

The initial developmental changes are due to the aggregation and organization of a portion of the germinal cells of the lower ectoderm that have been programmed to give rise to the mammary structures.

As development proceeds, the primitive cells form *mammary buds*, spherical structures that sink back into the mesenchyme except for a *pit*, that will eventually give rise to the teat. At this time, some 50 days after conception, the embryo is about 2 cm long, has formed limbs, and has assumed a distinctive quadruped shape. The male and female begin to develop a little differently after this stage, so the remainder of the description will be confined to the female fetus.

A phase of rapid proliferation of the mammary bud causes the tissue to push up under the ventral skin surface, and the most superficial end of the bud begins to open. By about 90 days, when the fetus is some 15 cm long and weighs about 200 gm, the teat and cistern structures start to form by invagination of the mammary bud. The teat now has a distinct lumen, and the cistern gives rise to primitive ducts that arborize back into the deeper tissue mass. The laying down of connective tissues and adipocytes at the base of the developing gland becomes evident at this stage. The connective tissues form into ligamentous sheets that will later support the secretory tissue. The other form of connective tissue, developing from the adipocytes, is known as the *mammary fat pad*. This will eventually be replaced by secretory tissue during postpuberal development. During the remainder of gestation and prepuberal development, the glandular structure expands at about the same rate as growth of the body in general. It has a primitive blood and lymphatic supply and has the basic architecture needed for subsequent maturation.

Prepuberal Development

Prepuberal development of the mammary tissue is unimpressive. There is some general growth, at much the same rate as the rest of the body. Such growth is called *isometric*. The duct system develops and the four glands start to grow together. There are still no alveolar units, so the internal mass of the gland remains essentially as a fat fad.

Figure 11–4. The dissected mammary gland. In this view, the left forequarter and teat are sectioned saggitally to show the parenchymal mass in section (MP$_{ss}$), the cistern (c), teat lumen (tl), and streak canal (sc). The mammary arteries and veins (MA&V) are shown at the base of the udder. The vein supplies the abdominal mammary vein (MV$_{ab}$) and the mammary vein (MV) that becomes the external pudic vein (EPV). The hindquarter is partially skinned, and sectioned in the transverse plane (tp) just behind the forequarter to show the cut surface of the parenchyma. The skin (S) overlies spongy connective tissue and the curved mass of the quarter is defined by the lateral suspensory ligament (LSL). Tributary lymphatics (L$_t$) pass to the lymph node (LN) which is drained dorsally. (Redrawn with modifications from W. Mosimann, Zentralverband schweizerischer Milchproduzenten, copyright © 1979.)

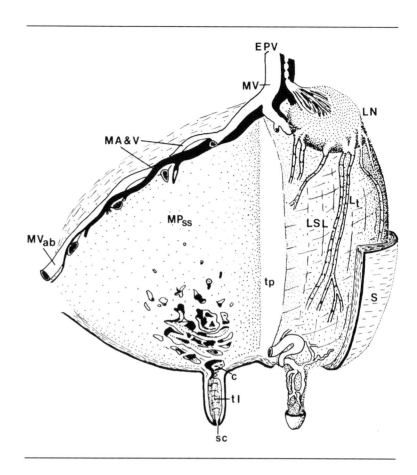

Puberal Development

At the time of puberty, hormones of the ovary begin to be secreted and, together with the pituitary hormones, lead to accelerated growth of mammary tissue. By a variety of criteria, mammary growth now proceeds much faster than growth of the body as a whole. Differential growth such as this is called *allometric* (meaning "not the same"). The ovarian steroids, estrogen and progesterone, and the pituitary hormones, especially growth hormone and prolactin, seem to be most important. The major ducts give rise to a series of branches, and buds of tissue proliferate into the fat pad. With each estrous cycle, there seems to be a phase of accelerated cell division, followed by some loss of cells. Each cycle, however, results in a net accumulation of parenchymal cells. These events result in invasion of the fat pad with an extensive branching system of ducts and primitive alveolar units. However, the fat pad is still the most obvious tissue mass in the gland at this time.

Pregnancy

During the early stages of pregnancy the cyclical changes in plasma estrogen and progestin concentrations are interrupted, and the gland is exposed to a fairly constant influence of progesterone. In domestic animals, there is little estrogen present during the first half of pregnancy. Only after about midway through pregnancy are major developmental changes evident in the mammae. The gland cistern begins to expand and secretory tissue proliferates off the terminal branches of the duct system. The alveolar units are quite discernible at this time and the vascular system develops fully. These changes probably reflect the gradual, but now continuous, exposure of the tissue to estrogens being produced by the placenta. Although there is some uncertainty about the cow, in other ruminants, placental lactogen probably stimulates the continuing development of the gland that characterizes pregnancy. Of the various domestic species, most is known about the goat. The number of fetuses relates to the total mass of placental tissue and then to the concentrations of placental lactogen (see Figure 10–20) present in the maternal plasma. During late pregnancy the mass of parenchymal tissue seems to relate closely to the concentrations of placental lactogen. This is another fascinating biologic adaptation that provides a mechanism whereby the fetuses dictate the degree of maternal preparation for lactation. The fetuses therefore partly control the ability of the dam to provide for postnatal nourishment of the young.

In the final stages of pregnancy, the beginnings of secretory function are apparent. There is limited synthesis of certain milk components and they accumulate, along with proteins selectively transported across the alveolar wall from the blood, in the alveolar lumen. The secretion has a high content of solids, particularly protein and cellular debris from the breakdown of alveolar epithelial cells. This product is called *colostrum* and it is noteworthy because of its high content of immune globulins, which confer passive immunity on the newborn.

Early Lactation

During established lactation, after parturition, there is still proliferation of mammary tissue, although the vast bulk of mammary growth is completed before parturition. The secretory cells perform at an incredible rate during lactation and it seems that considerable turnover of epithelial cells continues well into lactation. In part, epithelial cell turnover may reflect replacement and regeneration of the alveolar lining, but part of the cell division may result in a slight additional increase in total secretory mass. The turnover of cells is believed to continue throughout lactation, but gradually loss begins to surpass replacement and there is a net loss of secretory mass. There is reasonable evidence that the gland's secretory cell mass reaches its peak a few weeks after parturition, a time when milk production is also maximal.

11.2 • The Cell Biology of Milk Synthesis and Secretion

The synthesis of milk components imposes a great burden on the secretory epithelium and all of the support systems needed to deliver substrates to the cells. The cells are continuously replacing parts of their organelles as many of them leave the cells along with the secreted product. Central to all of this activity is the feature that mammary epithelial cells are specialized for the export of lipid, because the solids in milk contain as much as 50% by weight as fat.

The fat synthesized in the mammary gland is of course hydrophobic and it accumulates within the epithelial cell as a naked droplet within the cytoplasm. This enlarges in size as more triglycerides are synthesized and are incorporated into the droplet. Eventually the droplet dominates the volume of the cell and presses against the apical plasmalemma (Figure 11–5). The apical portion of the cell is on the luminal or free surface of the alveolus, opposite the basement membrane side. Biophysical forces cause the droplet to press the apical membrane out on the free surface, then this membrane closes in behind the lipid droplet and eventually causes it to be pinched off.

The lipid droplet is then released into the lumen of the alveolus, enclosed in a membrane derived from the secretory cell. This is the *milk fat membrane* and it contains the polar lipid fraction of milk fat. All typical plasmalemma constituents, described in Chapter 2, are present in this unique secretory product. Obviously, continued loss of plasmalemma cannot be tolerated by the secretory cell unless there is provision for the membrane to be replenished. This is achieved as part of the secretory mechanism for other milk constituents.

Milk proteins are secreted from granules packaged in the Golgi apparatus and thereby are enclosed in Golgi-derived membrane that eventually gets incorporated into the plasmalemma. The nature of this type of secretory mechanism, whereby secretory vesicles fuse into the plasmalemma as their contents are ejected, was noted earlier, and examples were provided for neurotransmitters (see Figure 3–10).

Milk fat is a unique biological product consisting of a bulk volume of triglycerides enclosed in a lipoprotein membrane. The triglycerides are unusual in structure, as noted in the initial discussion of digestion (see Chapter 6). Typically they consist of one short chain fatty acid, such as butyric acid ($C_{4:0}$), one medium chain acid, such as palmitic acid ($C_{16:0}$) and one longer chain acid that may or may not be unsaturated. In ruminants, few dietary unsaturated fatty acids escape hydrogenation before absorption from the gut, and this longer chain acid may be stearic acid ($C_{18:0}$) or a monounsaturated acid formed within the animal. Usually this is oleic acid ($C_{18:1}$) or palmitoleic acid ($C_{16:1}$) formed by desaturation of the corresponding saturated acid. This desaturase activity is an enzymic property of the mammary cell and it may function to provide the cell with reducing equivalents in the form of the hydrogens removed from the saturated acids.

The synthesis of milk lipid can be considered in several parts. There is some new synthesis, or de novo synthesis, of the short to medium chain fatty acids that takes place within the cell (see below). Some of the medium chain fatty acids and virtually all of the long chain fatty acids are taken up from lipid fractions in the blood. As noted above, some of these may be-

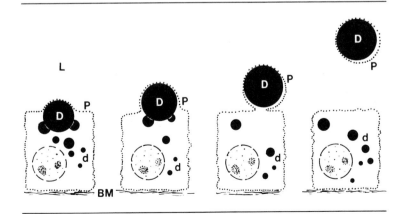

Figure 11–5. Secretion of milk fat. These views show small droplets (d) of fat coalescing into a major droplet (D) under the plasmalemma (P) on the apical pole of the cell adjacent to the lumen (L) of the alveolus. The basal pole contacts the basement membrane (BM), as shown in Figure 11–1. When the droplet (D) pinches off, it is surrounded by cell-derived plasmalemma.

come unsaturated within the epithelial cell. The fatty acids are incorporated from their activated, or coenzyme A (CoA-) ester form, into triglycerides, described in the section on triglyceride synthesis.

Fatty Acid Synthesis

As briefly introduced in Chapter 7, fatty acids can be synthesized from two-carbon units (acetyl-CoA) by a series of condensations resulting in the formation of longer chain length acids, or their CoA esters. These usually have an even number of carbons. If the condensation of 2C units is onto a 3C acid (propionic acid) as the initial substrate, the final product will be an odd-numbered fatty acid. These odd chain length acids do occur but only in very minor amounts.

The basic incremental unit is from acetyl-CoA. As emphasized earlier, ruminants directly activate acetic acid to acetyl-CoA so they do not need to expend scarce glycolytic substrates to obtain acetyl-CoA. Chain elongation proceeds to a variable degree before fatty acid synthesis is terminated. In mammary tissue, a substantial portion of the fatty acids synthesized de novo is of intermediate chain length. More striking is the fact that many of the acids are merely 4, 6, or 8 carbons in length.

The mammary gland is also capable of taking up ketone bodies, particularly beta-hydroxybutyric acid, and converting them into butyric acid for milk fat synthesis. The process of fatty acid synthesis consumes large amounts of reducing equivalents in the form of hydrogen, carried on a coenzyme NADP, in the form of NADPH. The reduced form, NADPH, is generated by metabolism of glucose, so even though in ruminants glucose does not contribute carbon to the fatty acid chain, it does provide these essential reducing equivalents.

Many of the fatty acids are obtained from blood lipids. Triglycerides in the blood are hydrolyzed by the enzyme lipoprotein lipase, an extracellular enzyme of the capillary endothelium. Nonesterified fatty acids, which are readily available during extensive mobilization of adipose tissue reserves, particularly early in lactation, can also be extracted from the plasma and used by the mammary tissue. During times of excessive fat mobilization, the fatty acid composition of the milk fat more closely resembles that of adipose depots.

Triglyceride Synthesis

The triglycerides are assembled by esterification of fatty acyl-CoA esters onto α-glycerophosphate. This is a triose product of glycolysis (see Chapter 7). Each glucose molecule entering glycolysis can give rise to two molecules of α-glycerophosphate. Some use may also be made of free glycerol, obtained from the blood, and ultimately derived from the hydrolysis of blood triglycerides by the action of lipoprotein lipase. Provision exists in the mammary glands of some species to phosphorylate the glycerol into the activated form, α-glycerophosphate, as required for triglyceride synthesis.

During esterification, a short chain acid is incorporated along with two longer chain acids. The three CoA moieties, from the three fatty acyl CoAs, are made available again for further synthesis of fatty acids. When triglyceride synthesis is slowed down, perhaps because of insufficient glucose to form α-glycerophosphate, or because of excessive accumulation of milk within the gland, fatty acid synthesis will also slow down, possibly because the availability of CoA becomes limiting.

As triglyceride molecules are assembled, they are attracted hydrophobically to other triglycerides and gradually coalesce into lipid droplets. The minute droplets fuse with each other to form large droplets in an attempt to minimize their surface area relative to volume. This is entirely predictable behavior related to surface properties of immiscible substances. The droplet leaves the cell enclosed within apical plasmalemma (see Figure 11–5).

Milk Proteins

Milk proteins are a diverse mixture of components, some of which are directly transferred across the endothelial-epithelial barrier from the plasma, others of which are synthesized de novo within the secretory epithelial cell. The most important of the latter fraction is the group of proteins called *casein*. Caseins are phosphoproteins in which many of the serine residues are phosphorylated. The mixture of casein subtypes is aggregated as micelles in milk. The aggregates include a large portion of the total content of the calcium in milk, and they give milk its characteristic opacity. Caseins have minimal solubility in the acidic range of pH and they are also precipitated by the abomasal enzyme called rennin. It was noted in Chapter 6 that milk proteins are clotted by rennin, possibly to delay their passage from the abomasum so that peptic digestion can proceed to completion.

Other important milk proteins include the broad classes of *lactoglobulins* and *lactalbumins*. These names merely describe physicochemical properties of the proteins. For example, proteins that are soluble in isotonic salt solutions, about 0.15M NaCl, but not in water are called globulins. One of the lactalbumins, α-lactalbumin, has special importance. It is one of the two subunits that make up the important mammary enzyme called *lactose synthetase*. This enzyme is unique to mammary tissue and milk, and it accounts for the unique occurrence of the disaccharide, *lactose*, in milk. Milk proteins have high biologic value, meaning that they provide an ideal balance of amino acids to support the growth of young mammals. The amino acid composition is the major factor determining the nutritive quality of proteins.

The milk proteins that are synthesized within the secretory cells are assembled from amino acids taken up from blood plasma. The amino acid sequence of the proteins is genetically coded and assembly takes place in aggregations of ribosomes, called polysomes, in the rough endoplasmic reticulum. The assembly is directed by codes provided by mRNA, in turn transcribed from DNA within the nucleus. The highly differentiated state of mammary epithelium is reflected in the unique expression of genes controlling synthesis of proteins found only in milk.

There is limited production of nonessential amino acids within the secretory epithelium using the transamination mechanisms, noted briefly in Chapter 7.

Lactose

Lactose, the disaccharide unique to milk, consists of two monosaccharides, one glucose and one galactose. The enzyme *lactose synthetase* is present only in lactating tissue. Its appearance in mammary tissues signals the onset of lactation, the process known as *lactogenesis*. Actually, it is the appearance of one of the two subunits of the enzyme, α-lactalbumin, that is the critical event for initiating lactose synthesis. The formation of the milk sugar takes place in the Golgi apparatus using monosaccharides obtained exclusively from blood glucose. Glucose is converted in part to galactose prior to its condensation to form lactose, but both monosaccharides are ultimately derived from glucose.

Lactose is osmotically active, so the secretion of lactose into the alveolar lumen draws along water. This is so effective that the concentration of lactose, expressed in mass per unit volume of fat-free milk, or the exclusively aqueous component, is remarkably constant. From this it should be obvious that any adjustment resulting in more lactose being synthesized will also result in more milk volume being secreted. The limiting factor for lactose synthesis in ruminants is unquestionably glucose availability. Of course, in ruminants, glucose availability is largely a reflection of the availability for gluconeogenesis of suitable substrates from the gut. When animals are fed diets enabling larger amounts of propionic acid to be produced by fermentation, more glucose can be synthesized by the liver, more lactose can be synthesized in the mammary gland, and milk volume increases. Diets containing soluble sugars, such as lush young pasture, or those containing ample amounts of starch, such as corn, favor this process.

Most important at this time is the concept that glucose is a critical substrate for milk synthesis. The bulk of the glucose is consumed for lactose synthesis, but some must be broken down to provide NADPH for fatty acid synthesis, and some must be used to produce α-glycerophosphate for synthesis of triglycerides. Mammary utilization of glucose during lactation is enormous and poses a heavy metabolic burden on the animal. Not suprisingly, as the animal attempts to meet the substrate needs of the mammary gland, a variety of metabolic adjustments are needed around the time when lactation is initiated. Sometimes the adjustments compromise the well-being of the animal, and there are a number of lactation-associated pathophysiologic disorders. These metabolic burdens carried by the lactating animal will be described further toward the end of this chapter.

11.3 • Endocrine Control of Mammogenesis and Lactogenesis

Mammary function can be considered in terms of a number of phases. The development of mammary tissue was described earlier in the section on mammogenesis. The initiation of secretory function is called lactogenesis. The maintenance of lactation, once it is established, is called *galactopoiesis* and includes aspects of milk synthesis and secretion, along with the distinct process of milk ejection. Eventually lactation ceases and a process of mammary *involution* takes place. The phenomena of galactopoiesis and mammary involution are discussed in the last section of this chapter.

Several of the hormones involved in preparing mammary tissue for lactation have already been described, either in the introductory material on endocrinology or in relation to reproductive function in Chapter 10. The sex steroids, pituitary prolactin and growth hormone, and placental lactogen were implicated in the total process of mammogenesis.

Estrogens and progesterone are largely responsible for the postpuberal growth of the gland and then the more striking development that accompanies pregnancy. Even so, in domestic animals the degree of development that occurs prior to a few days before parturition is superficially unimpressive. The steroids can not achieve development of the tissue without the cooperation of the protein hormones, or in the absence of hormones from the thyroid and adrenal cortex. The thyroid hormones seem to act permissively rather than in any specific way in the developing gland. Adrenal cortex hormones are required for the necessary differentiation of more primitive cells into the more specialized secretory cells. Part of the role of the steroids, for progesterone especially, is to allow this broad complex of hormones to stimulate mammogenesis, while at the same time holding lactogenesis in check.

In most instances, the specific functions of

the various hormones are still unknown. For example, growth hormone, prolactin, and placental lactogen, in species producing the latter, share many general actions and so seem able to substitute for each other if necessary. Exactly what they do to permit mammary growth and differentiation into a highly specialized secretory tissue is poorly understood. It was noted earlier that the extent of mammary development achieved by the time of parturition relates to fetal number and, in some species, to the concentrations of placental lactogen in the maternal circulation. In sheep and goats, maternal levels of placental lactogen reflect the mass of placental tissue and therefore the number of conceptuses. Mammary development in sows similarly relates to fetal number, but this species lacks a placental lactogen, and the manner in which the sow senses how many fetuses she is carrying is certainly not known to the animal scientist.

A critical event in the development of the milk-secreting potential of the udder in cattle occurs around the time that allometric growth sets in at puberty. It has long been known that the rate of growth and the degree of fatness of puberal heifers have a long-lasting effect on the lifetime lactational performance of cattle. Heifers that are excessively fat at puberty tend to perform less than optimally, even several years later. It will be recalled that the mammary gland is dominated by its fat pad at this early stage; the ductal system is just beginning to arborize into the pad as the tissue cyclically comes under the influence of ovarian steroids. It may be possible to explain the negative effects of overfatness on mammary development by sequestration of steroid hormones in the various fat stores of the body, which would considerably dampen changes in blood concentrations of the steroids. The other possibility is that the positive energy balance of heifers in heavy condition suppresses secretion of growth hormone to the extent that this hormone becomes limiting for the optimal progress of mammogenesis.

The initiation of lactation is an abrupt event that is signaled by the beginning of synthesis of lactose. As noted earlier, this is brought about because the synthesis of α-lactalbumin is suddenly switched on.

In domestic ruminants, lactogenesis is signaled by the initiation of copious milk secretion and the accumulation of milk within the mammary gland. Before this rapid synthesis of milk, there has been slow accumulation of the constituents of colostrum. The change occurs, rather abruptly, shortly before parturition. The gland becomes noticeably distended and turgid. The skin on the gland may be reddened and very sensitive to touch. The changes described are due to the prepartum shift in relative amounts of estrogen and progesterone in the maternal circulation. In particular, it appears that the reduction in maternal plasma progesterone concentrations removes a chronic inhibition over mammary synthesis of α-lactalbumin. The synthesis of this enzyme subunit is dependent on the presence of prolactin, but expression of this action of prolactin only occurs in the absence of progesterone. Prolactin is of course involved in mammogenesis, but these actions of prolactin are not impaired by the presence of progesterone. Progesterone is present in the circulation in fairly consistent concentrations until about 24 hours before parturition. The marked change in plasma progesterone concentrations at parturition varies in timing for the different species. In domestic animals, this usually precedes parturition by a day or so (see Figure 10–22). In humans, most of the change occurs after the placenta is delivered, and lactogenesis in women usually occurs sometime during the day following parturition.

The increased production of estrogens shortly before parturition leads to enhanced secretion of prolactin, and both estrogen and prolactin cause increased mammary blood flow. There may be substantial accumulation of interstitial fluid within the mammary gland at the time of parturition. This may result from the increased blood flow that occurs before venous drainage is optimal. Additionally, the accumulation of milk in the unmilked gland may occlude the lymphatic drainage system.

11.4 • Galactopoietic Mechanisms

Milk Ejection

Milk removal from the gland is achieved by the young *sucking* or by manual *milking*. The dam *suckles* its young, but the young is said to *suck* its dam. The physical removal of milk from the teat and immediately adjacent cistern involves either of two basic physical mechanisms. Vacuum can be applied to the teat orifice, called the *streak canal* in animals with teats, or to the multiple openings in a nipple. Alternatively, in animals with a sizable lumen within the teat, the lumen can be occluded proximally, near its base, and the contents can be squeezed so that milk passes through the streak canal under positive pressure.

Interestingly, when an animal sucks, it employs both mechanisms. Contraction of facial muscles making up the walls of the buccal cavity does create some negative pressure, or vacuum. Elevation of the tongue to press the teat against the roof of the buccal cavity serves to apply positive pressure to the teat lumen. It is effective in recovering milk only because the young closes its lips around the base of the teat.

Machine milking is usually based on the negative pressure principle, with vacuum applied to the streak canal and alternating vacuum and atmospheric pressure applied to the body of the teat. There are variations on this scheme, and various principles are used in the design of milking equipment.

Removal of milk from the teat and cistern is just one part of the overall process, because the bulk of the milk is held in the duct system and even within the alveoli. During suckling or milking, reflex secretion of oxytocin from the posterior pituitary stimulates contraction of the myoepithelial cells to cause expulsion of alveolar contents. Some of the ducts are also surrounded by myoepithelium, so milk is expressed from the secretory tissue down into the largest ducts and the cistern, from which it can be removed by the milking process. The physiology of the milk ejection reflex was described in detail in Chapter 4 as an example of a neurohumoral mechanism. If necessary, review the description at this time. It is important to appreciate the general nature of the receptive fields, the afferent pathways to the CNS, the sites of synthesis and secretion of oxytocin, and factors affecting delivery of the hormone to its target tissues. The breadth of these important aspects requires the reader to be conversant with much of the foregoing material in this book.

Galactopoiesis

Another aspect of milk removal concerns the opportunity, at each milking, to reinforce the drive toward the continued secretion of milk. This is called galactopoiesis. In part, the mere relief of intramammary congestion by removing accumulated products from the alveoli and ducts enables further secretion to take place. This is particularly important for milk fat secretion, for fat droplets must be physically extruded from the cell. Any buildup of alveolar pressure will hinder this process. If fat droplets do not leave the cell, cellular integrity is compromised, and damage or death of the epithelial cell may result. In an extreme situation, this loss of synthetic tissue will lead to reduced capacity to synthesize milk. The specific rate of milk secretion is maximal shortly after each milking. The rate declines with time after milk ejection, and this is one of the factors underlying the practice on some farms of milking more than twice daily. Of course, if young animals are being nursed and machine milking is not used, there may be as many as a dozen feeding episodes in the course of a day.

None of these feedings is likely to completely evacuate the available milk, but each time the young sucks, the reflex mechanisms underlying galactopoiesis are activated.

During each milking, in addition to the secretion of oxytocin, the hypothalamus stimulates the anterior pituitary to release thyroid-stimulating hormone (TSH), growth hormone, prolactin, and adrenocorticotropin (ACTH). ACTH causes a phase of increased secretion of glucocorticoid hormones from the adrenal cortex. It is assumed that the secretion of TSH, growth hormone, and prolactin helps maintain milk secretion. Certainly the administration of thyroid hormones and growth hormone increases milk production. The role of prolactin during established lactation in ruminants is less well understood.

These so-called *galactopoietic hormones* may act directly at the mammary gland, or they may be more important in extramammary roles such as maintaining the flux of nutrients toward the mammary gland for its use. For example, the tendency for nutrients to accumulate in adipose tissue may be held in check, thus increasing their availability to the mammary gland in support of milk synthesis. This type of "umbrella" regulation was called homeorhesis in the discussion presented in Chapter 9. In support of the "indirect" nature of action of growth hormone is failure to demonstrate growth hormone receptors in mammary tissue from lactating cattle. Receptors for one of the somatomedins (IGF-I) are, however, present, making it likely that the striking effects of exogenous growth hormone in stimulating milk yield (Figure 11–6) are in part mediated by the growth factor.

Although the precise details remain unknown, it is reasonable to speculate that galactopoietic hormones may function in maintaining or even increasing the number of cells making up the population of secretory epithelial cells. From the description provided in Section 11.1, it would be expected that this mechanism is most important in the early stages of lactation. Because cells are continually lost, the total popu-

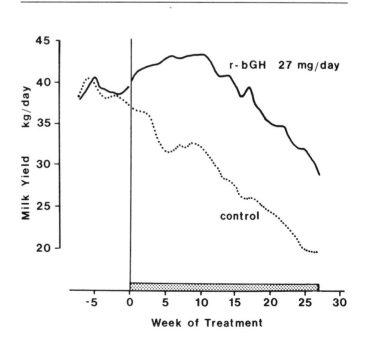

Figure 11–6. Milk yield responses to bovine growth hormone. The solid line shows the average daily milk yield from a group of 6 mature cows that were treated once daily with 27 mg of recombinantly-derived bovine growth hormone (r-bGH). The dotted line is the yield from 6 genetically similar cows from the same herd that were treated daily by injection of only the vehicle used to dissolve the GH (control). Treatment began on average 12 weeks into lactation and continued for 27 weeks (bar). Yields from the 2 groups before treatment were quite comparable for these highly productive cattle. The response to this dose of r-bGH was approximately a 36% increase in milk yield. (This figure was constructed from the data of Bauman, D.E., Eppard, P.J.; DeGeeter, M.J., and Lanza, G.M.: "Responses of High-Producing Dairy Cows to Long-Term Treatment with Pituitary Somatotropin and Recombinant Somatotropin," *Journal of Dairy Science* 1985; 68:1352–62.)

lation of secretory cells reflects the rate of loss and the rate of replenishment.

Another possible mode of action of these hormones could be in maintaining the synthetic capacity, or the integrity of the organelle and enzyme systems, of the existing cells.

The Metabolic Burden of Lactation

In cattle that have been highly selected for milk yield, the transition from pregnancy to lactation results in a sudden enormous additional metabolic load being placed on the cow. Relative to the needs of the conceptus, even when it is rapidly growing in very late pregnancy, the needs of the mammary gland in early lactation far outstrip the capacity for nutrient intake by the animal. The physiologic drive for lactation is such that animals mobilize body reserves to balance any energy deficit between what is leaving in milk and that obtained from the diet. The galactopoietic mechanisms noted in the preceding section are probably largely responsible for this driving force. This metabolic embarrassment during the critical early stage of lactation has been exacerbated in dairy animals by the efforts of man to genetically select animals of progressively superior lactation performance.

During early lactation, high-producing animals inevitably lose body weight by mobilizing fat reserves and depleting body reserves of carbohydrate, and possibly labile proteins. The animal will attempt to switch its metabolism to spare available glucose so that mammary tissue can extract all that it needs. The metabolic environment of the cow is now decidedly influenced by lipid catabolism and by ketogenesis, as outlined in Chapter 7. Coupled with the extraordinary consumption of glucose by the mammary gland, these changes place the cow in early lactation on the brink of metabolic disaster. It is not surprising that ketosis can be prevalent at this time. It is more surprising that many

animals can tolerate this profound metabolic challenge without displaying clinical signs of these disorders.

It is clear that the high-producing cow is in negative energy balance during early lactation. Milk production in cattle usually increases from calving until about 5 to 8 weeks into lactation, and then it starts a slow decline that continues over the remainder of lactation. The term *persistence* is used to describe how well milk yield is sustained after the peak of lactation. Under conditions of optimal feeding management, the total milk yield during a lactation is largely determined by the magnitude of the peak yield. Thus, selection for high lactation yield almost certainly selects for the ability of animals to reach high peak yields. The ability to reach these high peak levels of production despite the negative energy status, and without succumbing to the stress imposed by excessive fat catabolism, is probably the mark of the genetically superior individual.

When milk yield is increasing at the start, body weight continues to decline as energy reserves are mobilized. The mobilization of energy-rich depot lipids is reflected in the composition of milk. The content of fat in milk is highest in very early lactation. In addition, the milk fat has a fatty acid composition that reflects the makeup of the depot fats.

Feed intake of the cow increases throughout this early phase but is usually not sufficient to meet the needs of maintenance plus milk production until a few weeks into lactation. From the foregoing discussion, it should be obvious that different diets will differ in their suitability to meet the lactational needs of the animal. Depending on a variety of animal and dietary factors, feed intake will be sufficient by midlactation to enable a positive energy balance to be established. The animal will then set to and regain its body reserves (Figure 11–7).

Management factors determine when this is desirable, and the level of feeding, relative to calculated animal needs, determines if the animal is allowed to regain weight. Often, feeding is adjusted to just meet requirements so that zero energy balance, neither positive nor negative, is

Figure 11–7. *Energy status of highly productive cattle.* This figure shows mean data for a group of six animals that averaged about 10,000 kg milk yield during their lactation. The top curve shows the pattern of change in milk yield, with the peak in this case occurring at week 3. The middle curve shows one measure of their nutrient intake, in this case the net energy intake in Mcals per day. The lower curve is the calculated net energy balance also in Mcals per day. This is a measure of how well the cows' requirements are being met by intake. In early lactation, the animals are in negative energy balance and must be mobilizing stored reserves. This would be reflected in body weight loss. In mid-lactation, energy balance is attained and in late lactation the animals are in positive energy balance and so will be recovering the body weight and degree of fatness that was lost earlier. The curved dotted line shows a phase of overfeeding that is often used in late lactation so that animals are in good condition by the time they enter the dry period before next calving. (From Bauman, D.E. and Currie, W.B.: "Partitioning of Nutrients During Pregnancy and Lactation: A Review of Mechanisms Involving Homeostasis and Homeorhesis," *Journal of Dairy Science* 1980;63:1514–29.)

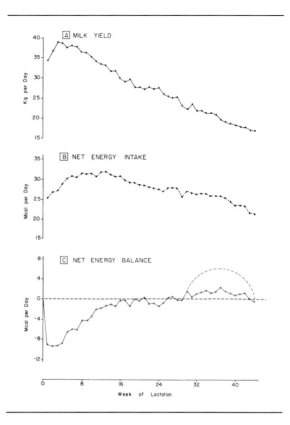

achieved. In these circumstances, the animal does not recover its original weight loss until after lactation is terminated, usually about 60 days before the next calving date. A controlled degree of weight gain is then permitted, in preparation for the demands of the next lactation.

The analysis provided in this last section is a little simplistic and has focused on milk yield, with little regard for other body functions. The optimal requirements for lactation may conflict with other vital functions. The reader is referred to the description of calcium metabolism in Box 8–1, in which a variety of neuromuscular disturbances were related to excessive mammary consumption of calcium.

The highly selected dairy animal seems to be remarkably well adjusted to deal with the stresses associated with the production of up to 20 to 25 times her own weight as milk during the course of each 10-month lactation. In addition, she is required to maintain the integrity of all of her vital systems, to ward off threats from disease and parasite loads, and to maintain thermal equilibrium, often despite inclement ambient conditions. Finally, she is expected to resume normal reproductive function in timely fashion so that she will continue to calve at regular intervals, ideally about every 12 months.

11.5 • Exercises

1. Write a brief description of the milk ejection reflex using all of the terms from the following list:

hypothalamic axons
posterior pituitary
intramammary
   pressure
oxytocin in arterial
   blood
dorsal roots of spinal
   cord

milk ejection
tactile stimulation of
   the teats
ascending spinal
   cord tracts
integration in the
   thalamus
myoepithelial cells

2. What is the origin (proximate or ultimate) of the following milk components?

Milk fat globule membrane

Galactose contained in lactose

Milk leukocytes

Casein

Alpha-lactalbumin

3. A diet known to favor glucose production by ruminant animals is fed in early lactation. Which of the following changes in milk could be expected?

No change because the cow will use the extra nutrients to lay down more adipose tissue.

Increased percentage of lactose in milk because more glucose is available for its synthesis.

Increased fat content in milk because glucose will permit nonesterified fatty acids to be used for mammary lipogenesis instead of ketogenesis.

Increased milk yield because lactose synthesis will increase and percentage of lactose stays fairly constant, so milk volume must increase.

4. Speculate on the function of the rather unusual dual vascular supply and drainage of the bovine mammary gland. Consider what might happen when the cow lies down and the abdominal mammary vein is occluded by the animal's weight.

5. Mammary tissue has a high capacity to use acetate for synthesis of short and medium chain fatty acids for incorporation into milk fat. In the section on digestion it was noted that protecting dietary lipids from ruminal hydrogenation could drastically modify the properties of milk fat. Can you reconcile these statements?

6. Write a brief statement about the magnitude of mammary glucose consumption. Indicate what processes consume glucose and how the animal obtains the substrate.

7. Exogenous growth hormone is galactopoietic in cattle. What does this statement say in everyday language? When the hormone is introduced to farm use, what key aspect of management of the cattle will need critical attention? What can be expected to occur if this aspect is neglected?

8. What is lactation ketosis, when is it most prevalent, and why does it occur? Integrate your understanding of digestion, milk synthesis and secretion, and negative energy balance in ruminants to assemble a simple statement about the need to carefully balance an animal's needs with appropriate feeding.

Epilogue

The mechanisms and phenomena described in this book provide an introduction to the flexibility, or plasticity, of normal animal function. When one body system functions less than optimally, the others are affected, but there is usually the flexibility for the latter to compensate and offset the problem. The highly productive animal, be it the dairy cow just described, a heavily worked thoroughbred horse, a sow that spends her life after puberty either pregnant or lactating, and so on, provides endless opportunity to prompt inquisitive people to ask: "But why?" "But how?" "What if?"

It should be quite apparent from the approach taken in this text that many questions remain to be asked and researched about the structure and normal function of domestic animals. With the benefit of more complete knowledge about normal function, abnormal function, as in stress and disease, can be approached more intelligently and rationally.

The pragmatic application, of course, is in being able to raise and care for animals with appropriate regard for their welfare and the economic realities prevailing in the agricultural industries. No less legitimate, however, is the possibility that the reader will go on to add to the store of knowledge that underlies what is studied as others learn about animals. The motivation for such effort is, first, simply one of curiosity. It is rewarding if the answers help solve real-world problems, but no less rewarding if they simply expose more of the seemingly endless examples of the way by which animals apply the fundamental principles of chemistry and physics to preserve their integrity.

Appendix A • Atoms and Ions

Atoms are made up of a nucleus of positively charged particles *(protons)* and uncharged particles *(neutrons)*, surrounded by orbiting *electrons*. The electrons are negatively charged and arranged in shells. The innermost shell of electrons is most stable when it is occupied by two electrons. The next shell is most stable with eight electrons, made up of four pairs. The third shell can be stabilized with a variable number of pairs of electrons. The change required to stabilize the outermost shell, by either giving up electrons or accepting them, involves different numbers of charged electrons. The number is called the *valence*.

Sodium, with a filled inner shell (two electrons) and a filled second shell (eight electrons) has only a single electron in the third shell. It yields up this electron to some other atom in order to stabilize. In so doing, it loses one negative charge and the residue (the sodium ion) carries a single positive charge and is said to have a valence of $+1$. In contrast, chlorine with 17 electrons arranged as an inner shell of two, a middle shell of eight, and an outer shell of seven, will readily accept an electron from some donor atom in order to stabilize. In so doing, it becomes more negative by the charge of one electron and hence has a valence of -1. When atoms combine to form molecules, they do so by sharing electrons in their incomplete or unstable shells. Sodium and chlorine combine to form sodium chloride. This molecule (common salt) has considerable biological significance.

Water ranks first among the array of substances of importance to living things. The water molecule has very special characteristics that are described in detail in Section 2.2. Many of these properties result from the hydrogens each having a single orbiting electron whereas oxygen has eight, two in the inner shell and six in the outer shell. The oxygen lacks two electrons for stability, but obtains them from two atoms of hydrogen within the water molecule. The oxygen is said to be *electronegative* as a result of its drawing electrons away from the hydrogen atoms. This sharing of electrons between two atoms is the basis for the covalent bond. Other forms of bond occur and will be shown to be of importance. When four electrons, rather than two, are shared the bond is called an *olefinic* or double bond, as in the case of a carbon = carbon $(C = C)$ bond. Numerous examples of rather specialized molecules with double bonds are noted in the text.

Many, but by no means all, substances dissociate into charged particles called ions when they dissolve in water. Such compounds are called electrolytes because their ions are capable of conducting electric currents. Depending on the degree to which they dissociate, it is convenient to classify electrolytes as being weak or strong. Strong electrolytes are completely dissociated in aqueous solution. The parent compound actually disappears and is totally replaced by the constituent ionic species. The example is a little pedantic, but it is actually incorrect to speak of a solution of sodium chloride. It is really a solution of sodium ions and chloride ions because the molecular form, sodium chloride, does not exist upon solution formation. In contrast, weak electrolytes only partially dissociate upon solution and they form more complex mixtures made up of some of the parent compound and the remainder in the form of ions. At any instant, some of the parent molecules are dissociating while some of the already dissociated ions are coming together to reform the original molecule. Equilibrium requires that the rate of dissociation equals the rate of association, as represented by the double-headed arrows in the equilibrium equation:

$$HA \rightleftharpoons H^+ + A^-$$

The equilibrium can be expressed in a more useful way in terms of the concentration of the three components:

$$[H^+] \times [A^-] = K_d \times [HA],$$

where square brackets [ ] signify concentrations and K_d is the equilibrium dissociation constant.

When the preceding equation is rearranged, it becomes immediately apparent that the dissociation constant indicates the value of the ratio of the dissociated species to the associated form, as:

$$K_d = \frac{[H^+] \times [A^-]}{[HA]}$$

The amount of charge carried by the ions is far more important than is their mass, so it is usual to express the concentration in terms of the charge, or numbers of electrons, carried in excess by anions, or by which they are deficient (in the case of cations). One equivalent of an anion carries 6×10^{23} electrons. For univalent ions such as Na^+ or Cl^-, the concentration in equivalents is exactly the same as the molar concentration. For an n-valent ion it is n times the molar concentration. From this it can be noted that 1 molar (1 M) solutions of the strong acids HCl and H_2SO_4 each contain 1 gram-mole per liter, but the SO_4^{2-} ions contribute twice the charge that is carried by the Cl^- ions. There are also twice as many H^+ ions in the solution formed from H_2SO_4 compared to those formed from the HCl.

With this simple background, it is now possible to provide some definitions concerning acids and bases. All uses of these terms will be consistent with the following statements:

- A solution is acidic (or acid) if the concentration of H^+ exceeds that of the OH^-.

- A solution is basic (or alkaline) if the concentration of H^+ is less than that of the OH^-.

- A solution is neutral, or more correctly is acid-base neutral, if the concentrations of H^+ and OH^- are equal.

- An acid is any substance that, when added to a solution, causes an increase in the concentration of H^+ relative to that of OH^-. Conversely, a base is any substance that has the reverse effect when it is added to a solution.

The reader who is well acquainted with chemistry may question these seemingly simplistic definitions because he or she may be comfortable with the concept of an acid being any proton donor while a base is any proton acceptor. The definitions provided here are far more useful for understanding physiological processes. For example, by virtue of the definition above, the biologist has no difficulty with the reality that carbon dioxide (CO_2) behaves as an acid because, as it dissolves in water, it increases the concentration of hydrogen ions (H^+) over that of hydroxide (OH^-) ions. The following equilibrium reaction shows that carbon dioxide actually reacts with water as it dissolves to form carbonic acid (H_2CO_3), which then equilibrates with the constituent ions H^+ and HCO_3^-. The last mentioned is the very important bicarbonate ion:

$$H_2O + CO_2 \rightleftharpoons H_2CO_3 \rightleftharpoons H^+ + HCO_3^-$$

This simple equation appears repeatedly in the text and, if understood, can provide the reader with the basis for comprehending an amazing number of physiological phenomena. It is of greatest importance that the reader understand what this equation means. Following the reactions from left to right, the addition of more carbon dioxide to the solution consumes water and produces more carbonic acid than was originally present. Now, because of the second equilibrium, the carbonic acid proceeds to dissociate, giving rise to increased concentrations of hydrogen ions and bicarbonate ions. Addition of carbon dioxide, therefore, has increased the concentration of hydrogen ions, which satisifies the definition given above for a substance to be classified as an acid. Now consider the reverse sequence, applicable when an acid is added to the solution described by this equation. Additional hydrogen ions, obtained from the added acid, consume bicarbonate ions and shift the overall reaction to the left. The equilibrium between carbonic acid and carbon dioxide and water is disturbed so carbon dioxide comes out of the solution. If the disturbance is of sufficient magnitude, the carbon dioxide will form bubbles and may even effervesce. This example can be observed by squeezing a few drops of citrus juice (a source of the weak citric acid) into a glass containing "flat" soda. A very similar process to your adding acid to the soda is a key part of the mechanism of gas exchange that occurs in the lung with every breath, as seen in Chapter 5.

There are a few additional definitions worth noting at this stage:

- Aqueous or watery solutions of appreciable volume always display electrical neutrality.

The sum of anions (negative charges) equals the sum of all cations (positive charges), which is why emphasis was placed earlier on expressing the concentration of ions in terms of charge equivalents.

- Mass is conserved, so the concentration of any substance in solution stays constant unless the substance is removed or more is added. Alternatively, and more important physiologically, the concentrations will stay the same unless reactions within the solution either generate or consume that substance.

- Concentration can be changed, without addition or removal of the solute, by variation in the volume of solvent. Selective addition or removal of water will either dilute or concentrate a solution.

Appendix B • Introduction to Organic Compounds

One definition of *organic chemistry* is the nature and reactions of the compounds of carbon, hydrogen, and their derivatives. The molecules making up living animals are dominated by organic substances—those containing carbon, hydrogen, oxygen, and nitrogen, along with some sulfur and phosphorus. These elements account for 68 kg of a 70-kg individual.

The simplest organic compounds are the hydrocarbons, made up exclusively of carbon and hydrogen. The atoms are held together by bonds that are sufficiently strong that they are preserved under a variety of conditions. The bonds are due to the sharing of pairs of electrons and their simultaneous attraction by the positive charges in the nuclei of the atoms that are bonded. Double bonds exist when four electrons are shared by two nuclei and triple bonds when six electrons are involved. These bonds will be represented here by single, double, and triple dashes:

$$— \qquad = \qquad \equiv$$

Hydrocarbons fall into three major classes. *Aliphatic* hydrocarbons are made from open-ended chains of carbon atoms.

is heptane (C_7H_{16}), a seven-carbon aliphatic hydrocarbon.

Alicyclic hydrocarbons are similar to the open-ended molecules except the chains form cyclic compounds and they lack two hydrogens when compared to the aliphatic relative.

is cyclohexane (C_6H_{12}), a six-carbon alicyclic molecule.

Aromatic hydrocarbons consist of six-carbon ring structures that characteristically contain three double bonds. These double bonds make the compound unsaturated with respect to hydrogen and result in greater reactivity.

is benzene (C_6H_6), the fundamental aromatic hydrocarbon. The double bonds are given locations within the molecule purely for convenience in drawing the structure. In reality, all six $C=C$ bonds are equivalent:

403

The following simpler structure represents either or both of the formal structures that have been shown.

The aliphatic hydrocarbons are divided into *alkanes*, saturated compounds with the maximum number of hydrogens; *alkenes*, containing one or more double or olefinic bonds; and *alkynes*, containing triple bonds. Alkenes and alkynes are unsaturated; that is, they are capable of reacting with hydrogen by the process of hydrogenation.

Alkanes range upward in size from methane, the single carbon compound.

H
|
H—C—H   CH$_4$ (methane)
|
H

H H
| |
H—C—C—H   CH$_3$CH$_3$ (ethane)
| |
H H

H H H
| | |
H—C—C—C—H   CH$_3$CH$_2$CH$_3$
| | | (propane)
H H H

Note the simpler formulas provided to the right. While the carbon chain is written along a horizontal line, the molecules actually occupy three dimensions and the chains may assume a variety of shapes. When all of the carbons occur in a continuous sequence, the molecules are *normal* and are shown in formulas by the prefix *n-*. If branching occurs, the term *isomeric* is applied, usually by means of the prefix *iso-*.

Simple alkanes include:

Methane	CH$_4$		
Ethane	C$_2$H$_6$	or	CH$_3$CH$_3$
Propane	C$_3$H$_8$	or	CH$_3$CH$_2$CH$_3$
n-Butane	C$_4$H$_{10}$	or	CH$_3$(CH$_2$)$_2$CH$_3$
iso-Butane	C$_4$H$_{10}$	or	CH$_3$CHCH$_3$

CH$_3$

n-Pentane	C$_5$H$_{12}$	or	CH$_3$(CH$_2$)$_3$CH$_3$
iso-Pentane	C$_5$H$_{12}$	or	CH$_3$CHCH$_2$CH$_3$

CH$_3$

Note that the formula to the left is identical for the normal and isomeric forms; the simple structural formulas to the right show the distinction between the forms. The only alkane of direct interest in animal science is methane because it is a product of microbial fermentation in the gut. Far more important are the alkyl groups (the roots of the parent structures). Numerous substituents can be found attached to these parent structures. Alcohol, for example, is the hydroxy derivative of ethane and is correctly called ethyl alcohol, or ethanol.

Alkyl groups include:

Methyl	CH$_3$—
Ethyl	CH$_3$CH$_2$—
Propyl	CH$_3$CH$_2$CH$_2$—
iso-Propyl	CH$_3$CH—

CH$_3$

and so on.

The simple substituted alkanes fall into several major classes such as:

Halides

R'—X

where R' means any alkyl group as above, and **X** can be

CL = chloride
F = fluoride
I = iodide
Br = bromide

for example, CH_3CH_2—**Cl** (ethyl chloride).

Alcohols

R'—OH

for example, CH_3CH_2—**OH** (ethanol).

Amines

R'—NH₂

for example, $CH_3(CH_2)_3$—**NH₂** (n-butylamine).

Acids

R'—C—OH
‖
O

for example, CH_3—**C**—**OH** (acetic acid).
                      ‖
                      O

Aldehydes

R'—C—H
‖
O

for example, CH_3—**C**—**H** (acetaldehyde).
                      ‖
                      O

Mercaptans

R'—SH

for example, $CH_3(CH_2)_3$—**SH** (n-butyl mercaptan), an odoriferous molecule, is used effectively by skunks!

Substitutions, such as those noted above, are also found on alkenes and alkynes, as well as on aromatic compounds. The following examples are derivatives of benzene and are shown using the simplified aromatic ring structure presented earlier:

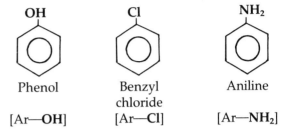

Phenol   Benzyl chloride   Aniline
[Ar—**OH**]   [Ar—**Cl**]   [Ar—**NH₂**]

Multiple substitutions are commonly found, both on aliphatic and aromatic molecules:

```
CH₂—OH    CH₂—COOH           NH₂
 |         |                  |
CH—OH     CH₂—COOH    CH₃—CH—COOH
 |
CH₂—OH
```

Glycerol   Succinic acid   Aminopropionic
                           acid (alanine)

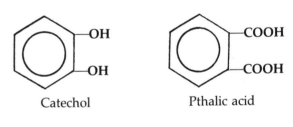

Catechol   Pthalic acid

Phenylalanine

Rather complex multi-ring compounds, related to benzene, and nitrogen-containing, or heterocyclic, compounds occur in nature. The parent structures are not so important at this time, but many of their derivatives are shown in Chapter 4 to have special functions in animals. A few of the basic structures are:

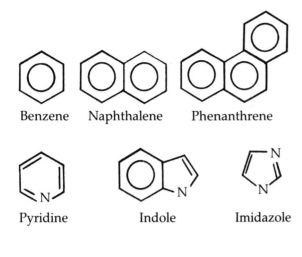

Benzene   Naphthalene   Phenanthrene

Pyridine   Indole   Imidazole

$CH_3(CH_2)_3$—COOH	valeric acid	(valeryl-)
$CH_3(CH_2)_4$—COOH	caproic acid	(caproyl-)
$CH_3(CH_2)_6$—COOH	caprylic acid	(caprylyl-)
$CH_3(CH_2)_8$—COOH	capric acid	(capryl-)
$CH_3(CH_2)_{10}$—COOH	lauric acid	(lauryl-)
$CH_3(CH_2)_{12}$—COOH	myristic acid	(myristyl-)
$CH_3(CH_2)_{14}$—COOH	palmitic acid	(palmityl-)
$CH_3(CH_2)_{16}$—COOH	stearic acid	(stearyl-)
$CH_3(CH_2)_{18}$—COOH	arachidic acid	(arachidyl-)

The Carboxylic Acids

The carboxylic acid derivatives of the aliphatic hydrocarbons (also known as fatty acids) are energy-rich constituents of lipids, both oils and fats. The shorter chain members are water soluble and relatively volatile while the longer fatty acids are neither. A fairly large list of fatty acids is provided and most are noted in the text. The names given to these acids are the trivial or common names and the same applies to the acid group (or acyl-) names. These common names are widely used in the literature of physiology and nutrition, but the systematic names are easily deduced. For example, stearic acid is a normal, saturated, 18-carbon fatty acid, which is formally called octadecanoic acid. This means the carboxylic acid of octadecane (*octa* meaning 8 and *deca* meaning 10 with *-ane* signifying an alkane). A shorthand designation that will be used periodically is $C_{18:0}$, which indicates a total of 18 carbons and 0 double bonds.

With the exception of the shortest of these acids, most of the above can be found in triglyceride molecules. Triglycerides are tri-acyl esters of glycerol and they form the bulk of animal and plant fats and oils.

$$
\begin{array}{lll}
CH_2\text{—OH} & HOOC\text{—}R^1 & CH_2\text{—O—}OC\text{—}R^1 \\
| & & | \\
CH\text{—OH} \quad + & HOOC\text{—}R^2 & \rightarrow CH\text{—O—}OC\text{—}R^2 \\
| & & | \\
CH_2\text{—OH} & HOOC\text{—}R^3 & CH_2\text{—O—}OC\text{—}R^3 \\
\end{array}
$$

Glycerol   Three fatty acids   Triglyceride

For example,

Normal Saturated Fatty Acids

CH_3—COOH	acetic	(acetyl-)
CH_3CH_2—COOH	propionic acid	(propionyl-)
$CH_3(CH_2)_2$—COOH	butyric acid	(butyryl-)

$$
\begin{array}{l}
\quad\quad\quad\quad\quad O \\
\quad\quad\quad\quad\quad \| \\
CH_2\text{—O—C—}(CH_2)_{16}CH_3 \\
\quad\quad\quad\quad\quad O \\
| \quad\quad\quad\quad \| \\
CH\text{—O—C—}(CH_2)_{14}CH_3 \\
\quad\quad\quad\quad\quad O \\
| \quad\quad\quad\quad \| \\
CH_2\text{—O—C—}(CH_2)_2CH_3 \\
\end{array}
$$

In this case, R^1 is $C_{18:0}$ (stearic acid), R^2 is $C_{16:0}$ (palmitic acid), and R^3 is $C_{4:0}$ (butyric acid). This particular triglyceride is a common constituent of milk fat.

In the formulas above, the ester links between the carboxylic acids and the hydroxyls are emphasized. This type of bond is so important that it is worth emphasizing again:

$$R-\overset{\displaystyle O}{\overset{\|}{C}}-OH \ + \ HO-R^* \rightarrow R-\overset{\displaystyle O}{\overset{\|}{C}}-O-R^*$$

Acid   Alcohol   Ester

For the special case of triglycerides, the glycerol provides three hydroxyls for esterification, hence the term tri-acyl esters of glycerol. In the discussion of digestive processes, the intermediate degraded products of dietary lipids are shown to include diglycerides and monoglycerides. These have one or two of the fatty acids removed and so have free hydroxyls.

Special properties result if the fatty acids are partially unsaturated (usually by having one or more double bonds) or if the acids are isomeric (i.e., they are branch chained).

Normal	*Isomers*
$CH_3CH_2CH_2COOH$	$CH_3\overset{\textstyle |}{\underset{\textstyle CH_3}{C}}HCOOH$
Butyric acid	Iso-butyric acid
$CH_3CH_2CH_2CH_2COOH$	$CH_3\overset{\textstyle |}{\underset{\textstyle CH_3}{C}}HCH_2COOH$
Valeric acid	Iso-valeric acid
	$CH_3CH_2\overset{\textstyle |}{\underset{\textstyle CH_3}{C}}HCOOH$
	2-Methyl butyric acid

These branch-chained acids are very volatile and odoriferous. They account for the characteristic odor of rumen contents.

Unsaturated Long-Chain Fatty Acids

Monoenes have a single double bond. The shorthand notation introduced earlier, with designations $C_{14:1}$, $C_{16:1}$, and $C_{18:1}$ could be used, though this method fails to indicate the location of the double bond within the aliphatic chain.

myristoleic	$CH_3(CH_2)_3CH{=}CH(CH_2)_7COOH$
palmitoleic	$CH_3(CH_2)_5CH{=}CH(CH_2)_7COOH$
oleic	$CH_3(CH_2)_7CH{=}CH(CH_2)_7COOH$

More information is obtained from the following:

cis-9-tetradecenoic acid	*c*-9-14:1
cis-9-hexadecenoic acid	*c*-9-16:1
cis-9-octadecenoic acid	*c*-9-18:1

The number indicates which carbon, numbered back from the carboxylic carbon as 1, is the first involved in an unsaturated bond. The *cis* provides information about the orientation of the bond. Bearing in mind the shortcomings of trying to represent a three-dimensional molecule on paper in two dimensions, consider a *cis* bond to angle off the paper toward you. A bond that is bent in the opposite direction (i.e., into or through the thickness of the paper) is called *trans*. Finally, the careful reader will have noticed that the acyl- root of these compounds is spelled *enoic* rather than *anoic* as used earlier. This indicates an *alkene* rather than *alkane* structure.

The bond angle at the carbons involved in the double bond is quite different from that at fully saturated carbons. The chain is decidedly kinked at this location, either into or out of the plane of the paper. Very complex shapes result if there are multiple double bonds. The various C_{18} fatty acids, which are extremely important to animals and man, illustrate this point. Again, the limitations of two-dimensional presentation require that you mentally picture these molecules in space.

Unsaturated 18-Carbon Fatty Acids

Monoenes:

> *c*-9-18:1   oleic acid
>
> *t*-9-18:1   elaidic acid

Diene:

> *c,c*-9,12-18:2   linoleic acid

$$CH_3(CH_2)_4CH{=}CHCH_2CH{=}CH(CH_2)_7COOH$$

Triene:

> *c,c,c*-9,12,15-18:3   linolenic acid

$$CH_3CH_2CH{=}CHCH_2CH{=}CHCH_2{-}$$
$$CH{=}CH(CH_2)_7COOH$$

Triglycerides containing a high proportion of unsaturated fatty acids or polyunsaturated fatty acids (PUFAs), cannot be packed together as tightly as can those with fully saturated fatty acids. The difference in packing results in a depression of the melting point of the unsaturated compounds so such lipids are liquid or oils at room temperature. Plant lipids such as refined corn oil contain large amounts of *c,c*-9,12-18:2 and *c,c,c*-9,12,15-18:3 and remain liquid even at refrigerator temperatures. In contrast, lard or rendered beef fat, which contains large amounts of $C_{18:0}$, moderate amounts of $C_{16:0}$ and *c*-9-18:1, but only small amounts of PUFAs is solid at room temperature and melts only upon heating.

In Chapter 6, an explanation is provided for these marked differences between corn fat and beef fat, despite the fact that the cow or steer may have obtained most of its dietary fat from corn products.

Complex lipids containing sugars and nitrogenous and phosphorous groups will be encountered numerous times. They have special properties, many of which are related to their ability to carry charges, which make these molecules especially useful to living tissues. A detailed description of the compounds is beyond the scope of this introduction.

Amino Acids and Proteins

A physiologically important group of bifunctional molecules includes the amino acids, the monomeric units from which proteins are made. Amino acids have the general form:

$$\begin{array}{c} NH_2 \\ | \\ R{-}CH \\ | \\ COOH \end{array}$$

R can represent any of a large number of structures. Amino acids are broadly classified into acidic, neutral, and basic compounds. Acidic amino acids exhibit negative charges at physiological pH, while basic amino acids are positively charged at this pH. In the simple generic structure just shown, two ionizable groups are present, the amino (—NH₂) and the carboxylic (—COOH) groups. It is said that such molecules are *amphoteric*, meaning that they can behave as acids or bases. Such molecules are often shown in their ionized forms because, depending upon the prevailing pH, they change readily from one state to the other:

$$\begin{array}{c} NH_3^+ \\ | \\ R{-}CH \\ | \\ COOH \end{array} \overset{\nearrow H^+}{\underset{\searrow H^+}{\rightleftharpoons}} \begin{array}{c} NH_3^+ \\ | \\ R{-}CH \\ | \\ COO^- \end{array} \overset{\nearrow H^+}{\underset{\searrow H^+}{\rightleftharpoons}} \begin{array}{c} NH_2 \\ | \\ R{-}CH \\ | \\ COO^- \end{array}$$

Sometimes the side chains contain additional ionizable groups, for example, an additional carboxylic group as in the cases of aspartic acid and glutamic acid. The converse is also true in the case of lysine, a basic amino acid that has an additional amino residue on the side chain. Some important amino acids are shown to illustrate the chemical diversity of the molecules. The structure of the side chain also determines the polarity character of the molecule. If there are many functional groups, the molecule will tend to be *polar* and it will interact readily with water. In contrast, if the side chain is relatively devoid of such groups and has the form of a simple hydrocarbon or alkyl chain, the molecule will be *apolar* or hydrophobic and interactions with water are less likely. Such apolar molecules tend to interact with each other rather than with the solvent. These properties, polarity and acidity or basicity, of the amino acids largely determine the chemical behavior of the proteins made from them.

Examples of Amino Acids

Name and type

alanine (neutral) $CH_3-CH\begin{smallmatrix}COO^-\\NH_3^+\end{smallmatrix}$

leucine (neutral) $\begin{smallmatrix}CH_3\\CH_3\end{smallmatrix}CH-CH_2-CH\begin{smallmatrix}COO^-\\NH_3^+\end{smallmatrix}$

phenyl-alanine (apolar) $\bigcirc-CH_2-CH\begin{smallmatrix}COO^-\\NH_3^+\end{smallmatrix}$

serine (polar) $^+H\ ^-O-CH_2-CH\begin{smallmatrix}COO^-\\NH_3^+\end{smallmatrix}$

cysteine (polar) $^+H\ ^-S-CH_2-CH\begin{smallmatrix}COO^-\\NH_3^+\end{smallmatrix}$

lysine (basic, cationic) $^+NH_3-(CH_2)_3-CH_2-CH\begin{smallmatrix}COO^-\\NH_3^+\end{smallmatrix}$

glutamic acid (anionic) $^-OOC-CH_2-CH_2-CH\begin{smallmatrix}COO^-\\NH_3^+\end{smallmatrix}$

These properties of proteins are very important in many ways to physiologic mechanisms.

The two major functional groups shown above, the amino group and the carboxyl group, facilitate polymerization of amino acids into larger molecules called peptides and proteins. Amide bonds are formed between the amino residue of one molecule and the carboxyl residue of another:

$$R'-C\begin{smallmatrix}O\\OH\end{smallmatrix} + NH_2-R'' \rightarrow R'-C\begin{smallmatrix}O\\N-R''\\H\end{smallmatrix}$$

Because each amino acid can enter into an amide bond (also called a *peptide bond*) at both sides, polymer formation is possible. The result can be an enormous molecule of hundreds of amino acids, each connected at both sides except the first and last amino acids. The peptide bond has a characteristic bond angle and this along with other noncovalent attractions between the atoms of a protein enable the large molecules to take on characteristic shapes. These structures are, of course, three dimensional with twisting and coiling within the molecule. Even very complex conformations can be quite stable under physiological conditions. When the stabilizing linkages are disrupted, the native structures are lost and the protein is said to be denatured, usually with the loss of its typical properties.

The vast array of functional groups present, their organization into stable three-dimensional structures, and the ability of other large molecules to recognize these features enable peptides and proteins to carry information as hormones. The flexibility in structure underlies the ability of some proteins to wrap about other molecules thereby providing binding sites and, in many cases, favorable positioning of the bound molecule to enable enzymatic processes to take place. Proteins are best considered to be very fluid in shape, flexible, and capable of interacting with other molecules.

The polymeric compounds are broadly classified by size into peptides or oligopeptides, with just a few amino acids; polypeptides, with more (up to about 100 amino acids), and proteins, the larger polymers.

Carbohydrates

Carbohydrates comprise the other major class of substances to be described at this stage. In their simple form, all are made of carbon, hydrogen, and oxygen, and they typically take the generic form:

$$C(H_2O)_n$$

The basic monomeric units are called *monosac-charides,* further divided into the important subgroups of *pentoses* (5 carbons) and *hexoses* (6 carbons). There are others that have some physiological importance, but they can be ignored for the present.

Monosaccharides occur widely in all living systems as intermediates in metabolism and as constituents of macromolecules such as nucleic acids and coenzymes. In the nucleic acids, the pentose called *ribose* is a key part of ribonucleic acid (RNA), while the deoxy form of this sugar, called *deoxyribose,* is its equivalent for the genetic material, deoxyribonucleic acid (DNA).

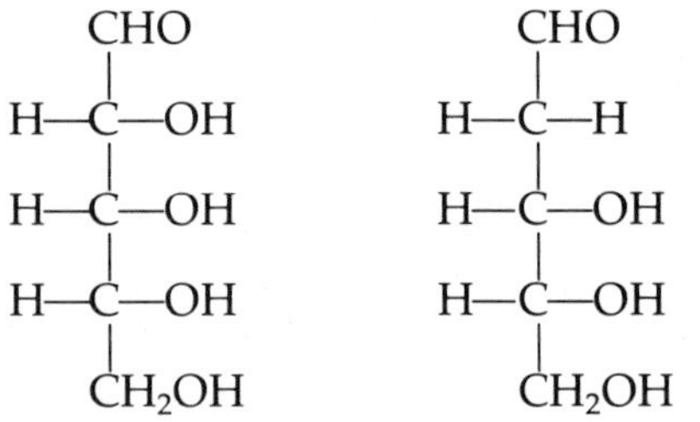

```
    CHO        1
     |
 H—C—OH        2
     |
 H—C—H         3
     |
 H—C—OH        4
     |
 H—C—OH        5
     |
 H—C—H         6
     |
    OH
```

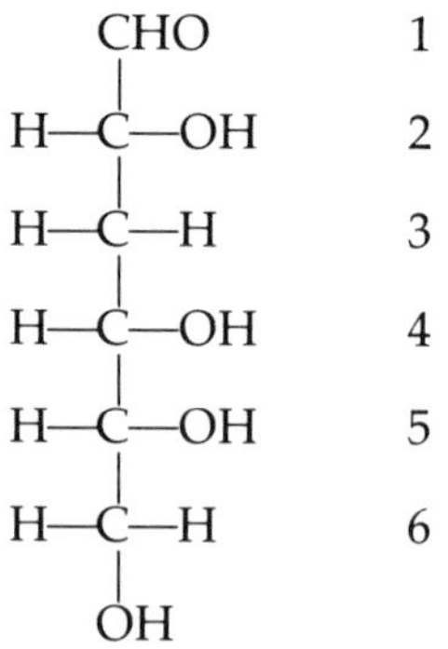

Because the aldehyde group (CHO) involving C_1 in reality reacts with the hydroxyl (OH) on C_5, the molecule is best viewed as being a closed ring structure:

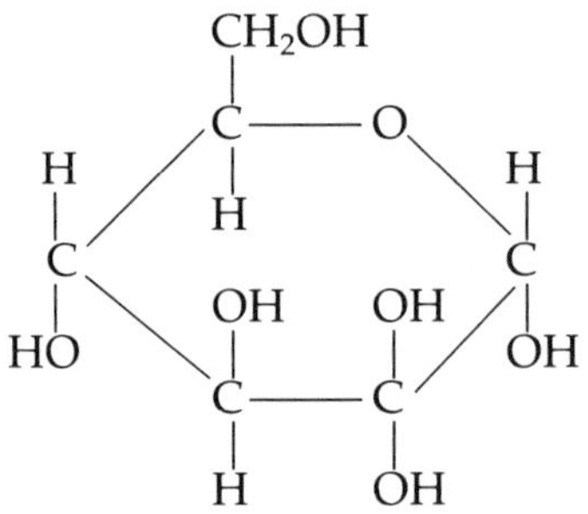

```
    CHO              CHO
     |                |
 H—C—OH          H—C—H
     |                |
 H—C—OH          H—C—OH
     |                |
 H—C—OH          H—C—OH
     |                |
   CH₂OH            CH₂OH
   Ribose          Deoxyribose
```

The hexoses, with the general formula of $C_6H_{12}O_6$, are made up of about 15 molecules representing various arrangements of the CHOH groups within the monosaccharide skeleton. The most important member, with regard to physiological processes, is glucose, but others such as galactose, fructose, and mannose are produced in metabolism and have important functions in a variety of molecules in which they are contained. Using the form of representation shown above for the pentoses (an *open-chain, linear form*), the hexoses can be shown with the CHOH groups oriented to the left or to the right. These different forms are called stereoisomers, and to fully distinguish among them requires some systematic numbering of the carbons:

The carbons are numbered as follows:

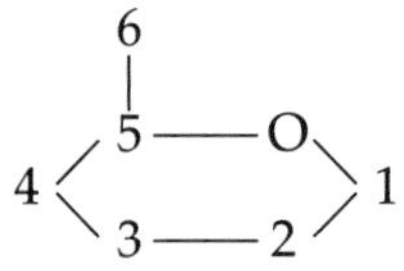

Disaccharides are made up of two monosaccharides linked by a *glycosidic* bond. This is a —C—O—C— (*ether*) linkage formed between a hydroxyl group of one sugar unit with the carbonyl carbon of another. The sugar units can be the same, as in the case of maltose where both units are glucose, or they can differ, as in the case of milk sugar (lactose), where one is glucose and the other is galactose (see Figure B–1). Depending on the steric (spatial) configuration at C_1, the glycosidic linkage is called alpha

Figure B–1. Monosaccharides. Glucose and galactose, the constituent monomeric units of lactose, form an epimeric pair; note that the orientation of the hydroxyl group on carbon 4 is the only structural difference between the two sugars. Fructose, one of the monomers of sucrose, is considerably different in structure.

glucose   **galactose**   **fructose**

or beta. This is important because animals are capable of degrading only the alpha linkages.

Polysaccharides are best considered to be long chains of sugar units joined by glycosidic links. The various forms differ according to the number and type of monosaccharides in the chain, the degree of branching of the chains, and the nature of the glycosidic bonds. Animals use a polymer of glucose, linked with alpha glycosidic bonds and with considerable branching, as a storage form of glucose. It is called *glycogen*, a molecule of enormous size ranging from about 300,000 to 1,000,000,000 daltons (Figure B–2). The equivalent energy storing molecule in plants is *starch* (Figure B–3), again a polymer of glucose but is a mixture of a linear polymer called *amylose*, linked [1–4] with the highly branched *amylopectin*, linked [1–4] and [1–6], and found as granules in plant cells. Plants have structural carbohydrates as well. There are various types but *cellulose* will be most familiar, and it is a polymer of glucose but is linked with beta-glycosidic [1–4] bonds.

Intermediate in size to the carbohydrate groups already described are small polymers, often of mixed sugars, that decorate certain proteins to form *glycoproteins*. These carbohydrate portions are very highly charged, making the glycoproteins ideal surface components for cells that exist in a watery environment. One especially important class of such compounds con-

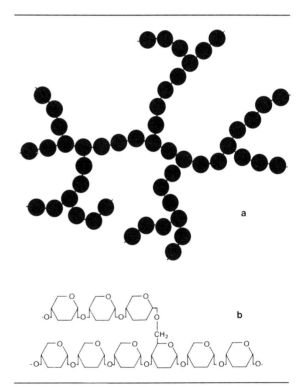

Figure B–2. Branched polymers of glycogen. Extensive branching, by means of 1–6 glycosidic bonds, is a characteristic of the storage carbohydrate of animals. The individual glucosyl units are depicted by closed circles in part *a*, while part *b* shows, in abbreviated form, the distinction between the 1–4 bonds forming the linear polymers and the 1–6 bonds providing the branches.

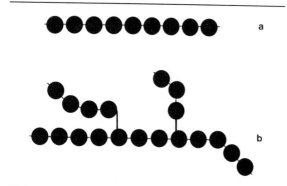

Figure B–3. *Structure of Starch.* Glucosyl units are linked by 1,4 glycosidic bonds to form linear polymers of amylose (part *a*). The other major component of starch (depicted in part *b*) is amylopectin, which possesses 1,6 linked branches on the otherwise linear chain. The nature of these bonds in amylopectin is quite similar to those of glycogen, shown in the previous figure.

sists of the blood-type antigens found on erythrocytes. Similar molecules are also responsible for different tissue types or histocompatability antigens. These are very important markers used to screen potential tissue or organ donor candidates prior to transplant operations.

Another group of physiologically important carbohydrates includes additional charged regions, often involving sulfate groups, that are extremely hydrophilic. These complex molecules make up much of the *ground substance* of connective tissues. They attract large amounts of water, keeping the tissue matrix in a state of hydration. This water-holding property aids in cushioning and lubricating the articulating joints.

Index

Numbers in boldface indicate definitions. Numbers followed by *f* or *s* indicate figures or chemical structures, respectively.